Breast Cancer

Home Exercise Guide
& Workbook

Plus

Exercise Benefits & Precautions

Lost Temple Fitness & Rehab

Karen Cutler: LPTA, ACE Certified Personal Trainer,

Cancer Exercise Specialist & Cert. Lymphedema Therapist

It is advised that you always check with your medical doctor or physical therapist before starting an exercise program or change in diet.

Websites

LostTempleFitness.com

LostTempleFitnessCancer.com

LostTemplePets.com

LostTempleArt.com

Cancer and Exercise

It is beneficial for people who are currently undergoing treatment for cancer or survivors to engage in an exercise program. As shown in the second part of this book, exercise can help with endurance, muscle strengthening and flexibility. It is advised that you glance through the chapters *Safety First* and *Components of a Conditioning Program*, before starting an exercise program. There are hundreds of pictures for beginner, intermediate and advanced exercise programs, as well as a list of equipment that you can use in the home. This section also includes worksheets and exercise precautions for those at risk for peripheral neuropathy or lymphedema.

Although this book is focused on breast cancer, most of the recommendations can be applied to other cancers, regarding side effects or late effects with treatments, such as radiation and chemotherapy.
The majority of the research is from the *National Cancer Institute* Please see *References*.

This book is not meant to substitute an exercise program prescribed by a health care professional, but designed to accompany their recommendations.
Please consult with your oncologist or team before starting any exercise program.

This book is for:
- Those that currently have or are cancer survivors that:
    - Are currently or may have had treatments, such as chemotherapy or radiation
    - Are planning or have had surgeries and/or at risk for lymphedema or peripheral neuropathy
- The beginner who has never exercised before or the individual that has mastered the basics but wants to know how to advance to the next level.
- The personal trainer, physical therapist, or other coaches who would like to know more about precautions with cancer patients or clients.

This book is not for or may need modification:
- Chronic or acute disorders/injuries that is not being followed by a health care professional. This book can be used in conjunction with a rehab program.
- If you are over 40 and have never exercised before, it is advised that a physician clears you first.
- Undiagnosed pain.
- The person that does not feel they can safely modify their individual program, although can be used in conjunction with rehab or coaches/personal trainers.
- People going through current treatments, lymphedema or other medical issues that have not been cleared by an MD for an exercise program. Other issues that may be addressed in future volumes: Cancer, Cardiac Disease, Respiratory Disease , Arthritis & Osteoporosis and Diabetes.

What is covered in this book?

- **Cancer / Breast Cancer / Lymphedema**
  - Breast Cancer: *What is breast cancer?*
  - Breast Cancer Types
  - Screening
  - Pathology
  - Staging
  - Prognostic Markers
  - Genes
  - Breast Surgeries
  - Breast Reconstruction
  - Breast Implants and Tissue Expanders
  - Tissue Flap Surgery
  - Sentinel And Axillary Lymph Nodes / Dissection
  - Lymph Nodes and Lymphedema
  - Risks After Breast Surgery
- **Home Exercise Program & Worksheets**.
  - Myofascial release
  - Flexibility – Stretching
  - Core Stability
  - Strengthening - Lower extremity (Lying and Seated) and Upper extremity
  - Balance with progression to Standing Strengthening exercises
  - Agility and Endurance
- Benefits and Factors to consider before starting an exercise program
- Vital signs and how to monitor exercise intensity
- Temperature – Heat and Cold; Dehydration
- Equipment needed for home exercise
- Warm up/cool down
- Duration, Frequency, Intensity and Primary Movement Patterns
- Anatomy
- Self-tests

BREAST CANCER / LYMPHEDEMA

INTRODUCTION

HOME EXERCISE PROGRAM
See Section for Specific TOC

REFERENCES

Quick Summary this Section

Cancer:

- Cancer is a disease in which some of the body's cells grow uncontrollably and spread to other parts of the body.

Cancer and Exercise:

- Exercise in Healthy Adults versus Cancer Patients
- Guidelines
- Risks for Cancer Patients
- Starting an Exercise Program

Lymph Nodes & Lymphedema & Exercises/ROM:

- Lymph nodes are part of the lymphatic and immune system, which protects your body against infection and disease.

Sentinel and Axillary Lymph Nodes:

- Sentinel Lymph Node Biopsy (SLNB)
- Axillary Lymph Node Dissection (ALND) - *see Lymphedema*

Breast Cancer:

- What is Breast Cancer, Stage Groups, Risk Factors, Protective Factors,

Types:

- DCIS, LCIS, IDC, ILC, Rare, Inflammatory, Paget Disease

Screening

- Mammogram, Diagnostic Mammography, Ultrasound, MRI, Biopsy, PET scan

Pathology: Testing and Diagnosis

- Tumor Grade/Differentiating Cells, Nottingham Grading System

Staging:

- TMN Staging, Stage 0-IV, Localized, Regional, Distant, Unknown

Prognostic Markers:

- Margins or Ink, HER2/neu Gene, Estrogen Receptor (ER), Progesterone Receptor (PR), Ki-67, S-Phase Fraction, Lymphovascular Invasion, Multigene Test, Molecular Subtypes

Genes:

- Tumor Suppressor Gene, BRCA1 and BRCA 2, PALB2, CHEK2, ATM

Surgeries:
- Mastectomy, Lumpectomy, Nipple Sparing Mastectomy, Total or Simple Mastectomy, Considerations, Comparisons

Reconstruction:
- Factors - Timing and Choice
- Reconstruction: Implants or Autologous Tissue

Breast Implants:
- Implants
- Tissue Expanders

Tissue Flap Surgeries:
- Autologous Tissue & Reconstruction
- TRAM, DIEP, SIEA, LAT, Gluteal, TUG, IGAP
- Nipple Reconstruction

Risks after Breast Surgery:
- Axillary Web Syndrome - AWS (Cording), Scar Tissue / Adhesions, Seroma / Compression

Exercise Contraindications / Precautions After Breast Surgery

Things to Avoid, Post Op Healing & Mastectomy:
- Avoid 2 - weeks Post op, Post op healing concerns, Recommendations post mastectomy

Exercise Examples - Post Mastectomy:
- Examples of Exercises, Stretches or Edema Control after Mastectomy

Home Exercise Guide Breast and / or Lymphedema:
- Home Exercise Guide For Post Surgery and / or Lymphedema

Therapies for Cancer:
- Therapy includes, but not limited to, chemotherapy, radiation, hormone, targeted, immunotherapy, stem cell

Side Effects and Late Side Effects:
- Side Effects and Late Side Effects of therapies and surgeries

Eating Hints: Before, during, and after Cancer Treatment:
Clear Liquids, Full Liquid Diet, Foods and Drinks that are Easy on the Stomach, Low Fiber, High Fiber, High Protein, Foods and Drinks that are Easy to Chew and Swallow

References

HOME EXERCISE GUIDE & WORKSHEETS

CANCER

Information and pictures from *National Cancer Institute* unless otherwise specified

Definition	Cancer is a disease in which some of the body's cells grow uncontrollably and spread to other parts of the body. • Cancer can start almost anywhere in the human body, which is made up of trillions of cells. Normally, human cells grow and multiply (through a process called cell division) to form new cells as the body needs them. When cells grow old or become damaged, they die, and new cells take their place. • Sometimes this orderly process breaks down, and abnormal or damaged cells grow and multiply when they shouldn't. These cells may form tumors, which are lumps of tissue. Tumors can be cancerous or not cancerous (benign). • Cancerous tumors spread into, or invade, nearby tissues and can travel to distant places in the body to form new tumors (a process called metastasis). Cancerous tumors may also be called malignant tumors. Many cancers form solid tumors, but cancers of the blood, such as leukemias, generally do not. • Benign tumors do not spread into, or invade, nearby tissues. When removed, benign tumors usually don't grow back, whereas cancerous tumors sometimes do. Benign tumors can sometimes be quite large, however. Some can cause serious symptoms or be life threatening, such as benign tumors in the brain.

How Does Cancer Develop?	Cancer is a genetic disease—that is, it is caused by changes to genes that control the way our cells function, especially how they grow and divide.
	
	 • Genetic changes that cause cancer can happen because:
	      o of errors that occur as cells divide.
	      o of damage to DNA caused by harmful substances in the environment, such as the chemicals in tobacco smoke and ultraviolet rays from the sun. (Our Cancer Causes and Prevention section has more information.)
	      o they were inherited from our parents.
	
	 • The body normally eliminates cells with damaged DNA before they turn cancerous. But the body's ability to do so goes down as we age. This is part of the reason why there is a higher risk of cancer later in life.
	
	 • Each person's cancer has a unique combination of genetic changes. As the cancer continues to grow, additional changes will occur. Even within the same tumor, different cells may have different genetic changes.

How Cancer Spreads	**Tissue.** The cancer spreads from where it began by growing into nearby areas **There are three ways that cancer spreads in the body** **Blood.** The cancer spreads from where it began by getting into the blood. The cancer travels through the blood vessels to other parts of the body **Lymph system.** The cancer spreads from where it began by getting into the lymph system. The cancer travels through the lymph vessels to other parts of the body
When Cancer Spreads	A cancer that has spread from the place where it first formed to another place in the body is called metastatic cancer. The process by which cancer cells spread to other parts of the body is called metastasis. Metastatic cancer has the same name and the same type of cancer cells as the original, or primary, cancer. For example, breast cancer that forms a metastatic tumor in the lung is metastatic breast cancer, not lung cancer. Under a microscope, metastatic cancer cells generally look the same as cells of the original cancer. Moreover, metastatic cancer cells and cells of the original cancer usually have some molecular features in common, such as the presence of specific chromosome changes. In some cases, treatment may help prolong the lives of people with metastatic cancer. In other cases, the primary goal of treatment for metastatic cancer is to control the growth of the cancer or to relieve symptoms it is causing. Metastatic tumors can cause severe damage to how the body functions, and most people who die of cancer die of metastatic disease.
References	National Cancer Institute (NCI) - What is Cancer? *https://www.cancer.gov/about- cancer/understanding/what-is-cancer*

Cancer and Exercise

It is beneficial for people who are currently undergoing treatment for cancer or survivors to engage in an exercise program. As shown in the first part of this book, exercise can help with endurance, muscle strengthening and flexibility. It is advised that you glance through the following sections: *Safety First* and *Components of a Conditioning Program*, before starting an exercise program. The Home Exercise Guide has general information regarding myofascial release, flexibility/stretches/ROM, core stability, strengthening, balance, agility, and endurance.

Things you should know before starting a program:
* If you had any number lymph nodes removed or radiation, this puts you at risk for lymphedema.
* What type of surgery, if any, was performed.
* If you are currently or have had radiation or chemotherapy, you may want to know the side effects and precautions, i.e. chemo can cause peripheral neuropathy (increases risk of falling) and radiation can put you at risk for lymphedema (swelling in the neck, arm, legs or trunk depending on the area treated).
* Any other risk factors, such as, but not limited to, diabetes, cardiac or pulmonary issues, neurological issues, poor bone density/osteopenia/arthritis or autoimmune disorders.

Most of the research is from the **National Cancer Institute** – Please see *References*.

This book is not meant to substitute an exercise program prescribed by a health care professional but is designed to accompany their recommendations.

Please consult with your oncologist or team before starting any exercise program.

Who is this section recommended for?

- Patients currently undergoing treatment for cancer to be used in conjunction with the oncologist or other health care provider and/or physical therapist recommendations.
- Cancer survivors that are trying to get back into a healthy exercise program.
- Physical therapists and other health care providers, such as a cancer exercise specialist, to be used to prescribe a home exercise program.

Who is this section not for?

- Those who are not able to follow or modify a program without supervision.
- Those who have other medical issues, such as respiratory, cardiac, fracture risks or other acute/chronic issues that have not been cleared by an MD.
- *Also see Introduction*

Exercise in Healthy Adults versus Cancer Patients

Fitness and exercise is the same for cancer patients as it is for the average adult. You can follow the exercise routines suggested in the first section of this book prior to, during and after treatments. In fact, it is recommended that you start reading or at least scanning this section, as suggestions for muscle strengthening, endurance, flexibility, and balance will be the same.

What makes the program different are the various side effects from chemotherapy, surgery, radiation, and other cancer treatments. For example, after a mastectomy you will need to get range back in the arm and have precautions, as well as possible complications, such as lymphedema. Chemotherapy can cause excessive fatigue where you may have to push yourself to get off the couch and make a meal. Radiation can also cause fatigue, and puts you at risk for lymphedema, as well as having localized pain or burning. Everybody's treatment and reaction will be different. This will all depend on the treatment itself, your physical condition prior to treatment and any other issues, such as diabetes or heart disease that may cause other complications.

Although this book is about Home Exercise Programs, it is extremely important to follow your oncology team's prescription, especially after surgery. All cancer treatments are different, and each doctor will have their particular protocol to follow. It may be necessary to participate in physical therapy first and use this book as a guide along with their program. It is also very important to be cleared from a specialist for other complications, such as, but not limited to, heart disease, pulmonary disease, diabetes, bone disease, immune disorders, obesity or neurological conditions.

If you had lymph nodes removed or radiation this puts you at risk for lymphedema, no matter how long ago. Please consult with a certified lymphedema specialist, esp. before adding resistance to your exercise routine.

About me, and the importance of keeping a chart of your daily symptoms.

In 2017 I was diagnosed with breast cancer with a right mastectomy followed by chemotherapy for 16 weeks, and then radiation, and finally reconstruction over a year later. I was exercising 6 days a week and was on fairly healthy diet prior to getting the cancer diagnosis. With that said, chemotherapy wiped me out where I had to push myself to walk in the driveway and eat, as I had no appetite. One of the best things I did was make myself a daily chart to see my ups and downs between chemotherapy treatments, which were every two weeks. Below is an example of a chart I did to show my mental and physical symptoms and how much I did each day. This does not show what I did around the house, but you can certainly make a chart that shows this as well. Again, this example is only my first two weeks of chemo treatments. As the treatments went on and they changed my medication, my symptoms also changed, some for the better, some for the worse.

First 2 weeks of Chemotherapy:

Day	Walk/Time of Day	Other	Eat	Info
Thursday		**First Session**	Grilled cheese and crackers	**Chemo 1**
Friday	Chemo Center	Neulasta Injection	Most crackers, grilled cheese, Jello	Nausea – extreme
Saturday	Driveway 10 & 1		Most crackers, grilled cheese, Jello	Nausea
Sunday	Driveway 11& 1		Most crackers, grilled cheese, Jello	Nausea
Monday		Went to oncology chemo center due to nausea / dehydration	Added soup	Added Zofran for nausea and took off Compazine (caused nausea / tremors) Went to oncology due to nausea / dehydration – put on Saline IV
Tuesday	Driveway 1:00		Crackers & soup, cereal grilled cheese	Nausea
Wednesday			Crackers & soup, cereal, grilled cheese, egg whites	Nausea, increased fatigue
Thursday	½ mile 3:00		Prior & peanut butter on toast	Nausea
Friday	1 mile 1:00	Bicep 5 lbs./Triceps 3 lbs.	Prior	Nausea
Saturday	1 mile 3:00		Prior	Decreased nausea
Sunday	2 miles 5:00		Spinach quiche ½ chicken breast	No nausea
Monday	2 ½ mile 5:00		Normal eating – non spicy, eggs	No nausea
Tuesday	2 ½ mile 1:00 1 mile 5:00	Biceps 5 lbs. Triceps 3 lbs. & 5 lbs.	Chicken, rice, broccoli, eggs	Started noticing hair falling out
Wednesday	3 miles 4:30		Turkey Burger Sweet potato pancakes	Hair falling out – depressed Food starting to taste burnt.

Exercise Guidelines

The following information includes research from:
> **American Cancer Society** - *Physical Activity and the Cancer Patient*
> **Cancer Research UK -** *Exercise guidelines for Cancer Patients*

Benefits for Cancer Patients

- May help to decrease nausea during chemotherapy
- May relieve constipation by stimulating digestion and elimination systems
- Increases endurance due to fatigue
- Help to keep or improve your physical abilities (how well you can use your body to do things)
- Improve balance, which may lower risk of falls and broken bones
- Keep muscles from wasting due to inactivity
- Decrease the risk of heart disease
- Decrease the risk of osteoporosis – helps to strength bones
- Improving blood flow to the legs, reducing the risk of blood clots
- Make you less dependent on others for help with normal activities of daily living
- Lower the risk of being anxious and depressed
- Help you control your weight

What Is your Current Activity Level or Was your Activity Level before Treatment?

This makes a big difference in deciding how you will proceed with your exercise program. If you lead a sedentary lifestyle before the cancer, this is not the time to start a moderate aerobic exercise program. This does not mean you should not start an exercise program at all; you will just need to start at a basic level. On the other hand, if you were an athlete before your diagnosis, this will mean you need to cut back during treatment and eventually move forward to regain your strength.

Pain, fatigue and possibly nausea are the most limiting factors during your treatment. Other factors could be peripheral neuropathy, which may alter your balance, dehydration, or lymphedema, etc. Some people also have a pre- existing, or cancer caused comorbidities, (*the presence of one or more additional diseases or disorders co-occurring with a primary disease or disorder*), which could include heart disease, pulmonary disease, obesity, diabetes, neurological conditions, or bone disease, among others. In this instance, you will have to speak to the team of doctors to discuss which exercises will be best suited for not only the cancer, but any other comorbidity.

What is your current performance level? (Chart adapted from *Clinical Exercise Physiology*, pg. 440)

Activity level	Exercise Duration	Exercise Frequency
Active, no limitations	15-20 min	Daily
Able to walk. Decreased leisure activity. Can perform self-care	15-20 min	Daily
Able to walk more than 50% of the time. Moderate fatigue. Limited assistance with ADL's (activity of daily living)	5-10 min	Two sessions daily
Able to walk less than 50% of the time. Fatigue with mild exertion. Requires assistance with ADL	5-10 min	Daily
Confined to bed *******Italic not from Clinical Exercise Physiology chart*	*******May be able to do ROM in bed with or without assistance.*	*******ROM (Range of Motion) Daily*

Guideline for Type of Exercise. Remember to always warm up before exercising and cool down if needed. This is especially true with flexibility training.

Type	Purpose / Benefit	Intensity / Frequency / Duration	Suggestions
Endurance / Aerobic *How to Monitor Heart Rate (HR) Intensity*	*Improves blood flow *Increases stamina *Reduces fatigue *Boosts mood *Controls body weight	*Low - Based on symptoms – can do walking everyday *Moderate 40-60% of HR * 3-5 days a week * 20-60 min. sessions	*Start with walking if possible, outside or on treadmill *Stationary bike if available, especially with neuropathy or balance issues *See balance for standing endurance exercises. *See strengthening exercises without resistance for general movements and Range of Motion (ROM)
Strength Lower *(Resistance information)*	*Improves muscle and contractile strength *Improves bone, tendon & ligament strength *Improves nervous system function	*Limited by Symptoms and Precautions *40-60% of 1 RM *2-3 days per week – Alternate days for UE/LE. *1-3 sets / 3-5 reps. Progress to 8-12 reps as tolerated	**It is important to follow a regiment designed by the oncology team during treatment due to risk of injury, especially after surgery.** *Start by not using any weight and complete Range of Motion if you have never used resistance before. *Increase to light hand weights or resistance bands as tolerated. *During treatment it is better to do high reps with light weights instead of trying to 'bulk up' with heavy weights. Your body needs to heal and should not be focused on repairing a torn muscle.
Strength – Upper *(Resistance information)*	*Improves function for ADLs (Activity Daily Living)		
Strength – Core	*Strengthens trunk, which is your foundation *Maintaining a stable core will assist with balance	*Limited by Symptoms and Precautions *2-3 days per week *1-3 sets / 3-5 reps. Progress to 8-10 reps as tolerated	**It is important to follow a regiment designed by the oncology team during treatment due to risk of injury, especially after surgery.** *It is important to follow progression and understand any precautions you may have. *Breathing correctly during abdominal or core exercises are very important.
Flexibility / ROM	*Helps to maintain ROM *Increases flexibility / ROM after certain surgeries *Decreases stiffness & tension *Increases blood supply to joints *Increases neuromuscular coordination	*20-30 second hold *5-7 days a week *2-4 reps per stretch	*Always warm up before stretching a muscle *Dynamic stretching can be a part of your warmup or even be used in conjunction with your endurance exercises. *Try doing arm stretches while walking to increase intensity.
Balance *(Also see Core, Lower Extremity Strengthening, Agility, Endurance)*	*Decreases risk for falls *Helps improve gait pattern *See Purpose for Endurance and Strength above)	*Limited by symptoms and standing tolerance *5-7 days a week *1 set / 2-4 reps 5-10 second hold *Can also be used in place of some Endurance & Strengthening Exercises	*Follow progression program for Balance *Can be used in place of some endurance and strengthening exercises if able to tolerate standing. *Must be able to stand to perform balance. *Sitting balance can strengthen the core. *Make sure you have a chair or sturdy object to hold or nearby in case of loss of balance. *Requires leg strength for progression.

Risks for Cancer Patients

Avoid Exercise:

- Low red blood cell count (anemia).
- Low white blood cell counts or if you take medicines that make you less able to fight infection and impair your immune system. Stay away from public gyms and other public places until your counts are at a safe level.
- Abnormal levels of minerals in your blood, such as sodium and potassium. This can happen if you have had a lot of vomiting or diarrhea.
- Unrelieved pain, nausea/vomiting, or any other symptom that causes you concern. Call your doctor.
- Do not exercise above a moderate level of exertion without talking with your doctor first. Remember, moderate exertion is about as much effort as a brisk walk.
- If you have a catheter or feeding tube, do not do resistance training that uses muscles in the area of the catheter to keep from dislodging it. Talk with your cancer team about what's safe for you. Avoid pools, lakes, or ocean water and other exposures that may cause infections

Modification or Recommendations:

- Skin irritation - people getting radiation should not expose skin in the treatment area to chlorine in swimming pools. Avoid direct sunlight, even after radiation treatments are over due to burning. For radiation to the upper part of the body, suggest wearing a rash guard (shirt that has UV sun protection).
- Stay away from uneven surfaces or any weight-bearing exercises that could cause you to fall and hurt yourself.
- If you have cancer affecting your bones, you might be more at risk of a break or fracture. You must avoid putting too much strain on the affected bones. You could try swimming or exercising in water, as the water supports your body weight, so the skeleton isn't stressed.
- Watch for swollen ankles, unexplained weight gain, or shortness of breath while at rest or with a small amount of activity. Let your doctor know if you have any of these problems.
- Watch out for lymphedema *(see Lymphedema)*.
- Watch for bleeding, especially if you are taking blood thinners. Avoid any activity that puts you at risk of falling or injury. If you notice swelling, pain, dizziness, or blurred vision, call your doctor right away.
- Peripheral neuropathy - Loss of sensation or feelings of pins and needles in your hands and feet due to cancer treatments. Because this puts you at a higher risk of falling, it might be better to use a stationary bike than to do other types of weight bearing exercise. *(Also, see Balance section)*

CETI Contraindications or Recommendations for Exercise

PICC line
- Avoid resistance exercises around the PICC site
- Do not swim or play contact sports
- Avoid repetitive movements in the affected arm

Chemotherapy or Immunotherapy
- IV Chemotherapy – No exercise for 24 hours
- Hematocrit less than 25% - No Exercise
- Hemoglobin less than 24% 8g/dl due to anemia – No Exercise
- White blood cell counts less than 300 mm3 – No Exercise
- White blood cell counts – Avoid public gyms unless blood cell count is above 500 mm3
- Platelet count less than 5000 mm3 – No resistance training – risk of internal bleeding/hemorrhage
- Platelet count less than 30,000 mm3 – Gentle Active Range of Motion *(CETI)*

Starting an Exercise Program

Although this book is about Home Exercise Programs, it is extremely important to follow your oncology team's prescription, especially after surgery. All cancer treatments are different, and each doctor will have their particular protocol to follow.

It may be necessary to participate in physical therapy first and use this book as a guide along with their program. It is also very important to be cleared from a specialist for other complications, such as, but not limited to, heart disease, pulmonary disease, diabetes, bone disease, immune disorders, obesity or neurological conditions.

Exercise Guidelines for Cancer patients currently receiving treatment

The following information includes research from:
National Comprehensive Cancer Network (NCCN) – Exercising During Cancer
Treatments American Cancer Society - *Physical Activity and the Cancer Patient*

- American Cancer Society: *"To make your exercise effort most effective (give you the best results), it's important that you work your heart.*
    - o *Notice your heart rate, your breathing, and how tired your muscles get. If you get short of breath or very tired, rest for a few seconds, and start exercising again as you are able.*
    - o *When you first start, the goal is to exercise for at least 10 minutes at a time. Go slow at first, and over the next few weeks, increase the length of time you exercise.*
    - o *Be careful if you're taking blood pressure medicine that controls your heart rate. Your heart rate will not go up, but your blood pressure can get high. Ask your doctor, nurse, or pharmacist about this if you're not sure about your medicines.*
    - o *We don't know the best level of exercise for someone with cancer. The goal is to have your exercise program help you keep up your muscle strength and keep you able to do the things you want and need to do. The more you exercise, the better you'll be able to exercise and function. But even if planned exercise stops, it's good to keep being active by doing your normal activities as much as you can". (See How to Monitor Exercise Intensity)*
- Goal: At least 30 minutes of aerobic exercise five days a week or more.
- Start slowly and work your way up. For example, if you are taking a walk, try short periods and rest frequently. Start at a slow 5–10-minute walk, rest, and try a brisk 5 minutes. You can also split up your sessions into 10 minutes throughout the day to equal 30. You don't have to start out at 30 minutes but work up to it.
- Keep track of when your energy levels are at their highest. Pain and fatigue can change daily but take advantage of the times when you are feeling the best. Try to keep on a daily routine.
- When you are feeling moderately fatigued, try getting up and doing something around the house to help with your endurance. It can be something as simple as walking up and down the hallway.
- Try getting up and walking hourly for circulation when you are not sleeping/napping.
- Balance activity with rest that does not interfere with nighttime sleep.
- Be flexible and listen to your body. Although you should keep some type of a schedule, don't feel like you need to
follow it strictly. If you are feeling ill, extremely fatigued or running a fever let your body rest.
- If you don't feel like doing a regimented routine, try gardening, housework or any other physical hobby you may enjoy. Ask someone to walk with you or use headphones while exercising or walking.
- Drink about 8 to 10 glasses of water a day unless your doctor tells you not to. Unless you are told otherwise, eat a balanced diet that includes protein (meat, milk, eggs, and legumes such as peas or beans).
- Dress comfortably, especially in either cold or humid weather. *(See Temperature).*

Lymph Nodes & Lymphedema TOC / Quick Summary

Information and pictures from *National Cancer Institute* unless otherwise specified

Lymph nodes:

- Lymph nodes are part of the lymphatic and immune system, which protects your body against infection and disease.

Lymphatic System:

- The lymph system is a network of lymph vessels, tissues, and organs that carry lymph throughout the body.

Anatomy of Lymphatic System:

- When the lymph system is working as it should, lymph flows through the body and is returned to the bloodstream.

Lymphedema and Cancer:

- Lymphedema can occur after any cancer or treatment that affects the flow of lymph through the lymph nodes, such as removal of lymph nodes or radiation.

Stages of Lymphedema:

- *Stage 0:* A subclinical state where swelling is not evident despite impaired lymph transport..
- *Stage I or Reversible*: The limb (arm or leg) is swollen and feels heavy. Pressing on the swollen area leaves a pit (dent).
- *Stage II or Spontaneous Irreversible:* The limb is swollen and feels spongy. Pressing on the swollen area does not leave a pit.
- *Stage III or Lymphostatic Elephantiasis:* This is the most advanced stage. The swollen limb may be very large.

Possible Signs of Lymphedema:

- Other conditions may cause the same symptoms and when a doctor should be consulted.

Preventative Measures:

- Skin care
- Avoid blocking fluids/pooling.

Treatment:

- Complete Decongestive Therapy (CDT) or Combined therapy
- Manual Lymph Drainage
- Bandaging
- Pressure Garments / Compression Devices
- Exercise
- Axillary Reverse Mapping

Upper and Lower Extremity Lymphedema Exercises

References

Lymph nodes	Lymph nodes are part of the lymphatic and immune system, which protects your body against infection and disease. • Lymph nodes are small, round organs that are clustered in many areas of the body, such as the underarm. • It consists of a network of vessels and organs that contain lymph, a clear fluid that carries infection-fighting white blood cells as well as fluid and waste products from the body's cells and tissues. • Cancer cells can spread to lymph nodes and other parts of the body through lymph vessels. In a person with cancer, lymph can also carry cancer cells that have broken off from the main tumor. • Once lymph nodes are removed, they will be checked for cancer. Knowing whether cancer is in the underarm lymph nodes can help the doctor decide if you need any treatment in addition to surgery. *NIH NCI (11)* and *NIH NCI (13)*
Sentinel and Axillary Lymph Node / Dissection	**Please see Sentinel and Axillary Lymph Node / Dissection at the end of the Breast Cancer Section**

Lymphatic System – *National Cancer Institute*

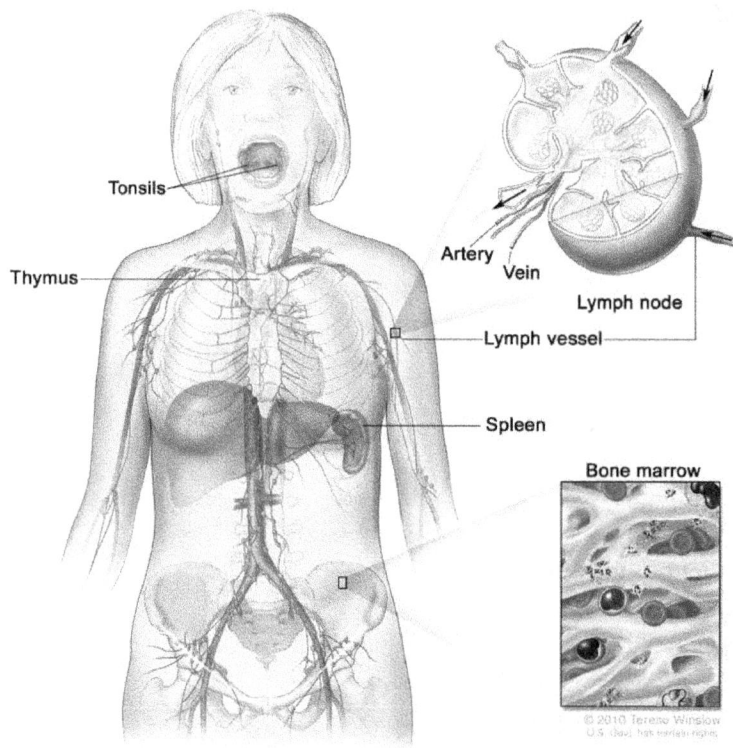

Tonsils

Thymus

Artery

Vein

Lymph node

Lymph vessel

Spleen

Bone marrow

NIH NCI (12) https://www.cancer.gov/about-cancer/treatment/side-effects/lymphedema/lymphedema-pdq)

Lymphatic System	The lymph system is a network of lymph vessels, tissues, and organs that carry lymph throughout the body.
	• The parts of the lymph system that play a direct part in lymphedema include the following:
	    o Lymph: Colorless, watery fluid that travels through the lymph vessels and carries T and B lymphocytes.
	        ▪ Lymphocytes are a type of white blood cell.
	    o Lymph vessels: A network of thin tubes that collect lymph from different parts of the body and return it to the bloodstream.
	    o Lymph nodes: Small, bean-shaped structures that filter lymph and store white blood cells that help fight infection and disease.
	        ▪ Lymph nodes are found along a network of lymph vessels throughout the body.
	        ▪ Groups of lymph nodes are found in the neck, underarm, mediastinum, abdomen, pelvis, and groin.
	• Lymph (clear fluid) and lymphocytes travel through the lymph vessels and into the lymph nodes where the lymphocytes destroy harmful substances. The lymph enters the blood through a large vein near the heart.
	• The spleen, thymus, tonsils, and bone marrow are also part of the lymph system but do not play a direct part in lymphedema.
	NIH NCI (12)

Anatomy of Lymphatic System	When the lymph system is working as it should, lymph flows through the body and is returned to the bloodstream.
	• Fluid and plasma leak out of the capillaries (smallest blood vessels) and flow around body tissues so the cells can take up nutrients and oxygen.
	• Some of this fluid goes back into the bloodstream. The rest of the fluid enters the lymph system through tiny lymph vessels.
	    o These lymph vessels pick up the lymph and move it toward the heart.
	    o The lymph is slowly moved through larger and larger lymph vessels and passes through lymph nodes where waste is filtered from the lymph.
	• The lymph keeps moving through the lymph system and collects near the neck, then flows into one of two large ducts:
	    o The right lymph duct collects lymph from the right arm and the right side of the head and chest.
	    o The left lymph duct collects lymph from both legs, the left arm, and the left side of the head and chest.
	• These large ducts empty into veins under the collarbones, which carry the lymph to the heart, where it is returned to the bloodstream.
	
	➢ **When part of the lymph system is damaged or blocked, fluid cannot drain from nearby body tissues.**
	➢ **Fluid builds up in the tissues and causes swelling/edema.**
	NIH NCI (12)

Cervical lymph nodes

Thoracic duct

Thymus

Lymphatics of the mammary gland

Axillary lymph nodes

Cisterna chyli

Spleen

Lumbar lymph nodes

Lymphatics of the upper limb

Pelvic lymph nodes

Lymphatics of the lower limb

Inguinal lymph nodes

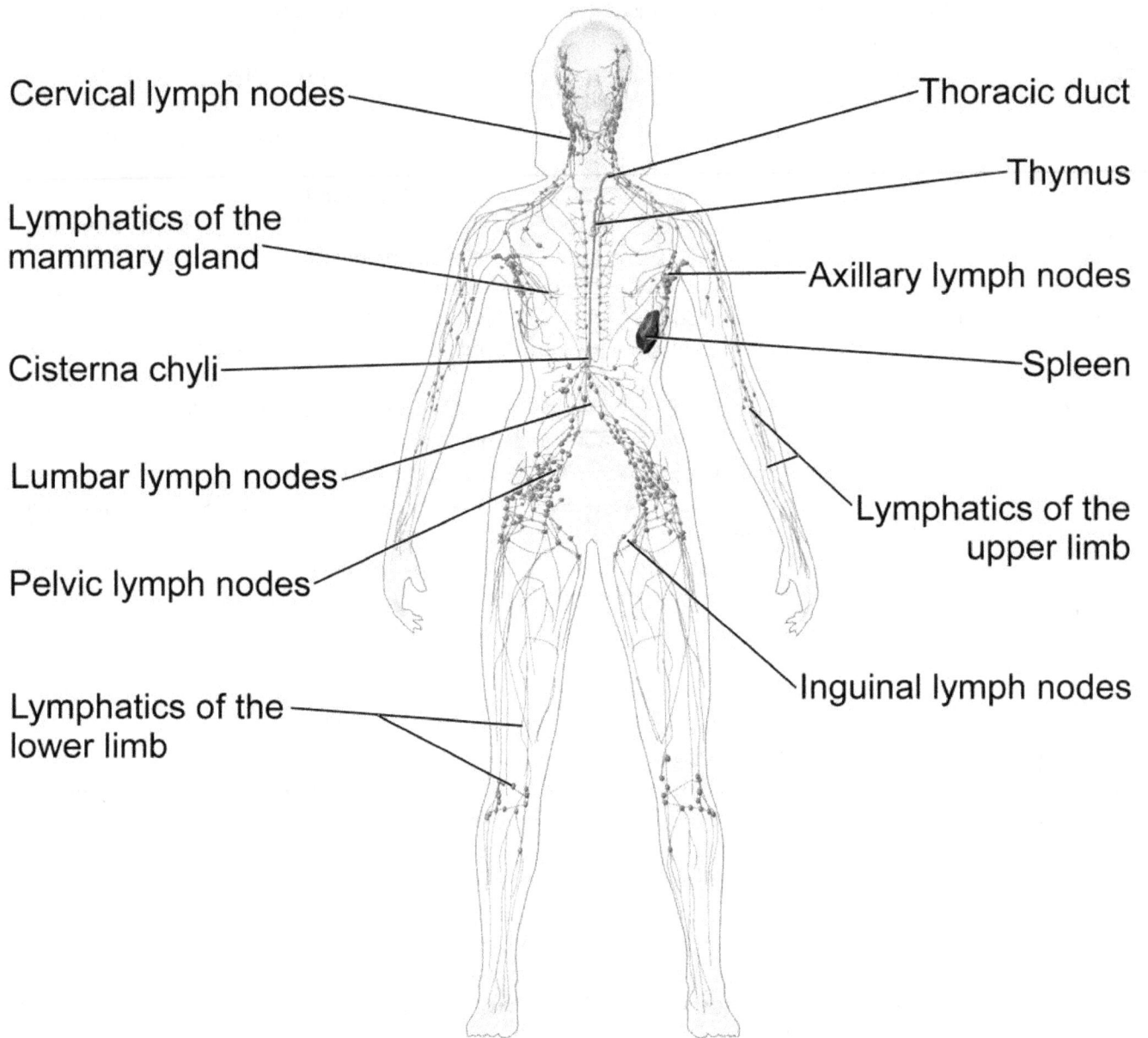

Medical gallery of Blausen Medical 2014". WikiJournal of Medicine

Lymphedema	**Lymphedema** is swelling caused by excess protein-rich lymph trapped within the interstitium and subcutaneous tissues. This is caused by dysfunction of the lymphatic system or pathology. Lymphedema occurs when the lymph system is damaged or blocked. Fluid builds up in soft body tissues and causes swelling. It is a common problem that may be caused by cancer and cancer treatment. Lymphedema usually affects an arm or leg, but it can also affect other parts of the body. Lymphedema can cause long-term physical, psychological, and social problems for patients. *NIH NCI (12)*

Lymphedema and Cancer	Lymphedema can occur after any cancer or treatment that affects the flow of lymph through the lymph nodes, such as removal of lymph nodes. It may develop within days or many years after treatment. Most lymphedema develops within three years of surgery.
	
	Risk factors for lymphedema include the following:
	• Removal and/or radiation of lymph nodes in the underarm, groin, pelvis, or neck.
	   o The risk of lymphedema increases with the number of lymph nodes affected.
	   o There is less risk with the removal of only the sentinel lymph node (the first lymph node in a group of lymph nodes to receive lymphatic drainage from the primary tumor).
	• Being overweight or obese.
	• Slow healing of the skin after surgery.
	• A tumor that affects or blocks the left lymph duct or lymph nodes or vessels in the neck, chest, underarm, pelvis, or abdomen.
	• Scar tissue in the lymph ducts under the collarbones, caused by surgery or radiation therapy.
	• Lymphedema often occurs in breast cancer patients who had all or part of their breast removed and axillary (underarm) lymph nodes removed. *(See below)*
	• Lymphedema in the legs may occur after surgery for uterine cancer, prostate cancer, lymphoma, or melanoma. It may also occur with vulvar cancer or ovarian cancer. Lymphedema occurs frequently in patients with cancers of the head and neck due to high-dose radiation therapy and combined surgery.
	NIH NCI (12)

Lymphedema and Breast Cancer	Lymphedema is swelling caused by a build-up of lymph. You may have this type of swelling in the hand, arm, chest, or back on the side of your body where lymph nodes were removed by breast cancer surgery or damaged by radiation therapy. Some important facts to know about lymphedema are: • Lymphedema can show up soon after surgery. • Sometimes, lymphedema can last for years. • Lymphedema can show up months or years after cancer treatment is over. • Lymphedema might develop after an insect bite, minor injury, or burn on the arm where lymph nodes were removed or damaged. • Lymphedema can cause pain and other problems. *NIH NCI (11)*

Stages of Lymphedema	• **Stage 0:** A subclinical state where swelling is not evident despite impaired lymph transport. This stage may exist for months or years before edema becomes evident.
	• **Stage I or Reversible:** The limb (arm or leg) is swollen and feels heavy. Pressing on the swollen area leaves a pit (dent).
	   o This stage of lymphedema may diminish with elevation.
	   o Subjective complaints are common.
	• **Stage II or Spontaneous irreversible**: The limb is swollen and feels spongy. Pressing on the swollen area does not leave a pit.
	   o A condition called tissue fibrosis may develop and cause the limb to feel hard.
	• **Stage III or Lymphostatic elephantiasis**: This is the most advanced stage. The swollen limb may be very large.
	   o Stage III lymphedema rarely occurs in breast cancer patients.
	     NIH NCI (12) and other

Possible Signs of Lymphedema	Other conditions may cause the same symptoms. A doctor should be consulted if any of the following problems occur: • Swelling of an arm or leg, which may include fingers and toes. • A full or heavy feeling in an arm or leg. • A tight feeling in the skin. • Trouble moving a joint in the arm or leg. • Thickening of the skin, with or without skin changes such as blisters or warts. • A feeling of tightness when wearing clothing, shoes, bracelets, watches, or rings. • Itching of the legs or toes. • A burning feeling in the legs. • Trouble sleeping. • Loss of hair. *NIH NCI (12)*
PREVENTATIVE MEASURES	Tell your doctor right away if you have any of the above symptoms. • The chance of improving the condition is better if treatment begins early. • Untreated lymphedema can lead to problems that cannot be reversed. *NIH NCI (12)*
Skin Care	Suggestions for Skin Care: • Keep skin and nails clean and cared for, to prevent infection. • Bacteria can enter the body through a cut, scratch, insect bite, or other skin injury. • Fluid that is trapped in body tissues by lymphedema makes it easy for bacteria to grow and cause infection. • Look for signs of infection, such as redness, pain, swelling, heat, fever, or red streaks below the surface of the skin. • Call your doctor right away if any of these signs appear. Careful skin and nail care helps to prevent infection: • Use cream or lotion to keep the skin moist. • Treat small cuts or breaks in the skin with an antibacterial ointment. • Avoid needle sticks of any type into the limb (arm or leg) with lymphedema. This includes shots or blood tests. • Use a thimble for sewing. • Avoid testing bath or cooking water using the limb with lymphedema. There may be less feeling (touch, temperature, pain) in the affected arm or leg, and skin might burn in water that is too hot. • Wear gloves when gardening and cooking. • Wear sunscreen and shoes outdoors. • Cut toenails straight across. See a podiatrist (foot doctor) as needed to prevent ingrown nails and infections. • Keep feet clean and dry and wear cotton socks. *NIH NCI (12)*

Avoid blocking fluids and pooling in Affected Limb	Avoid blocking the flow of fluids through the body. It is important to keep body fluids moving, especially through an affected limb or in areas where lymphedema may develop. • Do not cross your legs while sitting. • Change sitting position at least every 30 minutes. • Wear only loose jewelry and clothes without tight bands or elastic. • Do not carry handbags on the arm with lymphedema. • Do not use a blood pressure cuff on the arm with lymphedema. • Do not use elastic bandages or stockings with tight bands. Keep blood from pooling in the affected limb. • Keep the limb with lymphedema raised higher than the heart when possible. • Do not swing the limb quickly in circles or let the limb hang down. This makes blood and fluid collect in the lower part of the arm or leg. • Do not apply heat to the limb. *NIH NCI (12)*
Treatment	Possible Treatments: • Damage to the lymph system cannot be repaired. • Treatment is given to control the swelling caused by lymphedema and keep other problems from developing or getting worse. • Physical (non-drug) therapies are the standard treatment. • Treatment may be a combination of several physical methods. • The goal of these treatments is to help patients continue with activities of daily living, to decrease pain, and to improve the ability to move and use the limb (arm or leg) with lymphedema. • Drugs are not usually used for long-term treatment of lymphedema. *NIH NCI (12)*

Complete Decongestive Therapy or Combined Therapy	Combined physical therapy or complete decongestive therapy is a program managed by a certified lymphedema therapist to include:
	• Manual lymphatic drainage
	• Compression bandaging
	• Exercise
	• Skin care – *see skin care above*
	• Patient education
	• At the beginning of the program, the therapist gives many treatments over a short time to decrease most of the swelling in the limb with lymphedema.
	   • The patient then continues the program at home to keep the swelling down.
	    NIH NCI (12)

Manual Lymphatic Drainage **MLD**	**Manual Lymphatic Drainage (MLD)** • MLD (manual therapy) for lymphedema should begin with someone specially trained in treating lymphedema. • In this type of massage, the soft tissues of the body are lightly rubbed, tapped, and stroked. It is a very light touch, almost like dry brushing. • MLD may help move lymph out of the swollen area into an area with working lymph vessels. • Patients can be taught to do this type of massage therapy themselves by a certified lymphatic therapist. *NIH NCI (12)* **EFFECTS:** • Increases reabsorption of protein rich fluid • Increases lymphatic activity • Promotes relaxation • Creates and analgesic effect *(Klose Education)* When done correctly, massage therapy does not cause medical problems. **Massage should NOT be done on any of the following:** • Open wounds, bruises, or areas of broken skin. • Tumors that can be seen on the skin surface. • Areas with deep vein thrombosis (blood clot in a vein). • Sensitive soft tissue where the skin was treated with radiation therapy. *NIH NCI (12)* **CONTRAINDICATIONS:** • Acute infections, such as cellulitis • Untreated congestive heart failure (CHF) • Malignant disease – cancer • Renal dysfunction • Acute undiagnosed DVT *(Klose education)*

Bandages	**Bandages**
	• Once the lymph fluid is moved out of a swollen limb, bandaging (wrapping) can help prevent the area from refilling with fluid.
	• Bandages also increase the ability of the lymph vessels to move lymph along.
	• Lymphedema that has not improved with other treatments is sometimes helped with bandaging.
	NIH NCI (12)
	
	INDICATIONS:
	• Lymphedema
	• Chronic venous insufficiency (CVI)
	• Combination venous and lymphatic edema
	• Lipedema
	• Post-traumatic edema
	• Post-surgical edema
	• Acute DVT (*with* physician dx)
	
	CONTRAINDICATION:
	• Acute infections (MD must clear patient)
	• Arterial wounds
	• Arterial disease (ABI 0.8 or below)
	• Acute DVT (*without physician dx)*
	• Cardiac edema (untreated CHF)
	• Acute trauma without diagnosis
	
	PRECAUTIONS
	• Sensory deficits
	• Malignancy
	• Diabetes
	    – Small vessel (arteriole) and sensory deficits
	    – Toe bandaging may be contraindicated
	• Paralysis
	• Poor cognition or altered mental status
	• Sensitivity to the products used for bandaging
	(Klose Education)

Pressure Garments	**Pressure Garments** • Pressure garments are made of fabric that puts a controlled amount of pressure on different parts of the arm or leg to help move fluid and keep it from building up. • Some patients may need to have these garments custom-made for a correct fit. • Wearing a pressure garment during exercise may help prevent more swelling in an affected limb. • It is important to use pressure garments during air travel, because lymphedema can become worse at high altitudes. • Pressure garments are also called compression sleeves and lymphedema sleeves or stockings. *NIH NCI (12)*

Compression Device	**Compression Device** • Compression devices are pumps connected to a sleeve that wraps around the arm or leg and applies pressure on and off. The sleeve is inflated and deflated on a timed cycle. • This pumping action may help move fluid through lymph vessels and veins and keep fluid from building up in the arm or leg. • Compression devices may be helpful when added to complete decongestive therapy. • The use of these devices should be supervised by a trained professional because too much pressure can damage lymph vessels near the surface of the skin. *NIH NCI (12)*
Exercise *(Also see Exercise and Breast Cancer)*	**Exercise** Both light exercise and aerobic exercise (physical activity that causes the heart and lungs to work harder) help the lymph vessels move lymph out of the affected limb and decrease swelling. • Talk with a certified lymphedema therapist before beginning exercise. 　o Patients who have lymphedema or who are at risk for lymphedema should talk with a certified lymphedema therapist before beginning an exercise routine. 　o (*See the Lymphology Association of North America* (https://www.clt- lana.org/) *web site for a list of certified lymphedema therapists in the US*) • Wear a pressure garment if lymphedema has developed. 　o **Patients who have lymphedema should always wear a well-fitting pressure garment during all exercise that uses the affected limb or body part.** 　o When it is not known for sure if a woman has lymphedema, upper-body exercise without a garment may be more helpful than no exercise at all. 　o Patients who do not have lymphedema do not need to wear a pressure garment during exercise. • Breast cancer survivors should begin with light upper-body exercise and increase it slowly. 　o Some studies with breast cancer survivors show that upper-body exercise is safe in women who have lymphedema or who are at risk for lymphedema. 　o Weight-lifting that is slowly increased may keep lymphedema from getting worse. 　o Exercise should start at a very low level, increase slowly over time, and be overseen by the lymphedema therapist. 　o If exercise is stopped for a week or longer, it should be started again at a low level and increased slowly. 　o If symptoms (such as swelling or heaviness in the limb) change or increase for a week or longer, talk with the lymphedema therapist. 　o It is likely that exercising at a low level and slowly increasing it again over time is better for the affected limb than stopping the exercise completely. • More studies are needed to find out if weightlifting is safe for cancer survivors with lymphedema in the legs. *NIH NCI (12)*

Other Treatments	**Weight loss** • In patients who are overweight, lymphedema related to breast cancer may improve with weight loss. **Laser therapy** • Laser therapy may help decrease lymphedema swelling and skin hardness after a mastectomy. A hand-held, battery-powered device is used to aim low-level laser beams at the area with lymphedema. **Drug therapy** • Lymphedema is not usually treated with drugs. Antibiotics may be used to treat and prevent infections. Other types of drugs, such as diuretics or anticoagulants (blood thinners), are usually not helpful and may make the lymphedema worse. **Surgery** • Lymphedema caused by cancer is rarely treated with surgery. *NIH NCI (12)*

Axillary Reverse Mapping (ARM)

The axillary reverse mapping (ARM) technique has been developed to map and preserve arm lymphatic drainage during ALND and/or SLNB, thereby minimizing arm lymphedema. However, the success of ARM in reducing lymphedema has not been exactly determined.

• If ARM can be confirmed to be both effective and oncologically safe in preventing lymphedema, this technique should be recommended in the management of breast cancer treatment.
NIH – National Library of Medicine. Axillary Reverse Mapping (ARM): Where to Go

• Lymphedema is a major chronic morbidity that occurs in patients undergoing treatment for breast cancer (BC). Surgery for BC includes axillary surgery with either sentinel lymph node biopsy (SLNB) or axillary lymph node dissection (ALND).
• Lymphedema occurs due to removal or disruption of lymphatic drainage of the arm that overlaps with drainage of the breast. The risk of lymphedema increases significantly with adjuvant radiation.
• Axillary reverse mapping (ARM) is a technique where blue dye is injected into the upper arm at surgery, allowing direct visualization of arm lymphatics and nodes during either SLNB or ALND.
    • This allows preservation of arm lymphatics unless there is suspicion of metastatic disease in ARM lymphatics or if the ARM node is/are also the sentinel lymph node.
• Studies to date have largely been observational cohort studies, and mainly with low-risk patients undergoing SLNB only. There is only one published randomized controlled trial, and this included only patients undergoing modified radical mastectomy.
NIH – National Library of Medicine. Axillary Reverse Mapping (ARM) Technique (ARM)

• Traditionally, the rates of arm swelling after sentinel node biopsy range from 3-8%[1] and from 13-40%[2] after axillary dissection surgery. The studies that looked at ARM show a lymphedema rate that is lower, around 1-3% for the sentinel node surgery and 4-9%[3] for the axillary dissection surgery.
• Sometimes, it is not always possible to do ARM, and the surgeon needs to inject the blue dye in the breast to help identify the correct lymph nodes. This may be the case if you have had previous chemotherapy in the breast, or if the lymph nodes are not accurately found with other methods.
• Additionally, it is possible that the blue lymph nodes and the channels that are identified to drain the arm need to be removed to treat your cancer safely. If this is the case, you may be placed in a special group to watch your arm swelling closely or even have the option of having these channels reconnected. This is usually done by surgeons who are well experienced in lymphatic surgery and may include plastic surgeons also.
Summit Education: Oncology Rehab Dec 12, 2019

UPPER EXTREMITY LYMPHEDEMA EXERCISES

This routine of 10-12 repetitions should always be done prior to exercises for those with lymphedema or at risk, including those that have had *any* amount of lymph nodes remove in the upper extremity and/or radiation.

Description	Pictures
Other information at beginning of book. UE = Upper Extremity Section Flex = Flexibility Section	See UE or Flex section of book for other pictures
FIST CLENCH *Lymphedema control and circulation* Hands on thighs, open and close hand	
FIST CLENCH *Lymphedema control and circulation* Open and close your hand 15-20x with arm elevated above heart to prevent edema	
FIST CLENCH *Lymphedema control and circulation* Open and close your hand 15-20x with arm elevated above heart to prevent edema **NOT OVERHEAD first 1-2 weeks and/or until drains are out**	
SHRUGS UE #87 Raise your shoulders upward towards your ears as shown. Shrug both shoulders at the same time. Inhale up/exhale down	

Description	Pictures
Other information at beginning of book. UE = Upper Extremity Section Flex = Flexibility Section	See UE or Flex section of book for other pictures
SHOULDER ROLLS - Backwards UE #89 Move your shoulders in a circular pattern so that you are moving in an up, back and down direction. Perform small circles if needed for comfort.	
NECK ROTATION and SIDE BENDS Flex #47 SIDE BENDS: (*Top*) Tilt your head as if you are trying to touch your ear to your shoulder. ROTATION: (*Bottom*) Turn you head to the side as if looking over your shoulder.	
NECK FLEXION AND EXTENSION Flex #48 EXTENSION: Look up as if you are looking at the sky moving your neck only. FLEXION: Look down as if you are looking at the floor. For an extra stretch gently put both hands behind your head to move chin towards the chest and hold.	
SHOULDER RAISE / ELBOW CIRCLES Place your fingertips onto your shoulders. Slowly raise the elbow up to the side, then move it forwards, gently circling your arm. You are aiming to get your elbow level with your shoulder. Try to increase the height each time you do the exercises until you get level with your shoulder.	
ISOMETRIC CHEST PRESS Place the palms of your hands together with your elbows bent and arms at shoulder level or below. Exhale while pushing hands together and inhale and relax. 5-10x.	

Diaphragmatic Breathing

Lie either on your back with your knees bent or sit up

Inhale through your nose; as you do so, allow your stomach to rise. Limit movement in your chest. Attempt to push your bottom ribs out to the side as you breathe in.

Exhale through your mouth; as you do so, allow your stomach to fall. Limit movement in your chest.

Diaphragmatic breathing 6x a day for 5-10 repetitions

REFERENCES

American Cancer Society - Lymph Node Surgery for Breast Cancer *https://www.cancer.org/cancer/breast-cancer/treatment/surgery-for-breast-cancer/lymph-node-surgery-for-breast-cancer.html*

Medical gallery of Blausen Medical 2014". WikiJournal of Medicine

NIH NCI (11) https://www.cancer.gov/types/breast/surgery-choices/lymphedema

NIH NCI (12) https://www.cancer.gov/about-cancer/treatment/side-effects/lymphedema/lymphedema-pdq NIH

NCI (13) https://www.cancer.gov/about-cancer/diagnosis-staging/staging/sentinel-node-biopsy-fact-sheet

NIH – National Library of Medicine. Axillary Reverse Mapping (ARM): Where to Go *https://pubmed.ncbi.nlm.nih.gov/29961238/*

NIH – National Library of Medicine. Axillary Reverse Mapping (ARM) Technique (ARM) *https://clinicaltrials.gov/ct2/show/NCT03109522*

Pink Ribbon Program©

Summit Education: Oncology Rehab Dec 12, 2019

UPMC Axillary Lymph Node Dissection *https://www.upmc.com/locations/hospitals/magee/services/magee-womens-cancers/breast-cancer-program/treatment/breast-cancer-surgery/axillary-lymph-node*

Wikipedia – Axillary Lymph Nodes - *https://en.wikipedia.org/wiki/Axillary_lymph_nodes*

Wiki McMaster: *Breast Cancer https://wiki.mcmaster.ca/LIFESCI_4M03/_detail/screen_shot_2017-10-02_at_5.51.59_pm.png?id=group_1_presentation_1_-_breast_cancer*

SENTINEL AND AXILLARY LYMPH NODES / DISSECTION
Information and pictures from *National Cancer Institute* unless otherwise specified

Quick Summary of Section

Sentinel Lymph Node:

- A sentinel lymph node is defined as the first lymph node to which cancer cells are most likely to spread from a primary tumor.

Sentinel Lymph Node (SLNB):

- A sentinel lymph node biopsy (SLNB) is a procedure in which the sentinel lymph node is identified, removed, and examined to biopsy determine whether cancer cells are present.

Surgery:

- The surgeon injects a dye, a radioactive tracer, or both into the breast near the tumor. This helps the surgeon see which lymph nodes the lymph from that area of the breast flows to first.

SLNB and Breast Cancer:

- Breast cancer cells are most likely to spread first to lymph nodes located in the axilla, or armpit area, next to the affected breast.

Benefits of SLNB:

- SNLB helps doctors stage cancers and estimate the risk that tumor cells have developed the ability to spread to other parts of the body.

Risks of SLNB:

- All surgery to remove lymph nodes, including SLNB, can have harmful side effects, although removal of fewer lymph nodes is usually associated with fewer side effects, particularly serious ones such as lymphedema.

Axillary Lymph Nodes Dissection (ALND):

- The axillary lymph nodes or armpit lymph nodes are lymph nodes in the human armpit.

Risks of ALND:

- Anywhere from about 10 to 40 (though usually less than 20) lymph nodes are removed from the area under the arm (axilla)and checked for cancer spread.

3 Levels of ALND:

- Least aggressive to most aggressive.

Nerves that may be Damaged during Surgery:

- Several structures, including vessels and muscles with their nerve supply, are related to the breast and should be preserved during mastectomy or axillary node dissection.

Sentinel Lymph Node	A sentinel lymph node is defined as the first lymph node to which cancer cells are most likely to spread from a primary tumor. Sometimes, there can be more than one sentinel lymph node. • Lymph nodes are small round organs that are part of the body's lymphatic system. The lymphatic system is a part of the immune system. It consists of a network of vessels and organs that contains lymph, a clear fluid that carries infection-fighting white blood cells as well as fluid and waste products from the body's cells and tissues. • In a person with cancer, lymph can also carry cancer cells that have broken off from the main tumor. *NIH NCI (13)*

Sentinel lymph Node Biopsy (SLNB)

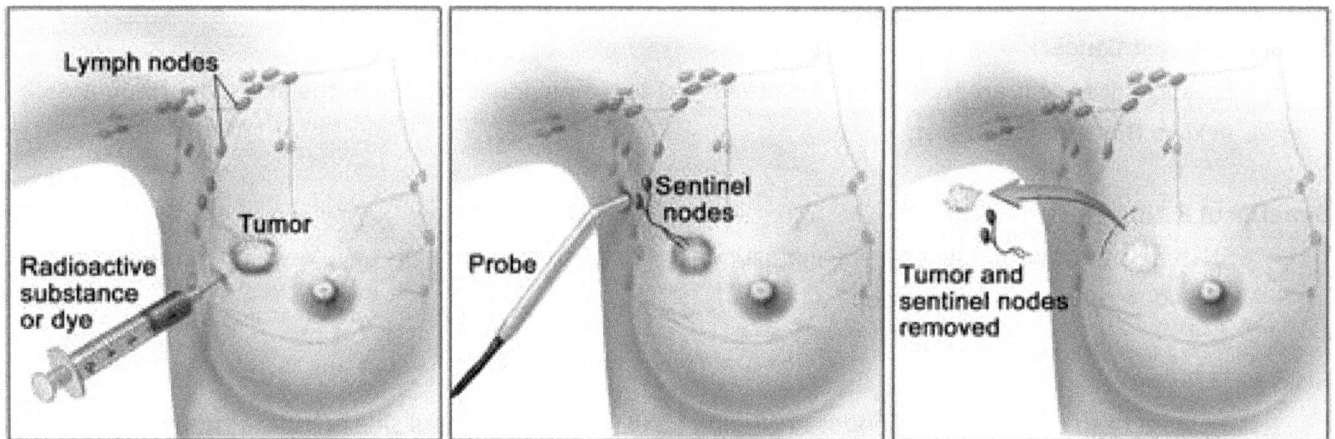

NIH NCI (13) https://www.cancer.gov/about-cancer/diagnosis-staging/staging/sentinel-node-biopsy-fact-sheet

Sentinel Lymph Node Biopsy (SLNB)	A sentinel lymph node biopsy (SLNB) is a procedure in which the sentinel lymph node is identified, removed, and examined to determine whether cancer cells are present. • It is used in people who have already been diagnosed with cancer. • A negative SLNB result suggests that cancer has not yet spread to nearby lymph nodes or other organs. • A positive SLNB result indicates that cancer is present in the sentinel lymph node and that it may have spread to other nearby lymph nodes (called regional lymph nodes) and, possibly, other organs. o This information can help a doctor determine the stage of the cancer (extent of the disease within the body) and develop an appropriate treatment plan. *NIH NCI (13)*

Surgery	• First, the surgeon injects a dye, a radioactive tracer, or both into the breast near the tumor. This helps the surgeon see which lymph nodes the lymph from that area of the breast flows to first.
	• Then, he or she removes the node or nodes that contain the dye or radioactive tracer to see if they have cancer.
	    ○ If they do not contain cancer, it is not likely that the other nodes under the arm have cancer. This means that the surgeon usually doesn't have to remove any other lymph nodes.
	    ○ If cancer is found, the surgeon may remove additional lymph nodes, either during the same biopsy procedure or during a follow-up surgical procedure. SLNB may be done on an outpatient basis or may require a short stay in the hospital. *NIH NCI (13)*
	• Fewer lymph nodes are removed with sentinel lymph node biopsy than with standard lymph node surgery.
	• Having fewer lymph nodes removed helps lower the chances that you will develop lymphedema and other problems caused by damage to lymph vessels and lymph nodes.
	NIH NCI (11)

SLNB and Breast Cancer	Breast cancer cells are most likely to spread first to lymph nodes located in the axilla, or armpit area, next to the affected breast. However, in breast cancers close to the center of the chest (near the breastbone), cancer cells may spread first to lymph nodes inside the chest (under the breastbone, called internal mammary nodes) before they can be detected in the axilla.
	• The number of lymph nodes in the axilla varies from person to person; the usual range is between 20 and 40.
	• Historically, all of these axillary lymph nodes were removed (in an operation called axillary lymph node dissection, or ALND) in women diagnosed with breast cancer. This was done for two reasons:
	    ○ Help stage the breast cancer
	    ○ Help prevent a regional recurrence of the disease. (Regional recurrence of breast cancer occurs when breast cancer cells that have migrated to nearby lymph nodes give rise to a new tumor.)
	• However, because removing multiple lymph nodes at the same time increases the risk of harmful side effects, clinical trials were launched to investigate whether just the sentinel lymph nodes could be removed. Two NCI-sponsored randomized phase 3 clinical trials have shown that SLNB without ALND is sufficient for staging breast cancer and for preventing regional recurrence in women who have no clinical signs of axillary lymph node metastasis, such as a lump or swelling in the armpit that may cause discomfort, and who are treated with surgery, adjuvant systemic therapy, and radiation therapy.
	NIH NCI (13)

Benefits of SLNB	SNLB helps doctors stage cancers and estimate the risk that tumor cells have developed the ability to spread to other parts of the body. • If the sentinel node is negative for cancer, a patient may be able to avoid more extensive lymph node surgery, reducing the potential complications associated with having many lymph nodes removed. *NIH NCI (13)*

Risks of SLNB	All surgery to remove lymph nodes, including SLNB, can have harmful side effects, although removal of fewer lymph nodes is usually associated with fewer side effects, particularly serious ones such as lymphedema.
	The potential side effects include:
	
	• Lymphedema *(see lymphedema)*. During lymph node surgery, lymph vessels leading to and from the sentinel node or group of nodes are cut. This disrupts the normal flow of lymph through the affected area, which may lead to an abnormal buildup of lymph fluid that can cause swelling.
	  o The risk of lymphedema increases with the number of lymph nodes removed. There is less risk with the removal of only the sentinel lymph node.
	  o In the case of extensive lymph node removal in an armpit or groin, the swelling may affect an entire arm or leg.
	  o In addition, there is an increased risk of infection in the affected area or limb.
	  o Very rarely, chronic lymphedema due to extensive lymph node removal may cause a cancer of the lymphatic vessels called lymphangiosarcoma.
	• Seroma - a mass/ lump caused by the buildup of lymph fluid at the site of the surgery
	• Numbness, tingling, swelling, bruising, or pain at the site of the surgery, and an increased risk of infection
	• Difficulty moving the affected body part
	• Skin or allergic reactions to the blue dye used in SNLB
	• A false-negative biopsy result—that is, cancer cells are not seen in the sentinel lymph node even though they have already spread to regional lymph nodes or other parts of the body. A false-negative biopsy result gives the patient and the doctor a false sense of security about the extent of cancer in the patient's body.
	NIH NCI (13)

Axillary Lymph Nodes	The axillary lymph nodes or armpit lymph nodes are lymph nodes in the human armpit. • Between 20 and 49 in number. • They drain lymph vessels from the lateral quadrants of the breast, the superficial lymph vessels from thin walls of the chest and the abdomen above the level of the navel, and the vessels from the upper limb. • They are divided in several groups according to their location in the armpit. These lymph nodes are clinically significant in breast cancer, and metastases from the breast to the axillary lymph nodes are considered in the staging of the disease. • About 75% of lymph from the breasts drains into the axillary lymph nodes, making them important in the diagnosis and staging of breast cancer. • A doctor will usually refer a patient to a surgeon to have an axillary lymph node dissection to see if the cancer cells have been trapped in the nodes. • For clinical stages I and II breast cancer, axillary lymph node dissection should only be performed after first attempting sentinel node biopsy. *Wikipedia – Axillary Lymph Nodes*

Wikipedia – Axillary Lymph Nodes www.scientificanimations.com

Risks of Axillary Node Dissection	Anywhere from about 10 to 40 (though usually less than 20) lymph nodes are removed from the area under the arm (axilla) and checked for cancer spread.

	• ALND is usually done at the same time as a mastectomy or breast-conserving surgery (BCS), but it can be done in a second operation. ALND may be needed:
	    o If a previous SLNB has shown 3 or more of the underarm lymph nodes have cancer cells
	    o If swollen underarm or collarbone lymph nodes can be felt before surgery or seen on imaging tests and a FNA or core needle biopsy shows cancer
	    o If the cancer has grown large enough to extend outside the lymph node(s)
	    o If the SLNB is positive for cancer cells after chemotherapy was given to shrink the tumor before surgery. *American Cancer Society*
	• Compared with axillary sampling alone, partial or total mastectomy followed by full axillary lymph node dissection significantly increases a patient's chance of developing arm edema.
	• In one series of 100 women who underwent partial or total mastectomy and then full axillary lymph node dissection or axillary sampling, arm edema developed in more patients who underwent axillary lymph node dissection compared with sampling alone (30% vs. none). In addition, the extent of axillary lymph node dissection increases the risk for developing arm edema.

3 Levels of ALND	The three levels of an axillary lymph node dissection, from least aggressive to most aggressive, are: • Level I- The surgical removal of all tissue below the lower edge of the pectoralis minor muscle. • Level II- The surgical removal of the tissue lying underneath the pectoralis minor muscle. • Level III - The most aggressive dissection, and is the surgical removal of tissue lying above the pectoralis minor muscle. A traditional axillary lymph node dissection usually includes removal of the nodes in levels I and II from the "fat pad" under the arm. *UPMC- Axillary Lymph Node Dissection* Surgical Margin for Fat Pad: • Axillary vein – Superior • Thoracodorsal bundle – Lateral • Long thoracic nerve – Medial ## Axillary Lymph Nodes level III (high axilla) level II (mid axilla) level I (low axilla) armpit (axilla) Wiki McMaster: *Breast Cancer*

Nerves that may be Damaged during Surgery *Pink Ribbon Program©*	Several structures, including vessels and muscles with their nerve supply, are related to the breast and should be preserved during mastectomy or axillary node dissection. <ul><li>The **lateral pectoral nerve** passes medially around the medial pectoralis minor, and the medial pectoral nerve passes laterally around the pectoralis minor. These nerves can be severed during surgery. This results in ***numbness, motor atrophy, decreased sweat production in armpit and arm.***</li><li>The **medial pectoral nerve** innervates pectoralis minor and the lateral portion of the pectoralis major muscles. Preservation of this nerve is particularly important to prevent ***atrophy of the pectoral muscles*** if submuscular implant reconstruction is planned.</li><li>The **thoracodorsal nerve** is identifiable medial to the thoracodorsal vein. Injury may result in a ***weakening of the latissimus.***</li><li>The **long thoracic nerve** of Bell is located more medially in the axilla. It runs just beneath the fascia of the serratus anterior, medial to the thoracodorsal complex. Injury to this nerve will result in weakness in the serratus anterior muscle and cause ***winging of the scapula.***</li></ul> *Pink Ribbon Program©*

Latissimus dorsi

Pec Major

Pec Minor

Scapular – normal

Scapular – winging

BREAST CANCER

Information and pictures from *National Cancer Institute* unless otherwise specified

Quick Summary this Section

Breast Cancer:
- What is Breast Cancer, Stage Groups, Risk Factors, Protective Factors

Types:
- DCIS, LCIS, IDC, ILC, Rare, Inflammatory, Paget Disease

Screening
- Mammogram, Diagnostic Mammography, Ultrasound, MRI, Biopsy, PET scan

Pathology: Testing and Diagnosis
- Tumor Grade/Differentiating Cells, Nottingham Grading System

Staging:
- TMN Staging, Stage 0-IV, Localized, Regional, Distant, Unknown

Prognostic Markers:
- Margins or Ink, HER2/neu Gene, Estrogen Receptor (ER), Progesterone Receptor (PR), Ki-67, S-Phase Fraction, Lymphovascular Invasion, Multigene Test, Molecular Subtypes

Genes:
- Tumor Suppressor Gene, BRCA1 and BRCA 2, PALB2, CHEK2, ATM

Surgeries:
- Mastectomy, Lumpectomy, Nipple Sparing Mastectomy, Total or Simple Mastectomy, Considerations, Comparisons

Reconstruction:
- Factors - Timing and Choice
- Reconstruction: Implants or Autologous Tissue

Breast Implants:
- Implants
- Tissue Expanders

Tissue Flap Surgeries:
- Autologous Tissue & Reconstruction
- TRAM, DIEP, SIEA, LAT, Gluteal, TUG, IGAP
- Nipple Reconstruction

Risks after Breast Surgery:

- Axillary Web Syndrome - AWS (Cording), Scar Tissue / Adhesions, Seroma / Compression

Things to Avoid, Post Op Healing & Mastectomy:

- Avoid 2 - weeks Post op, Post op healing concerns, Recommendations post mastectomy

Exercise Examples - Post Mastectomy:

- Examples of Exercises, Stretches or Edema Control after Mastectomy

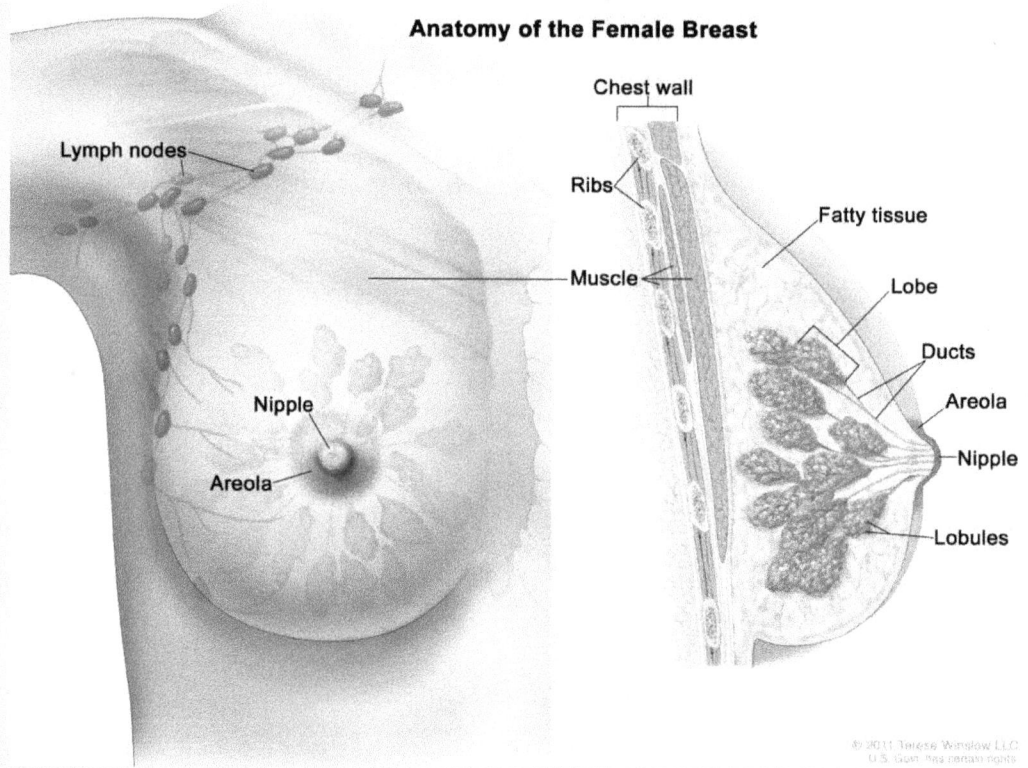

What is Breast Cancer?	Breast cancer is a disease in which cells in the breast grow out of control. There are different kinds of breast cancer. The kind of breast cancer depends on which cells in the breast turn into cancer. • Breast cancer can begin in different parts of the breast. A breast is made up of three main parts: lobules, ducts, and connective tissue. • The lobules are the glands that produce milk. The ducts are tubes that carry milk to the nipple. • The connective tissue (which consists of fibrous and fatty tissue) surrounds and holds everything together. • Most breast cancers begin in the ducts or lobules. • Breast cancer can spread outside the breast through blood vessels and lymph vessels. ○ When breast cancer spreads to other parts of the body, it is said to have metastasized. *CDC (1)* **Anatomy of the Female Breast** Chest wall Lymph nodes Ribs Fatty tissue Muscle Lobe Ducts Nipple Areola Areola Nipple Lobules © 2011 Terese Winslow LLC U.S. Govt. has certain rights *NIH - NCI (National Cancer Institute) https://www.cancer.gov/types/breast/patient/breast- treatment-pdq#_148*

Staging and Stage Groups	Stage refers to the extent of your cancer, such as how large the tumor is, and if it has spread.
	• A cancer is always referred to by the stage it was given at diagnosis, even if it gets worse or spreads.
	• New information about how a cancer has changed over time gets added on to the original stage. So, the stage doesn't change, even though the cancer might.
	
	Systems that Describe Stage
	There are many staging systems. Some, such as the TNM staging system, are used for many types of cancer. Others are specific to a particular type of cancer.
	
	Most staging systems include information about:
	• Where the tumor is located in the body
	• The cell type (such as, adenocarcinoma or squamous cell carcinoma)
	• The size of the tumor
	• Whether the cancer has spread to nearby lymph nodes
	• Whether the cancer has spread to a different part of the body
	• Tumor grade, which refers to how abnormal the cancer cells look and how likely the tumor is to grow and spread
	NIH – NCI (6)
	
	In breast cancer, stage is based on the size and location of the primary tumor, the spread of cancer to nearby lymph nodes or other parts of the body, tumor grade, and whether certain biomarkers are present.
	
	To plan the best treatment and understand your prognosis, it is important to know the breast cancer stage. *NIH – NCI (2)*
	
	• **Clinical Prognostic Stage** is used first to assign a stage for all patients based on health history, physical exam, imaging tests (if done), and biopsies
	    ○ The Clinical Prognostic Stage is described by the TNM system, tumor grade, and biomarker status (ER, PR, HER2).
	    ○ In clinical staging, mammography or ultrasound is used to check the lymph nodes for signs of cancer.
	
	• **Pathological Prognostic Stage** is then used for patients who have surgery as their first treatment.
	    ○ Prognostic Stage is based on all clinical information, biomarker status, and laboratory test results from breast tissue and lymph nodes removed during surgery
	
	• **Anatomic Stage** is based on the size and the spread of cancer as described by the TNM system.

| Risk Factors | **Risk Factors**
• A personal history of benign (non-cancer) breast disease.
• A family history of breast cancer in a first- degree relative (mother, daughter, or sister).
• Inherited changes in the BRCA1 or BRCA2 genes or in other genes (such as PALB2) that increase the risk of breast cancer.
• Breast tissue that is dense on a mammogram.
• Exposure of breast tissue to estrogen made by the body. This may be caused by:
   o Menstruating at an early age.
   o Older age at first birth or never having given birth.
   o Starting menopause at a later age.
• Taking hormones such as estrogen combined with progestin for symptoms of menopause.
• Treatment with radiation therapy to the breast/chest.
• Drinking alcohol.
• Obesity.

BRCA
Of all women with breast cancer, 5% to 10% may have a germline mutation of the genes BRCA1 and BRCA2. Specific mutations of BRCA1 and BRCA2 are more common in women of Jewish ancestry.
• The estimated lifetime risk of developing breast cancer for women with BRCA1 and BRCA2 mutations is 40% to 85%.
• Carriers with a history of breast cancer have an increased risk of contralateral disease that may be as high as 5% per year.
• Male BRCA2 mutation carriers also have an increased risk of breast cancer.
• Mutations in either the BRCA1 or the BRCA2 gene also confer an increased risk of ovarian cancer or other primary cancers.
• Once a BRCA1 or BRCA2 mutation has been identified, other family members can be referred for genetic counseling and testing. *NIH – NCI (1)* |
| **Protective Factors** | **Protective Factors**
Protective factors and interventions to reduce the risk of female breast cancer include the following:
• Estrogen use (after hysterectomy).
• Exercise.
• Early pregnancy.
• Breast feeding.
• Selective estrogen receptor modulators (SERMs).
• Aromatase inhibitors or inactivators.
• Risk-reducing mastectomy.
• Risk-reducing oophorectomy or ovarian ablation.
NIH – NCI (1) |

Quick Summary of Section

Ductal carcinoma in situ (DCIS):

- DCIS is considered a precursor lesion for the subsequent development of invasive carcinoma with a high-risk index factor than that expected in women without DCIS

Lobular carcinoma in situ (LCIS):

- Lobular carcinoma in situ (LCIS) is an uncommon condition in which abnormal cells form in the milk glands (lobules) in the breast. LCIS isn't cancer, but being diagnosed with LCIS indicates that you have an increased risk of developing breast cancer.

Invasive ductal carcinoma (IDC):

- The most common type of invasive breast cancer. It begins in the lining of the milk ducts (thin tubes that carry milk from the lobules of the breast to the nipple) and spreads outside the ducts to surrounding normal tissue. Invasive ductal carcinoma can also spread through the blood and lymph systems to other parts of the body.

Invasive lobular carcinoma (ILC):

- A type of invasive breast cancer that begins in the lobules (milk glands) of the breast and spreads to surrounding normal tissue. It can also spread through the blood and lymph systems to other parts of the body.

Rare cancers:

- For example, male breast cancer, medullary breast cancer, lymphoma of the breast

Inflammatory breast

- Inflammatory breast cancer is a rare and very aggressive disease in which cancer cells block lymph vessels in the skin of the breast. This type of breast cancer is called "inflammatory" because the breast often looks swollen and red, or inflamed.

Paget Disease of the Breast:

- Paget disease of the breast (also known as Paget disease of the nipple and mammary Paget disease) is a rare type of cancer involving the skin of the nipple and, usually, the darker circle of skin around it, which is called the areola.

Ductal Carcinoma in situ (DCIS)	DCIS is considered a precursor lesion for the subsequent development of invasive carcinoma with a high-risk index factor than that expected in women without DCIS Death due to DCIS is extremely rare, but death occurring after initial diagnosis of DCIS is either because of undetected invasive component or due to recurrence of invasive lesion after the treatment. *NCBI - Diversity of Breast Carcinoma* • 85% of breast cancer originates in the ducts • These cancers are considered benign, but eventually will become invasive with time **Symptoms:** DCIS doesn't typically have any signs or symptoms. However, DCIS can sometimes cause signs such as: • A breast lump • Bloody nipple discharge *Mayo Clinic: Ductal carcinoma in situ (DCIS)*
Lobular Carcinoma in situ (LCIS)	Lobular carcinoma in situ (LCIS) is an uncommon condition in which abnormal cells form in the milk glands (lobules) in the breast. LCIS isn't cancer, but being diagnosed with LCIS indicates that you have an increased risk of developing breast cancer. Women with LCIS have an increased risk of developing invasive breast cancer in either breast. • 15% of breast cancer originates in the lobules • These cancers are considered benign but eventually will become invasive with time. **Symptoms:** LCIS usually doesn't show up on mammograms. The condition is most often discovered as a result of a breast biopsy done for another reason, such as a suspicious breast lump or an abnormal mammogram. *Mayo Clinic: Lobular carcinoma in situ (LCIS)*
Invasive Ductal Carcinoma (IDC)	The most common type of invasive breast cancer. It begins in the lining of the milk ducts (thin tubes that carry milk from the lobules of the breast to the nipple) and spreads outside the ducts to surrounding normal tissue. Invasive ductal carcinoma can also spread through the blood and lymph systems to other parts of the body. Also called infiltrating ductal carcinoma. *NIH – NCI – IDC definition* • The cancer cells grow outside the ducts into other parts of the breast tissue. • Invasive cancer cells can also spread, or metastasize, to other parts of the body. **Symptoms:** • A lump in your breast. • Thickened breast skin. • Rash or redness on your breast. • Swelling in your breast. • New pain in your breast. • Dimpling on your breast or the skin of your nipple. • Nipple pain. • Inverted nipple.

Invasive Lobular Carcinoma (ILC)	A type of invasive breast cancer that begins in the lobules (milk glands) of the breast and spreads to surrounding normal tissue. It can also spread through the blood and lymph systems to other parts of the body. Also called infiltrating lobular carcinoma. *NIH- NCI – ILC definition* • Begins in the milk-producing glands (lobules) of the breast. • Cancer cells have broken out of the lobule where they began and have the potential to spread to the lymph nodes and other areas of the body. • Invasive lobular carcinoma makes up a small portion of all breast cancers. • Invasive lobular carcinoma is less likely than other forms of breast cancer to cause a firm or distinct breast lump. **Symptoms:** At its earliest stages, invasive lobular carcinoma may cause no signs and symptoms. As it grows larger, invasive lobular carcinoma may cause: • An area of thickening in part of the breast • A new area of fullness or swelling in the breast • A change in the texture or appearance of the skin over the breast, such as dimpling or thickening • A newly inverted nipple *Mayo Clinic: Invasive lobular carcinoma*
Rare Cancers – not limited to:	• Male Breast Cancer - Cancer that forms in tissues of the breast in men. Most male breast cancer begins in cells lining the ducts. It is very rare and usually affects older men. • Medullary breast cancer • Mucinous (mucoid or colloid) breast cancer • Tubular breast cancer • Adenoid cystic carcinoma of the breast • Metaplastic breast cancer • Lymphoma of the breast • Basal type breast cancer • Phyllodes or cystosarcoma phyllodes • Papillary breast cancer

Inflammatory Breast Cancer	Inflammatory breast cancer is a rare and very aggressive disease in which cancer cells block lymph vessels in the skin of the breast. This type of breast cancer is called "inflammatory" because the breast often looks swollen and red, or inflamed. • Inflammatory breast cancer is rare, accounting for 1 to 5 percent of all breast cancers diagnosed in the United States. Most inflammatory breast cancers are invasive ductal carcinomas, which means they developed from cells that line the milk ducts of the breast and then spread beyond the ducts. • Inflammatory breast cancer progresses rapidly, often in a matter of weeks or months. At diagnosis, inflammatory breast cancer is either stage III or IV disease, depending on whether cancer cells have spread only to nearby lymph nodes or to other tissues as well. • Compared with other types of breast cancer, inflammatory breast cancer tends to be diagnosed at younger ages. • More common and diagnosed at younger ages in African American women than in white women. • Inflammatory breast tumors are frequently hormone receptor negative, which means they cannot be treated with hormone therapies, such as tamoxifen, that interfere with the growth of cancer cells fueled by estrogen. • More common in obese women than in women of normal weight. *NIH – NCI – Inflammatory Breast*
Paget Disease of the Breast	• Paget disease of the breast (also known as Paget disease of the nipple and mammary Paget disease) is a rare type of cancer involving the skin of the nipple and, usually, the darker circle of skin around it, which is called the areola. • Most people with Paget disease of the breast also have one or more tumors inside the same breast. These breast tumors are either ductal carcinoma in situ or invasive breast cancer. • Paget disease of the breast occurs in both women and men, but most cases occur in women. Approximately 1 to 4 percent of all cases of breast cancer also involve Paget disease of the breast. • The average age at diagnosis is 57 years, but the disease has been found in adolescents and in people in their late 80s • Studies have shown that breast-conserving surgery that includes removal of the nipple and areola, followed by whole-breast radiation therapy, is a safe option for people with Paget disease of the breast who do not have a palpable lump in their breast and whose mammograms do not reveal a tumor The symptoms of Paget disease of the breast are often mistaken for those of some benign skin conditions, such as dermatitis or eczema. These symptoms may include the following: • Itching, tingling, or redness in the nipple and/or areola • Flaking, crusty, or thickened skin on or around the nipple • A flattened nipple • Discharge from the nipple that may be yellowish or bloody • Because the early symptoms of Paget disease of the breast may suggest a benign skin condition, and because the disease is rare, it may be misdiagnosed at first. • People with Paget disease of the breast have often had symptoms for several months before being correctly diagnosed. *NIH NCI – Paget*

CDC – Center of Disease Control and Prevention

CDC (1) – What is Breast Cancer? *https://www.cdc.gov/cancer/breast/basic_info/what-is-breast-cancer.htm*

Mayo Clinic: *Mayoclinic.org*

Mayo Clinic: Ductal carcinoma in situ (DCIS) *https://www.mayoclinic.org/diseases-conditions/dcis/symptoms-causes/syc-20371889*

Mayo Clinic: Invasive lobular carcinoma *https://www.mayoclinic.org/diseases-conditions/invasive-lobular-carcinoma/symptoms-causes/syc-20373973*

Mayo Clinic: Lobular carcinoma in situ (LCIS) *https://www.mayoclinic.org/diseases-conditions/lobular-carcinoma-in-situ/symptoms-causes/syc-20374529*

NCBI - Diversity of Breast Carcinoma *https://www.ncbi.nlm.nih.gov/pmc/articles/PMC4689326/*

NIH – NCI – National Cancer Institute

NIH – NCI - IDC definition *https://www.cancer.gov/publications/dictionaries/cancer-terms/def/invasive-ductal-carcinoma*

NIH – NCI (1) - Breast Treatment (professional) *https://www.cancer.gov/types/breast/hp/breast-treatment-pdq*

NIH – NCI (2) Treatment (patient) *https://www.cancer.gov/types/breast/patient/breast-treatment-pdq#_181*

NIH- NCI - ILC definition- *https://www.cancer.gov/publications/dictionaries/cancer-terms/def/invasive-lobular-carcinoma*

NIH NCI - Paget *https://www.cancer.gov/types/breast/paget-breast-fact-sheet*

NIH – NCI – Inflammatory Breast Cancer *https://www.cancer.gov/types/breast/ibc-fact-sheet*

SCREENING

Quick Summary of Section

Screenings

- High or low levels of certain substances in your body can be a sign of cancer, so, lab tests of your blood, urine, or other body fluids that measure these substances can help doctors make a diagnosis.

Screening Mammogram

- X-rays of the breasts taken to check for breast cancer in the absence of signs or symptoms.

Diagnostic Mammography

- A type of mammography in which more x-ray pictures of the breast are taken from different angles to allow a possible abnormality to be examined more closely.

Ultrasound

- A procedure that makes a picture (called a sonogram) of breast tissue in order to find out if a lump is solid or is filled with fluid (that is, a cyst).

MRI

- A procedure that uses a powerful magnet, radio waves, and a computer to take detailed pictures of areas inside the breast.

Ductography

- A procedure that takes pictures of the breast ducts, so that doctors can learn more about certain kinds of abnormal nipple discharge or masses.

PET Scan

- A PET scan is a type of nuclear scan that makes detailed 3-D pictures of areas inside your body where glucose is taken up.

Biopsy

- A procedure that removes a sample of breast tissue or an entire lump so that it can be checked for signs of disease.

Lab Tests	<ul><li>High or low levels of certain substances in your body can be a sign of cancer. So, lab tests of your blood, urine, or other body fluids that measure these substances can help doctors make a diagnosis.</li><li>Some lab tests involve testing blood or tissue samples for tumor markers. Tumor markers are substances that are produced by cancer cells or by other cells of the body in response to cancer.</li><li>Most tumor markers are made by normal cells and cancer cells but are produced at much higher levels by cancer cells. *NIH – NCI (4)*</li></ul>

Screening Mammogram	X-rays of the breasts taken to check for breast cancer in the absence of signs or symptoms.
	
	Possible mammogram findings include:
	
	• Lumps (mass or tumor). Lumps come in different sizes and shapes. Fluid-filled cysts are usually smooth and rounded, with clear, defined edges and are not cancer. Lumps that have a jagged outline and an irregular shape are of more concern.
	• Calcifications. There are two types of breast calcifications, or calcium deposits:
	    o Macrocalcifications, which look like small white dots on a mammogram. They are often caused by aging, an old injury, or inflammation and are usually benign.
	    o Microcalcifications, which look like white specks on a mammogram. If found in an area of rapidly dividing cells or grouped together in a certain way, they may be a sign of DCIS or breast cancer.
	• Dense breast tissue: A dense breast has relatively less fat and more glandular and connective tissue. This mammogram finding is both common and normal, especially among younger women and women who use menopausal hormone therapy. Dense breast tissue can make a mammogram more difficult to interpret because both dense breast tissue and breast tumors appear as solid white areas in the image.
	NIH – NCI (3)

Diagnostic mammography	A type of mammography in which more x-ray pictures of the breast are taken from different angles to allow a possible abnormality to be examined more closely. • X-ray of the breasts used to check for breast cancer after a lump or other sign or symptom of breast cancer has been found. *NIH – NCI (3)*
Ultrasound	A procedure that makes a picture (called a sonogram) of breast tissue in order to find out if a lump is solid or is filled with fluid (that is, a cyst). Pictures are made using sound waves. *NIH – NCI (3)*
MRI (also called Magnetic Resonance Imaging):	A procedure that uses a powerful magnet, radio waves, and a computer to take detailed pictures of areas inside the breast. • An MRI can be used to learn more about breast lumps or large lymph nodes that were found during a clinical breast exam or breast self-exam but were not seen on a mammogram or ultrasound. *NIH – NCI (3)*
Ductography AKA Galactography	A procedure that takes pictures of the breast ducts, so that doctors can learn more about certain kinds of abnormal nipple discharge or masses such as intraductal papilloma's (wart-like tumors that are benign). • Pictures of the breast ducts are taken using a contrast material that is given through an injection to help breast ducts show up clearly. *NIH – NCI (3)*

PET scan	A PET scan is a type of nuclear scan that makes detailed 3-D pictures of areas inside your body where glucose is taken up. • Because cancer cells often take up more glucose than healthy cells, the pictures can be used to find cancer in the body. • Before the scan, you receive an injection of a tracer called radioactive glucose. During the scan, you will lie still on a table that moves back and forth through a scanner. *NIH – NCI (4)*

Biopsy	A procedure that removes a sample of breast tissue or an entire lump so that it can be checked for signs of disease.
	
	• Imaging procedures (such as ultrasound, MRIs, or x-rays) are often used during a biopsy to guide the surgeon.
	
	• A pathologist then examines the sample under a microscope or performs other tests on it.
	
	Common types of breast biopsies include:
	
	• **Core needle biopsy:** The use of a wide needle to remove small tissue sample(s) that are about the size of a grain of rice. It may cause a temporary bruise. Also called core biopsy.
	• **Fine-needle aspiration biopsy:** The use of a thin needle to drain fluid and/or to remove cells.
	• **Surgical biopsy:** The removal of part, or all, of a lump so it can be checked for signs of cancer.
	   ○ An incisional biopsy removes a sample of breast tissue.
	   ○ An excisional biopsy removes an entire lump or suspicious area.
	   ○ Wire localization (also called needle localization and needle (wire) localization) may be used to mark the area of abnormal tissue before the biopsy.
	• **Vacuum-assisted biopsy:** The removal of a small sample of breast tissue using a probe that is connected to a vacuum device. The small cut made in the breast is much smaller than with surgical biopsy. This procedure causes little scarring, and no stitches are needed. It may also be called vacuum-assisted core biopsy.
	• A biopsy procedure that uses a computer and a 3-dimensional scanning device to find a tumor site and guide the removal of tissue for examination under a microscope.
	
	Biopsies are usually done in a doctor's office or a clinic on an outpatient basis. This means you will go home the same day as the procedure.
	• **Local anesthesia** is used for many biopsies, so you'll be awake but won't feel pain during the procedure.
	• **General anesthesia** is commonly used for surgical biopsies, which means you'll be asleep during the procedure.
	NIH – NCI (3)

NIH – NCI (3) Breast Changes and Conditions *https://www.cancer.gov/types/breast/breast-changes*
NIH – NCI (4) How Cancer Is Diagnosed *https://www.cancer.gov/about-cancer/diagnosis-staging/diagnosis*

PATHOLOGY: TESTING AND DIAGNOSIS

Quick Summary of Section

Tumor Grade/Differentiating Cells
- Tumor grade is the description of a tumor based on how abnormal the tumor cells and the tumor tissue look under a microscope.
- It is an indicator of how quickly a tumor is likely to grow and spread.

Nottingham Grading System
- Numbers are assigned to different features (gland formation, nuclear grade, and mitotic count) seen under the microscope and then added up to assign the grade".

Tumor Grade/

Differentiating Cells

Tumor grade is the description of a tumor based on how abnormal the tumor cells and the tumor tissue look under a microscope. It is an indicator of how quickly a tumor is likely to grow and spread.

Based on these and other differences in microscopic appearance, doctors assign a numerical "grade" to most cancers. The factors used to determine tumor grade can vary between different types of cancer. *NIH – NCI (5)*

Well differentiated:
If the cells of the tumor and the organization of the tumor's tissue are close to those of normal cells and tissue, the tumor is called "well-differentiated ." These tumors tend to *grow and spread at a slower rate.*

Poor or undifferentiated:
Tumors that are "undifferentiated" or "poorly differentiated," have abnormal-looking cells and may lack normal tissue structures and *grow at a faster rate.*

Nottingham grading system

AKA

Elston-Ellis modification of the Scarff-Bloom-Richardson grading system

"Numbers are assigned to different features (gland formation, nuclear grade, and mitotic count) seen under the microscope and then added up to assign the grade". *American Cancer Society*

Tubule formation: how much of the tumor tissue has normal breast (milk) duct structures

Nuclear grade: an evaluation of the size and shape of the nucleus in the tumor cells

Mitotic rate: how many dividing cells are present, which is a measure of how fast the tumor cells are growing and dividing

Each of the categories gets a score between 1 and 3.

A score of "1" means the cells and tumor tissue look the most like *normal* cells and tissue, and a score of "3" means the cells and tissue look the most *abnormal*.

The scores for the three categories are then added, yielding a total score of 3 to 9.

NIH – NCI (5)

Total score = 3–5: G1

Low grade or well differentiated

Total score = 6–7: G2

Intermediate grade or moderately differentiated

Total score = 8–9: G3

High grade or poorly differentiated

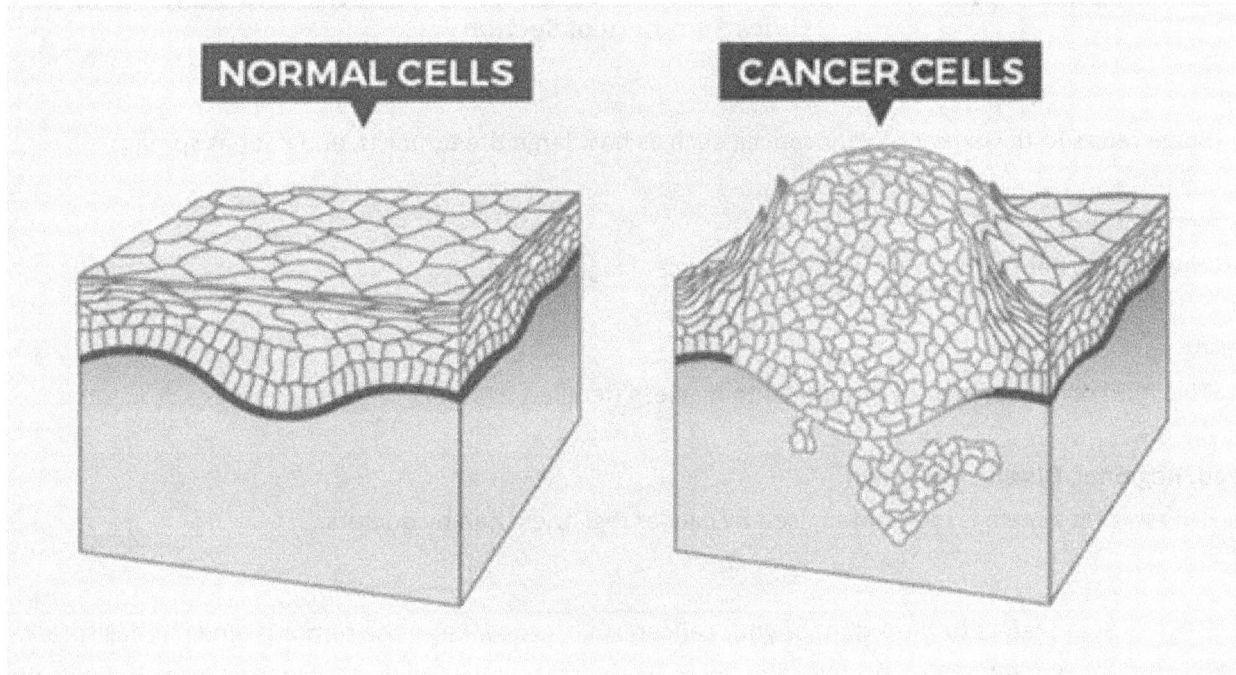

NIH – *NCI*

https://www.cancer.gov/about-cancer/understanding/what-is-cancer

STAGING

Quick Summary of Section

Staging
- Stage refers to the extent of your cancer, such as how large the tumor is, and if it has spread.

TNM Staging System
- The TNM system is the most widely used cancer staging system.

Stage 0-IV
- The TNM combinations are grouped into five less-detailed stages.

Localized, Regional, Distant, Unknown
- This staging system is more often used by cancer registries than by doctors.

Staging	Stage refers to the extent of your cancer, such as how large the tumor is, and if it has spread.
	• A cancer is always referred to by the stage it was given at diagnosis, even if it gets worse or spreads.
	• New information about how a cancer has changed over time gets added on to the original stage. So, the stage doesn't change, even though the cancer might.
	Systems that Describe Stage
	There are many staging systems. Some, such as the TNM staging system, are used for many types of cancer. Others are specific to a particular type of cancer.
	Most staging systems include information about:
	• Where the tumor is located in the body
	• The cell type (such as, adenocarcinoma or squamous cell carcinoma)
	• The size of the tumor
	• Whether the cancer has spread to nearby lymph nodes
	• Whether the cancer has spread to a different part of the body
	• Tumor grade, which refers to how abnormal the cancer cells look and how likely the tumor is to grow and spread
	NIH – *NCI (6)*

TNM Staging System	The TNM system is the most widely used cancer staging system.

The TNM system is the most widely used cancer staging system.

- The **T (Tumor)** refers to the size and extent of the main tumor. The main tumor is usually called the primary tumor.
- The **N (Nodes)** refers to the number of nearby lymph nodes that have cancer.
- The **M (Metastasis)** refers to whether the cancer has metastasized. This means that the cancer has spread from the primary tumor to other parts of the body.

When your cancer is described by the TNM system, there will be numbers after each letter that give more details about the cancer—for example, T1N0MX or T3N1M0.

The following explains what the letters and numbers mean:

Primary tumor (T)
- TX: Main tumor cannot be measured.
- T0: Main tumor cannot be found.
- T1, T2, T3, T4: Refers to the size and/or extent of the main tumor. The higher the number after the T, the larger the tumor or the more it has grown into nearby tissues. T's may be further divided to provide more detail, such as T3a and T3b.

Regional lymph nodes (N)
- NX: Cancer in nearby lymph nodes cannot be measured.
- N0: There is no cancer in nearby lymph nodes.
- N1, N2, N3: Refers to the number and location of lymph nodes that contain cancer. The higher the number after the N, the more lymph nodes that contain cancer.

Distant metastasis (M)
- MX: Metastasis cannot be measured.
- M0: Cancer has not spread to other parts of the body.
- M1: Cancer has spread to other parts of the body
  NIH – NCI (6)

Stage 0-IV

The TNM system helps describe cancer in great detail, but, for many cancers, the TNM combinations are grouped into five less-detailed stages. When talking about your cancer, your doctor or nurse may describe it as one of these stages:

- **Stage 0** or in situ- Abnormal cells are present but have not spread to nearby tissue.
  - Also called carcinoma in situ, or CIS. CIS is not cancer, but it may become cancer.
- **Stage I, Stage II, and Stage III** - Cancer is present. The higher the number, the larger the cancer tumor and the more it has spread into nearby tissues.
- **Stage IV** - The cancer has spread to distant parts of the body.
  NIH – NCI (6)

Localized, Regional, Distant, Unknown

Another staging system that is used for all types of cancer groups the cancer into one of five main categories. This staging system is more often used by cancer registries than by doctors.But, you may still hear your doctor or nurse describe your cancer in one of the following ways:

- **Localized**—Cancer is limited to the place where it started, with no sign that it has spread.
- **Regional**—Cancer has spread to nearby lymph nodes, tissues, or organs.
- **Distant**—Cancer has spread to distant parts of the body.
- **Unknown**—There is not enough information to figure out the stage. *NIH – NCI (6)*

PROGNOSTIC MARKERS

Quick Summary of Section

Margins or Ink

- When an entire tumor is removed, the outside edges (or margins) of the specimen are coated with ink, sometimes even with different colors of ink on different sides of the specimen.

HER2/neu Gene

- Some breast cancers have too much of a growth-promoting protein called HER2/neu (HER2). The HER2/neu gene instructs the cells to make this protein.
- Immunohistochemistry (IHC)
- Fluorescent in situ hybridization (FISH)
- Chromogenic in situ hybridization (CISH)

Estrogen Receptor (ER)

- A protein found inside the cells of the female reproductive tissue, some other types of tissue, and some cancer cells.
- The hormone estrogen will bind to the receptors inside the cells and may cause the cells to grow.

Progesterone Receptor (PR)

- A protein found inside the cells of the female reproductive tissue, some other types of tissue, and some cancer cells.
- The hormone progesterone will bind to the receptors inside the cells and may cause the cells to grow.

Ki-67

- Ki-67 is a way to measure how fast the cancer cells are growing and dividing.

S-Phase Fraction

- This number tells you what percentages of cells in the sample are in the process of copying their genetic information, or DNA.

Lymphovascular Invasion

- Lymphovascular invasion (LVI) is defined as the presence of tumor cells within a definite endothelial-lined space (lymphatics or blood vessels) in the breast surrounding invasive carcinoma.

Multigene Tests

- Tests in which samples of tissue are studied to look at the activity of many genes at the same time.
- These tests may help predict whether cancer will spread to other parts of the body or recur (come back).

Molecular Subtypes

- Four main breast cancer subtypes have been identified according to estrogen receptor (ER), progesterone receptor (PR), and HER2.
- These subtypes include luminal types A and B, basal-like, and HER2-enriched subtype.

Margins or Ink	When an entire tumor is removed, the outside edges (or margins) of the specimen are coated with ink, sometimes even with different colors of ink on different sides of the specimen.
	  • The pathologist looks at slides of the tumor under the microscope to see how close the cancer cells get to the ink (the edges or margins of the specimen).
	 American Cancer Society: Understanding Your Pathology Report
	
	  • The margin is described as negative or clean when the pathologist finds no cancer cells at the edge of the tissue, suggesting that all of the cancer has been removed.
	  • The margin is described as positive or involved when the pathologist finds cancer cells at the edge of the tissue, suggesting that all of the cancer has not been removed.
	 NIH – NCI (1)

HER2/neu Gene
 	
 IHC and FISH test
	Some breast cancers have too much of a growth-promoting protein called HER2/neu (HER2). The HER2/neu gene instructs the cells to make this protein.
	  • Tumors with increased levels of HER2/neu are referred to as HER2-positive.
	  • The cells in HER2-positive breast cancers have too many copies of the HER2/neu gene, resulting in greater than normal amounts of the HER2 protein. These cancers tend to grow and spread more quickly than other breast cancers.
	  • Women with HER2-positive cancers are much more likely to benefit from treatment with drugs that target the HER2 protein. If your cancer is HER2-positive, your doctor might add certain drugs to your treatment. How the results of your tests will affect your treatment is best discussed with your doctor.
	
	 Testing of the biopsy or surgery sample:
	  • ***Immunohistochemistry (IHC):*** In this test, special antibodies that will stick to the HER2 protein are applied to the sample, which cause cells to change color if many copies are present. This color change can be seen under a microscope.
	 The test results are reported as 0, 1+, 2+, or 3+.
	     o **0 or 1+: HER2- (negative).** Women with HER2- negative tumors are not treated with drugs that target HER2.
	     o **3+ : HER2 + (positive).** The person might benefit from treatment with drugs that target HER2.
	     o **2+: HER2 status** of the tumor is not clear and is called "equivocal." This means that the HER2 status needs to be tested with FISH to clarify the result.
	  • ***Fluorescent in situ hybridization (FISH):*** This test uses fluorescent pieces of DNA that specifically stick to copies of the HER2/neu gene in cells, which can then be counted under a special microscope.
	  • ***Chromogenic in situ hybridization (CISH):*** This test works similarly to FISH, by using small DNA probes to count the number of HER2/neu genes in breast cancer cells.
	
	 American Cancer Society: Understanding Your Pathology Report

Estrogen Receptor (ER)	**Estrogen:** A type of hormone made by the body that helps develop and maintain female sex characteristics and the growth of long bones. Estrogens can also be made in the laboratory.
	They may be used as a type of birth control and to treat symptoms of menopause, menstrual disorders, osteoporosis, and other conditions.

Moving content out of table structure for readability:

Estrogen: A type of hormone made by the body that helps develop and maintain female sex characteristics and the growth of long bones. Estrogens can also be made in the laboratory.

They may be used as a type of birth control and to treat symptoms of menopause, menstrual disorders, osteoporosis, and other conditions.

- **Estrogen receptor (ER):** A protein found inside the cells of the female reproductive tissue, some other types of tissue, and some cancer cells.
  - The hormone estrogen will bind to the receptors inside the cells and may cause the cells to grow.
  - Also called ER.
- **Estrogen receptor negative (ER-):** Describes cells that do not have a protein to which the hormone estrogen will bind.
  - Cancer cells that are estrogen receptor negative do not need estrogen to grow and usually do not stop growing when treated with hormones that block estrogen from binding.
  - Also called ER negative.
- **Estrogen receptor positive (ER+):** Describes cells that have a receptor protein that binds the hormone estrogen.
  - Cancer cells that are estrogen receptor positive may need estrogen to grow and may stop growing or die when treated with substances that block the binding and actions of estrogen.
  - Also called ER positive.
- **Estrogen receptor (ER) test:** A lab test to find out if cancer cells have estrogen receptors (proteins to which estrogen will bind).
  - If the cells have estrogen receptors, they may need estrogen to grow, and this may affect how the cancer is treated.
    NIH – NCI (2)

Results for ER are reported separately and can be reported in different ways:
- Negative, weakly positive, positive
- Percent positive
- Percent positive and whether the staining is weak, moderate, or strong.

Women with hormone receptor-positive cancers tend to have a better prognosis and are much more likely to respond to hormone therapy than women with cancers without these receptors.

American Cancer Society: Understanding Your Pathology Report

Progesterone Receptor (PR)	**Progesterone:** A type of hormone made by the body that plays a role in the menstrual cycle and pregnancy.
	Progesterone can also be made in the laboratory.
	It may be used as a type of birth control and to treat menstrual disorders, infertility, symptoms of menopause, and other conditions.
	
	• **Progesterone receptor (PR):** A protein found inside the cells of the female reproductive tissue, some other types of tissue, and some cancer cells.
	   ○ The hormone progesterone will bind to the receptors inside the cells and may cause the cells to grow.
	   ○ Also called PR.
	• **Progesterone receptor negative (PR-):** Describes cells that do not have a protein to which the hormone progesterone will bind.
	   ○ Cancer cells that are progesterone receptor negative do not need progesterone to grow and usually do not stop growing when treated with hormones that block progesterone from binding.
	   ○ Also called PR negative.
	• **Progesterone receptor positive (PR+):** Describes cells that have a protein to which the hormone progesterone will bind.
	   ○ Cancer cells that are progesterone receptor positive need progesterone to grow and will usually stop growing when treated with hormones that block progesterone from binding.
	   ○ Also called PR positive.
	• **Progesterone receptor (PR) test:** A lab test to find out if cancer cells have progesterone receptors (proteins to which the hormone progesterone will bind).
	   ○ If the cells have progesterone receptors, they may need progesterone to grow, and this can affect how the cancer is treated. *NIH – NCI (3)*
	
	Results for PR are reported separately and can be reported in different ways:
	• Negative, weakly positive, positive
	• Percent positive
	• Percent positive and whether the staining is weak, moderate, or strong.
	
	Women with hormone receptor-positive cancers tend to have a better prognosis and are much more likely to respond to hormone therapy than women with cancers without these receptors.
	
	American Cancer Society: Understanding Your Pathology Report

Ki-67	Ki-67 is a way to measure how fast the cancer cells are growing and dividing. • High values (over 30%) for Ki-67 mean that many cells are dividing, so the cancer is likely to grow and spread more quickly". *American Cancer Society: Understanding Your Pathology Report* • Less than 10% - low • 10-20/25% - borderline, • More than 20-25% - high ***The higher the percentage, the more aggressive the cancer is.*** *BreastCancer.org: Rate of Cell Growth*

S-Phase Fraction	This number tells you what percentages of cells in the sample are in the process of copying their genetic information, or DNA. This S-phase, short for "synthesis phase," happens just before a cell divides into two new cells. *BreastCancer.org: Rate of Cell Growth* • Less than 6% - low • 6-10% - intermediate • More than 10% - high.
Lymphovascular Invasion	Lymphovascular invasion (LVI) is defined as the presence of tumor cells within a definite endothelial-lined space (lymphatics or blood vessels) in the breast surrounding invasive carcinoma. • The presence of LVI is associated with an increased risk of axillary lymph node and distant metastases. • Although the mechanism of LVI has not been completely elucidated, LVI is considered as a prognostic factor in patients with operable breast cancer with or without metastatic axillary lymph nodes who are undergoing adjuvant treatment. *NCBI – PMC Lymphovascular invasion*

Multigene Tests	Tests in which samples of tissue are studied to look at the activity of many genes at the same time.
	These tests may help predict whether cancer will spread to other parts of the body or recur (come back).
	
	There are many types of multigene tests.
	The following multigene tests have been studied in clinical trials:
	
	• **Oncotype DX**: This test helps predict whether early-stage breast cancer that is estrogen receptor positive and node negative will spread to other parts of the body.
	   ○ If the risk that the cancer will spread is high, chemotherapy may be given to lower the risk.
	• **MammaPrint**: A laboratory test in which the activity of 70 different genes is looked at in the breast cancer tissue of women who have early-stage invasive breast cancer that has not spread to lymph nodes or has spread to 3 or fewer lymph nodes.
	   ○ The activity level of these genes helps predict whether breast cancer will spread to other parts of the body or come back.
	   ○ If the test shows that the risk that the cancer will spread or come back is high, chemotherapy may be given to lower the risk.
	NIH – NCI (2)

Molecular Subtypes	Four main breast cancer subtypes have been identified according to estrogen receptor (ER), progesterone receptor (PR), and HER2. These subtypes include luminal types A and B, basal-like, and HER2-enriched subtype.

Luminal A

30-74% of subtypes; most common;
good prognosis

* ER+ and/or PR+; HER2−

* Low Ki-67

* Tumor Grade 1-2

Luminal B

10-20% of subtypes; more aggressive;
larger tumor

* ER+ and/or PR+; HER2− or HER2 +

* High Ki-67

* Higher tumor grade

* Lymph node +

HER2 Type Enriched

5-15% of subtypes; more aggressive; cannot be given anti- estrogen drugs

* ER- and/or PR-; HER2+

* Lymph node +

* More common in younger women

Triple Negative / Basil Like

15-20% of subtypes

* ER- and/or PR-; HER2−

* More common in women with BRCA 1 gene: pre- menopausal

NCBI – NIH (1) and Breast Cancer Rehab

American Cancer Society: Understanding Your Pathology Report: Breast Cancer
https://www.cancer.org/treatment/understanding-your-diagnosis/tests/understanding-your-pathology-report/breast-pathology/breast-cancer-pathology.html

Breast Cancer Rehab Course – Klose

BreastCancer.org: Rate of Cell Growth https://www.breastcancer.org/symptoms/diagnosis/rate_grade

NCBI – NIH Ki-67 as a prognostic marker https://www.ncbi.nlm.nih.gov/pmc/articles/PMC5250608/

NCBI – PMC Lymphovascular invasion https://www.ncbi.nlm.nih.gov/pmc/articles/PMC6078671/

NIH – NCI (1) - Breast Treatment (professional) https://www.cancer.gov/types/breast/hp/breast-treatment-pdq

NIH – NCI (2) Treatment (patient) https://www.cancer.gov/types/breast/patient/breast-treatment-pdq#_181

NIH – NCI (5) Tumor Grade https://www.cancer.gov/about-cancer/diagnosis-staging/prognosis/tumor-grade-fact-sheet

NIH – NCI (6) Staging https://www.cancer.gov/about-cancer/diagnosis-staging/staging

GENES

Quick Summary of Section

Tumor Suppressor Gene
- Any of a class of genes that are normally involved in regulating cell growth but that may become cancer-causing when damaged.

BRCA1 and BRCA 2
- BRCA1 and BRCA2 are human genes that produce tumor suppressor proteins. These proteins help repair damaged DNA and, therefore, play a role in ensuring the stability of each cell's genetic material.

PALB2
- Inherited mutations in the ATM (Ataxia-Telangiectasia mutated) gene are associated with increased risk of certain cancers.
- The PALB2 gene is called the partner and localizer of the BRCA2 gene.

CHEK 2
- A tumor suppressor gene that encodes a serine/threonine kinase, the CHK2.

ATM
- Inherited mutations in the ATM (Ataxia-Telangiectasia mutated) gene are associated with increased risk of certain cancers.

Tumor Suppressor Gene, *AKA* **Anti-oncogene** *and* **Inherited Gene Changes**	Any of a class of genes that are normally involved in regulating cell growth but that may become cancer-causing when damaged. • Tumor suppressor genes encode for proteins that are involved in inhibiting the proliferation of cells, which is crucial to normal cell development and differentiation. • Because of this ability, tumor suppressor genes can also act to stem the uncontrolled growth of cancer cells. Genetic damage, or mutation, that occurs to these genes contributes to the development of a cancerous tumor. *Britannica: Tumor suppressor gene* **Inherited gene changes** Certain inherited DNA mutations (changes) can dramatically increase the risk for developing certain cancers and are linked to many of the cancers that run in some families. • For instance, the BRCA genes (BRCA1 and BRCA2) are tumor suppressor genes. • When one of these genes changes, it no longer suppresses abnormal cell growth, and cancer is more likely to develop. • A change in one of these genes can be passed from a parent to a child. *American Cancer Society: How Does Breast Cancer Start?* Other examples of inherited genes include PALB2, ATM and CHEK2.

NIH – NCI *https://www.cancer.gov/about-cancer/understanding/what-is-cancer*

BRCA1 and **BRCA 2**	**BRCA1 and BRCA2** are human genes that produce tumor suppressor proteins. These proteins help repair damaged DNA and, therefore, play a role in ensuring the stability of each cell's genetic material.

- When either of these genes is mutated, or altered, such that its protein product is not made or does not function correctly, DNA damage may not be repaired properly.
- As a result, cells are more likely to develop additional genetic alterations that can lead to cancer.
- Specific inherited mutations in BRCA1 and BRCA2 most notably increase the risk of female breast and ovarian cancers, but they have also been associated with increased risks of several additional types of cancer.
- People who have inherited mutations in BRCA1 and BRCA2 tend to develop breast and ovarian cancers at younger ages than people who do not have these mutations.
- A harmful BRCA1 or BRCA2 mutation can be inherited from a person's mother or father. Each child of a parent who carries a mutation in one of these genes has a 50% chance (or 1 chance in 2) of inheriting the mutation.
- About 12% of women in the general population will develop breast cancer sometime during their lives. By contrast, a recent large study estimated that about 72% of women who inherit a harmful BRCA1 mutation and about 69% of women who inherit a harmful BRCA2 mutation will develop breast cancer by the age of 80.
- There also is a higher risk of developing a new primary cancer in the opposite (contralateral) breast in the years following a breast cancer diagnosis.

Who should get tested:

Several screening tools are available to help health care providers with this evaluation:

- Breast cancer diagnosed before age 50 years
- Cancer in both breasts in the same woman
- Both breast and ovarian cancers in either the same woman or the same family
- Multiple breast cancers in the family
- Two or more primary types of BRCA1- or BRCA2-related cancers in a single family member
- Cases of male breast cancer
- Ashkenazi Jewish ethnicity *NHI – NCI (7) - BRCA Mutations*

PALB2	The **PALB2 gene** is called the partner and localizer of the BRCA2 gene. • Women with an abnormal PALB2 gene had a 14% risk of developing breast cancer by age 50 and a 35% risk of developing breast cancer by age 70. • Inheriting two abnormal PALB2 genes causes Fanconi anemia type N, which suppresses bone marrow function and leads to extremely low levels of red blood cells, white blood cells, and platelets. In women with an abnormal PALB2 gene, breast cancer risk was: • 8 to 9 times higher than average in women ages 20 to 39 • 6 to 8 times higher than average in women ages 40 to 60 • 5 times higher than average in women older than 60 • By age 70, women with an abnormal PALB2 gene: with no family history of breast cancer had a 33% risk of developing breast cancer. With two or more first-degree relatives (sister, mother, daughter) with breast cancer had a 58% risk of developing the disease • "On the basis of our estimates, the breast-cancer risk for a PALB2 mutation carrier, even in the absence of a family history of breast cancer, would be classified as high according to various guidelines." *BreastCancer.org: Abnormal PALB2*
CHECK 2	**CHEK2** is a tumor suppressor gene that encodes a serine/threonine kinase, the CHK2. This gene is involved in pathways such as DNA repair, cell cycle regulation and apoptosis in response to DNA damage. Mutations of CHEK2 have been implicated in various types of cancer including breast cancer. *NCBI: Current perspectives on CHEK2 mutations in breast cancer* Women with mutations in the CHEK2 gene have an increased risk for breast cancer, sometimes at relatively young ages. • This increase in risk is not as high as what is seen in women with mutations in the BRCA1 and BRCA2 genes, but it is high enough to consider ways to reduce cancer risk and to increase screening in an attempt to find any breast cancers that do develop as early as possible. • A woman who has a CHEK2 mutation, and who has already had breast cancer, has a high risk of developing a second breast cancer within the next 5 to 25 years. *My support 360: CHEK2 Gene Mutations*
ATM	Inherited mutations in the **ATM (Ataxia-Telangiectasia Mutated)** gene are associated with increased risk of certain cancers. • People who inherit a mutated copy of ATM from one parent are at increased risk of female breast cancer (up to 52% lifetime risk), and possibly pancreatic, prostate and other cancers. • Ongoing research may identify other cancer risk, such prostate and pancreatic cancer in people with inherited ATM mutations. *FORCE-Facing Our Risk of Cancer Empowered, Inc: No one should face hereditary cancer alone*
HER2/neu gene	*See Prognosis Markers*

American Cancer Society: How Does Breast Cancer Start? *https://www.cancer.org/cancer/breast-cancer/about/how-does-breast-cancer-form.html*

American Cancer Society: Understanding Your Pathology Report: Breast Cancer *https://www.cancer.org/treatment/understanding-your-diagnosis/tests/understanding-your-pathology-report/breast-pathology/breast-cancer-pathology.html*

BreastCancer.org: Abnormal PALB2 Gene Increases Breast Cancer Risk More Than Previously Thought *https://www.breastcancer.org/research-news/abnormal-palb2-gene-increases-risk*

Britannica: Tumor suppressor gene *https://www.britannica.com/science/tumor-suppressor-gene*

FORCE-Facing Our Risk of Cancer Empowered, Inc: No one should face hereditary cancer alone *https://www.facingourrisk.org/understanding-brca-and-hboc/information/hereditary-cancer/other-genes/basics/atm.php*

My support 360: CHEK2 Gene Mutations *https://mysupport360.com/associations/genes/chek2-gene-mutations/*

NCBI: Current perspectives on CHEK2 mutations in breast cancer *https://www.ncbi.nlm.nih.gov/pmc/articles/PMC5439543/*

NHI – NCI (7)- BRCA Mutations *https://www.cancer.gov/about-cancer/causes-prevention/genetics/brca-fact-sheet#what-are-brca1-and-brca2*

Breast Surgeries

Information and pictures from *National Cancer Institute* unless otherwise specified

Quick Summary of Section

Mastectomy:

- Surgical removal of the breast that has DCIS or cancer.

Breast Conserving Lumpectomy:

- Breast-sparing surgery means the surgeon removes only the DCIS or cancer and some normal tissue around it.

Considerations for Breast - Conserving surgery:

- Most women with DCIS or breast cancer can choose to have breast- sparing surgery, usually followed by radiation therapy: Choices, what will my breasts look and feel like, returning to activities, will I need more surgery, recurrence.

Nipple-Sparing Mastectomy:

- A nipple-sparing mastectomy is similar to the skin-sparing mastectomy. This procedure is more often an option for women who have a small, early-stage cancer near the outer part of the breast, with no signs of cancer in the skin or near the nipple.

Total Mastectomy or Simple Mastectomy:

- The surgeon removes your whole breast.

Modified Radical Mastectomy:

- Surgery for breast cancer in which the breast, most or all of the lymph nodes under the arm and the lining over the chest muscles are removed.

Considerations with Mastectomy:

- Most women with DCIS or breast cancer can choose to have a mastectomy: Choices, what will my breasts look and feel like, returning to activities, will I need more surgery, recurrence.

Considerations with Mastectomy and Reconstruction:

- If you have a mastectomy, you might also want breast reconstruction surgery.

Compare the Types of Breast Surgery:

- Mastectomy, Skin sparing mastectomy, Mastectomy with reconstruction:
    - Is this surgery right for me?
    - How long before I can return to normal activities?
    - What other problems might I have?
    - What will my breast look like?
    - Will my breast have feeling?
    - Will I need more surgery?
    - What are the chances that my breast cancer will return in the same area?

Mastectomy	Surgical removal of the breast that has DCIS or cancer. There are different types of mastectomies: • Total mastectomy (also known as simple mastectomy) • Skin-sparing mastectomy • Modified radical mastectomy. ***A mastectomy is most often recommended when:*** • There are multiple areas of cancer within your breast • The tumor is greater than 5cm (2inches) • Your breast is small or shaped such that removal of the entire cancer will leave little breast tissue or a deformed breast • You do not want or cannot have radiation therapy (sometimes radiation is necessary, even if you have a mastectomy). ***Possible Side Effects of Mastectomy*** • Infection, poor wound healing, a reaction to the drugs used in surgery (anesthesia) • A collection of fluid or blood under the skin may occur after a mastectomy *Department of Health NY: Breast Cancer Treatment*
Breast Conserving - Lumpectomy Also called breast-sparing surgery, partial mastectomy, quadrantectomy, and segmental mastectomy.	Breast-sparing surgery means the surgeon removes only the DCIS or cancer and some normal tissue around it. • If you have cancer, the surgeon will also remove one or more lymph nodes from under your arm. • Breast-sparing surgery usually keeps your breast looking much like it did before surgery. • After breast-sparing surgery, most women also receive radiation therapy. Some women will also need chemotherapy, hormone therapy, and/or targeted therapy. • The main goal of this treatment is to keep cancer from coming back in the same breast. *NIH NCI (8)*

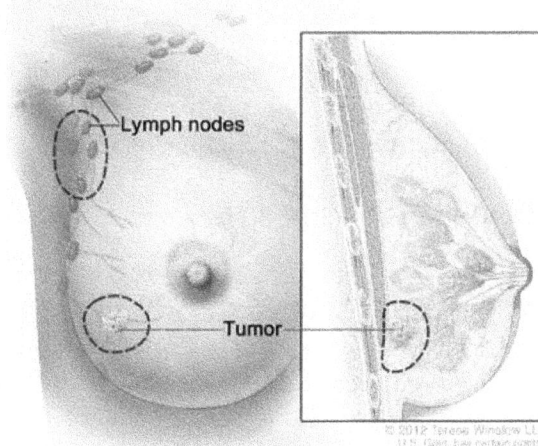

Breast-sparing Surgery

Lymph nodes

Tumor

NHI NCI (8) https://www.cancer.gov/types/breast/surgery-choices

Considerations for Breast-conserving surgery	*Is this surgery right for me?* • Most women with DCIS or breast cancer can choose to have breast-sparing surgery, usually followed by radiation therapy. *How long before I can return to normal activities?* • Most women are ready to return to most of their usual activities within 5 to 10 days. *What other problems might I have?* • You may feel very tired and have skin changes from radiation therapy. *What will my breast look like?* • Your breast should look a lot like it did before surgery. • But if your tumor is large, your breast may look different or smaller after breast-sparing surgery. • You will have a small scar where the surgeon cut to remove the DCIS or cancer. The length of the scar will depend on how large an incision the surgeon needed to make. *Will my breast have feeling?* • Yes. You should still have feeling in your breast, nipple, and areola (the dark area around your nipple). *Will I need more surgery?* • If the surgeon does not remove all the DCIS or cancer the first time, you may need more surgery. *What are the chances that my breast cancer will return in the same area?* • There is a chance that your cancer will come back in the same breast. But if it does, it is not likely to affect how long you live. • About 10% of women (1 out of every 10) who have breast-sparing surgery along with radiation therapy get cancer in the same breast within 12 years. If this happens, you can be effectively treated with a mastectomy. *NIH NCI (8)*
Nipple-sparing mastectomy	A nipple-sparing mastectomy is similar to the skin-sparing mastectomy. This procedure is more often an option for women who have a small, early-stage cancer near the outer part of the breast, with no signs of cancer in the skin or near the nipple. • The surgeon often removes the breast tissue beneath the nipple (and areola) during the procedure, to check for cancer cells. If cancer is found in this tissue, the nipple must be removed. *Department of Health NY: Breast Cancer Treatment*

Total Mastectomy or **Simple Mastectomy**	The surgeon removes your whole breast. • Sometimes, the surgeon also takes out one or more of the lymph nodes under your arm.

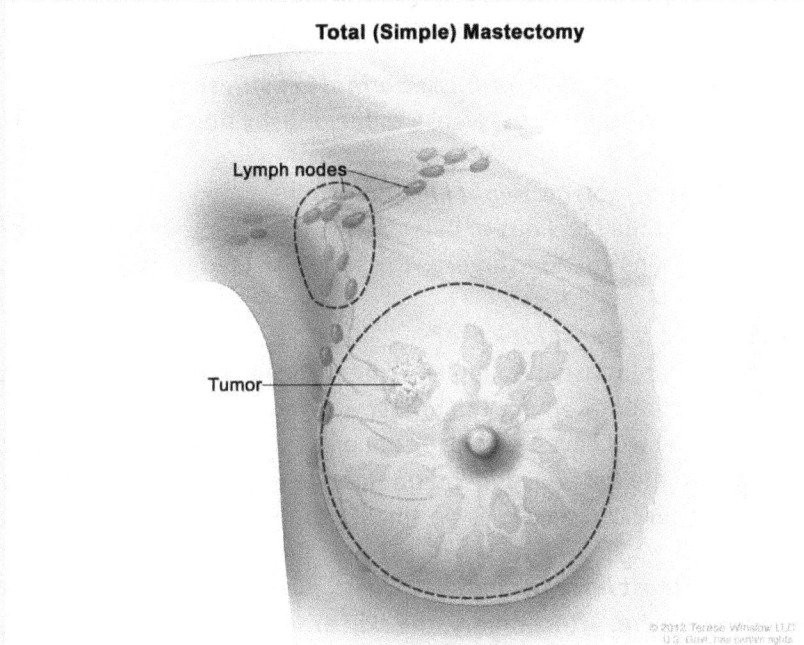

NHI NCI (8) https://www.cancer.gov/types/breast/surgery-choices

Modified Radical Mastectomy	Surgery for breast cancer in which the breast, most or all of the lymph nodes under the arm, and the lining over the chest muscles are removed. • Sometimes the surgeon also removes part of the chest wall muscles.

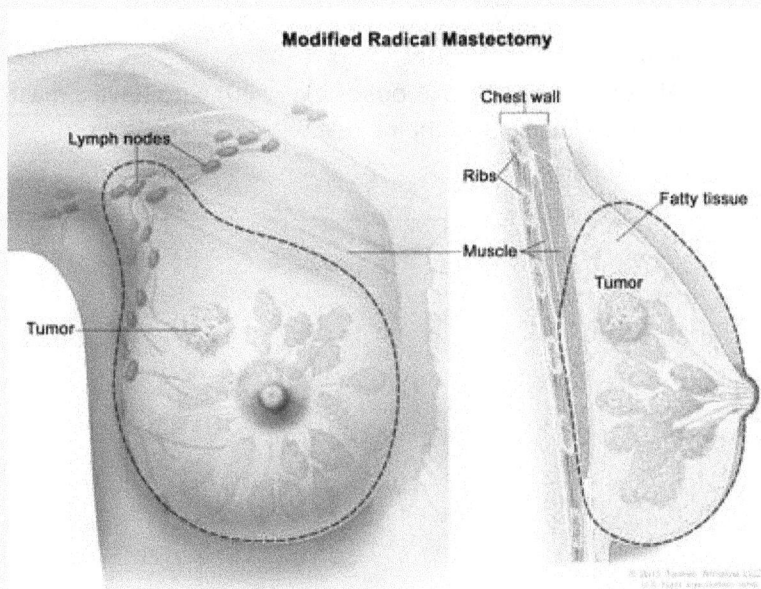

NHI NCI (8) https://www.cancer.gov/types/breast/surgery-choices

Considerations with Mastectomy	*Is this surgery right for me?* Most women with DCIS or breast cancer can choose to have a mastectomy. A mastectomy may be a better choice for you if: • You have small breasts and a large area of DCIS or cancer. • You have DCIS or cancer in more than one part of your breast. • The DCIS or cancer is under the nipple. • You are not able to receive radiation therapy. *How long before I can return to normal activities?* • It may take 3 to 4 weeks to feel mostly normal after a mastectomy. *What other problems might I have?* • You may feel out of balance if you had large breasts and do not have reconstruction surgery. This may also lead to neck and shoulder pain. *What will my breast look like?* • Your breast and nipple will be removed. You will have a flat chest on the side of your body where the breast was removed. • You will have a scar over the place where your breast was removed. The length of the scar will depend on the size of your breast. If you have smaller breasts, your scar is likely to be smaller than if you have larger breasts. *Will my breast have feeling?* • Maybe. After surgery, the skin around where the surgeon cut and maybe the area under your arm will be numb (have no feeling). • This numb feeling may improve over 1 to 2 years, but it will never feel like it once did. Also, the skin where your breast was may feel tight. *Will I need more surgery?* • If you have problems after your mastectomy, you may need more surgery. *What are the chances that my breast cancer will return in the same area?* • There is a smaller chance that your cancer will return in the same area than if you have breast-sparing surgery. • About 5% of women (1 out of every 20) who have a mastectomy will get cancer on the same side of their chest within 12 years. *NHI NCI (8)*

Considerations with Mastectomy and Reconstruction	*Is this surgery right for me?*
	• If you have a mastectomy, you might also want breast reconstruction surgery.
	• You can choose to have reconstruction surgery at the same time as your mastectomy or wait and have it later.
	
	How long before I can return to normal activities?
	• Your recovery will depend on the type of reconstruction you have. It can take 6 to 8 weeks or longer to fully recover from breast reconstruction.
	
	What other problems might I have?
	• You may not like how your breast-like shape looks.
	• If you have an implant:
	    o Your breast may harden and can become painful.
	    o You will likely need more surgery if your implant breaks or leaks.
	• If you have flap surgery, you may lose strength in the part of your body where a muscle was removed.
	
	What will my breast look like?
	• You will have a breast-like shape, but your breast will not look or feel like it did before surgery. And, it will not look or feel like your other breast.
	• You will have scars where the surgeon stitched skin together to make the new breast-like shape.
	• If you have tissue flap reconstruction, you will have scars around the new breast, as well as the area where the surgeon removed the muscle, fat, and skin to make the new breast-like shape.
	
	Will my breast have feeling?
	• No. The area around your breast will not have feeling.
	
	Will I need more surgery?
	• You will need more than one surgery to build a new breast-like shape. The number of surgeries you need will depend on the type of reconstruction you have and if you choose to have a nipple or areola added.
	• Some women may also decide to have surgery on the opposite breast to help it match the new breast-like shape better.
	• If you have an implant, you are likely to need surgery many years later to remove or replace it.
	
	What are the chances that my breast cancer will return in the same area?
	• Your chances are the same as mastectomy, since breast reconstruction surgery does not affect the chances of the cancer returning.
	
	NHI NCI (8)

Compare the Types of Breast Surgery

National Cancer institute (NHI NCI (8)

Is this surgery right for me?

Breast-Sparing Surgery	Most women with DCIS or breast cancer can choose to have breast-sparing surgery, usually followed by radiation therapy.
Mastectomy	Most women with DCIS or breast cancer can choose to have a mastectomy. A mastectomy may be a better choice for you if: • You have small breasts and a large area of DCIS or cancer. • You have DCIS or cancer in more than one part of your breast. • The DCIS or cancer is under the nipple. • You are not able to receive radiation therapy.
Mastectomy with Reconstruction	If you have a mastectomy, you might also want breast reconstruction surgery. You can choose to have reconstruction surgery at the same time as your mastectomy or wait and have it later.

How long before I can return to normal activities?

Breast-Sparing Surgery	Most women are ready to return to most of their usual activities within 5 to 10 days.
Mastectomy	It may take 3 to 4 weeks to feel mostly normal after a mastectomy.
Mastectomy with Reconstruction	Your recovery will depend on the type of reconstruction you have. It can take 6 to 8 weeks or longer to fully recover from breast reconstruction.

What other problems might I have?

Breast-Sparing Surgery	You may feel very tired and have skin changes from radiation therapy.
Mastectomy	You may feel out of balance if you had large breasts and do not have reconstruction surgery. This may also lead to neck and shoulder pain.
Mastectomy with Reconstruction	You may not like how your breast-like shape looks. If you have an implant: • Your breast may harden and can become painful. • You will likely need more surgery if your implant breaks or leaks. If you have flap surgery, you may lose strength in the part of your body where a muscle was removed.

What will my breast look like?

Breast-Sparing Surgery	Your breast should look a lot like it did before surgery. But if your tumor is large, your breast may look different or smaller after breast-sparing surgery. You will have a small scar where the surgeon cut to remove the DCIS or cancer. The length of the scar will depend on how large an incision the surgeon needed to make.
Mastectomy	Your breast and nipple will be removed. You will have a flat chest on the side of your body where the breast was removed. You will have a scar over the place where your breast was removed. The length of the scar will depend on the size of your breast. If you have smaller breasts, your scar is likely to be smaller than if you have larger breasts.
Mastectomy with Reconstruction	You will have a breast-like shape, but your breast will not look or feel like it did before surgery. And, it will not look or feel like your other breast. You will have scars where the surgeon stitched skin together to make the new breast-like shape. If you have tissue flap reconstruction, you will have scars around the new breast, as well as the area where the surgeon removed the muscle, fat, and skin to make the new breast-like shape.

Will my breast have feeling?

Breast-Sparing Surgery	Yes. You should still have feeling in your breast, nipple, and areola (the dark area around your nipple).
Mastectomy	Maybe. After surgery, the skin around where the surgeon cut and maybe the area under your arm will be numb (have no feeling).
	This numb feeling may improve over 1 to 2 years, but it will never feel like it once did. Also, the skin where your breast was may feel tight.
Mastectomy with Reconstruction	No. The area around your breast will not have feeling.

Will I need more surgery?

Breast-Sparing Surgery	If the surgeon does not remove all the DCIS or cancer the first time, you may need more surgery.
Mastectomy	If you have problems after your mastectomy, you may need more surgery.
Mastectomy with Reconstruction	You will need more than one surgery to build a new breast-like shape. The number of surgeries you need will depend on the type of reconstruction you have and if you choose to have a nipple or areola added.
	Some women may also decide to have surgery on the opposite breast to help it match the new breast-like shape better.
	If you have an implant, you are likely to need surgery many years later to remove or replace it.

What are the chances that my breast cancer will return in the same area?

Breast-Sparing Surgery	There is a chance that your cancer will come back in the same breast. But if it does, it is not likely to affect how long you live. About 10% of women (1 out of every 10) who have breast-sparing surgery along with radiation therapy get cancer in the same breast within 12 years. If this happens, you can be effectively treated with a mastectomy.
Mastectomy	There is a smaller chance that your cancer will return in the same area than if you have breast-sparing surgery. About 5% of women (1 out of every 20) who have a mastectomy will get cancer on the same side of their chest within 12 years.
Mastectomy with Reconstruction	Your chances are the same as mastectomy, since breast reconstruction surgery does not affect the chances of the cancer returning.

NIH NCI (8:) https://www.cancer.gov/types/breast/surgery-choices

Department of Health NY: Breast Cancer Treatment - What You Should Know
https://www.health.ny.gov/publications/0401/#treatment_options

Breast Reconstruction
Information and pictures from *National Cancer Institute* unless otherwise specified

Quick Summary of Section

Breast Reconstruction:
- Women who choose to have their breasts rebuilt have several options for how it can be done.
- Breasts can be rebuilt using implants (saline or silicone).
- They can also be rebuilt using autologous tissue (that is, tissue from elsewhere in the body).

Factors – Timing:
- What factors can affect the timing of breast reconstruction?.

Factors – Choice:
- What factors can affect the choice of breast reconstruction method?.

Reconstruction with Implants:
- Surgery and recovery; Possible complications.

Reconstruction with Autologous Tissue:
- Surgery and recovery; Possible complications.

Breast Reconstruction	Many women who have a mastectomy—surgery to remove an entire breast to treat or prevent breast cancer—have the option of having the shape of the removed breast rebuilt. • Women who choose to have their breasts rebuilt have several options for how it can be done. Breasts can be rebuilt using implants (saline or silicone). • They can also be rebuilt using autologous tissue (that is, tissue from elsewhere in the body). • Sometimes both implants and autologous tissue are used to rebuild the breast. Surgery to reconstruct the breasts can be done (or started) at the time of the mastectomy (which is called immediate reconstruction) or it can be done after the mastectomy incisions have healed and breast cancer therapy has been completed (which is called delayed reconstruction). • Delayed reconstruction can happen months or even years after the mastectomy. • In a final stage of breast reconstruction, a nipple and areola may be re-created on the reconstructed breast, if these were not preserved during the mastectomy. • Sometimes breast reconstruction surgery includes surgery on the other, or contralateral, breast so that the two breasts will match in size and shape. *NIH NCI (9)*

What factors can affect the timing of breast reconstruction?	• One factor that can affect the timing of breast reconstruction is whether a woman will need radiation therapy. 　○ Radiation therapy can sometimes cause wound healing problems or infections in reconstructed breasts, so some women may prefer to delay reconstruction until after radiation therapy is completed. However, because of improvements in surgical and radiation techniques, immediate reconstruction with an implant is usually still an option for women who will need radiation therapy. 　○ Autologous tissue breast reconstruction is usually reserved for after radiation therapy, so that the breast and chest wall tissue damaged by radiation can be replaced with healthy tissue from elsewhere in the body. • Another factor is the type of breast cancer. Women with inflammatory breast cancer usually require more extensive skin removal. This can make immediate reconstruction more challenging, so it may be recommended that reconstruction be delayed until after completion of adjuvant therapy. • Even if a woman is a candidate for immediate reconstruction, she may choose delayed reconstruction. For instance, some women prefer not to consider what type of reconstruction to have until after they have recovered from their mastectomy and subsequent adjuvant treatment. • Women who delay reconstruction (or choose not to undergo the procedure at all) can use external breast prostheses, or breast forms, to give the appearance of breasts. *NIH NCI (9)*
What factors can affect the choice of breast reconstruction method?	Several factors can influence the type of reconstructive surgery a woman chooses. These include the size and shape of the breast that is being rebuilt, the woman's age and health, her history of past surgeries, surgical risk factors (for example, smoking history and obesity), the availability of autologous tissue, and the location of the tumor in the breast. • Women who have had past abdominal surgery may not be candidates for an abdominally based flap reconstruction. Each type of reconstruction has factors that a woman should think about before making a decision. • All women who undergo mastectomy for breast cancer experience varying degrees of breast numbness and loss of sensation (feeling) because nerves that provide sensation to the breast are cut when breast tissue is removed during surgery. 　○ However, a woman may regain some sensation as the severed nerves grow and regenerate, and breast surgeons continue to make technical advances that can spare or repair damage to nerves. • Any type of breast reconstruction can fail if healing does not occur properly. In these cases, the implant or flap will have to be removed. If an implant reconstruction fails, a woman can usually have a second reconstruction using an alternative approach. *NIH NCI (9)* *Some of the more common considerations are listed below*

Reconstruction with Implants	**Surgery and recovery** • Enough skin and muscle must remain after mastectomy to cover the implants • Shorter surgical procedure than for reconstruction with autologous tissue; little blood loss • Recovery period may be shorter than with autologous reconstruction • Many follow-up visits may be needed to inflate the expander and insert the implant **Possible complications** • Infection • Accumulation of clear fluid causing a mass or lump (seroma) within the reconstructed breast • Pooling of blood (hematoma) within the reconstructed breast • Blood clots • Extrusion of the implant (the implant breaks through the skin) • Implant rupture (the implant breaks open and saline or silicone leaks into the surrounding tissue) • Formation of hard scar tissue around the implant (known as a contracture) • Obesity, diabetes, and smoking may increase the rate of complications • Possible increased risk of developing a very rare form of immune system cancer called anaplastic large cell lymphoma **Other considerations** • May not be an option for patients who have previously undergone radiation therapy to the chest • May not be adequate for women with very large breasts • Will not last a lifetime; the longer a woman has implants, the more likely she is to have complications and to need to have her implants removed or replaced • Silicone implants may feel more natural than saline implants to the touch • The Food and Drug Administration (FDA) recommends that women with silicone implants undergo periodic MRI screenings to detect possible "silent" rupture of the implants. *NIH NCI (9)* More information about implants can be found on *FDA's Breast Implants page.* *https://www.fda.gov/MedicalDevices/ProductsandMedicalProcedures/ImplantsandProsthetics/BreastImplants/default.html*

Reconstruction with Autologous Tissue	**Reconstruction with Autologous Tissue**
	
	• **Surgery and recovery**
	  ○ Longer surgical procedure than for implants
	  ○ The initial recovery period may be longer than for implants
	  ○ Pedicled flap reconstruction is usually a shorter operation than free flap reconstruction and usually requires a shorter hospitalization
	  ○ Free flap reconstruction is a longer, highly technical operation compared with pedicled flap reconstruction that requires a surgeon who has experience with microsurgery to re-attach blood vessels
	
	• **Possible complications**
	  ○ Necrosis (death) of the transferred tissue
	  ○ Blood clots may be more frequent with some flap sources
	  ○ Pain and weakness at the site from which the donor tissue was taken
	  ○ Obesity, diabetes, and smoking may increase the rate of complications
	
	• **Other considerations**
	  ○ May provide a more natural breast shape than implants
	  ○ May feel softer and more natural to the touch than implants
	  ○ Leaves a scar at the site from which the donor tissue was taken
	  ○ Can be used to replace tissue that has been damaged by radiation therapy
	  NIH NCI (9)

Breast Implants

Information and pictures from *National Cancer Institute* unless otherwise specified

Quick Summary of Section

Breast Implant:

- Implants are inserted underneath the skin or chest muscle following the mastectomy.
- Breast reconstruction with an implant is often done in steps with a tissue expander.
- In some cases, the implant can be placed in the breast during the same surgery as the mastectomy. That is, a tissue expander is not used to prepare for the implant.

Tissue Expanders:

- A breast tissue expander is an inflatable breast implant designed to stretch the skin and muscle to make room for a future, more permanent implant.

Breast Implant *(Also see below)*	Implants are inserted underneath the skin or chest muscle following the mastectomy. (Most mastectomies are performed using a technique called skin-sparing mastectomy, in which much of the breast skin is saved for use in reconstructing the breast.) Implants are usually placed in two parts: • The first step is called *tissue expansion*. This is when the plastic surgeon places a balloon expander under the chest muscle (*usually over the pectoralis minor and under the pectoralis major*). Over many weeks, saline (salt water) will be added to the expander to stretch the chest muscle and the skin on top of it by the plastic surgeon. This process makes a pocket for the implant. • After the chest tissue has relaxed and healed enough, the expander is removed and replaced with an implant (filled with saline or silicone gel). The chest tissue is usually ready for the implant 2 to 6 months after mastectomy. This creates a new breast-like shape. Although this shape looks like a breast, you will not have the same feeling in it because nerves were cut during your mastectomy. • In some cases, the implant can be placed in the breast during the same surgery as the mastectomy—that is, a tissue expander is not used to prepare for the implant. • Surgeons are increasingly using material called acellular dermal matrix as a kind of scaffold or "sling" to support tissue expanders and implants. ○ Acellular dermal matrix is a kind of mesh that is made from donated human or pig skin that has been sterilized and processed to remove all cells to eliminate the risks of rejection and infection. • Breast implants do not last a lifetime. If you choose to have an implant, chances are you will need more surgery later on to remove or replace it. • Implants can cause problems such as breast hardness, pain, and infection. The implant may also break, move, or shift. These problems can happen soon after surgery or years later. • Chemotherapy or radiation may be recommended to you by your surgical oncologist following your mastectomy. If you choose to have these treatments it will delay the tissue expansion process by approximately four to eight weeks. *John Hopkins Medicine - Tissue Expanders* *NIH NCI (9)* & (10)

Tissue Expander

John Hopkins Medicine (YouTube Video)

Tissue Expanders

Tissue expansion involves expansion of the breast skin and muscle using a temporary tissue expander. A few months later, the expander is removed and the patient receives either microvascular flap reconstruction, or the insertion of a permanent breast implant. This type of breast reconstruction requires two separate operations.

What is a breast tissue expander?
- A breast tissue expander is an inflatable breast implant designed to stretch the skin and muscle to make room for a future, more permanent implant.
- At the same time your mastectomy is done by our breast surgical oncologist, the breast plastic and reconstructive surgeon will insert a tissue expander beneath your skin and chest muscle.
- Through a tiny valve mechanism located inside the expander, the nurse practitioner will periodically inject a salt-water solution to gradually fill the expander over several weeks or months.
- You may feel a sensation of stretching and pressure in the breast area during this procedure, but most women find it is not too uncomfortable.
- This process will usually begin three to four weeks after your mastectomy, once your drains are removed, and will continue until the size is slightly larger than your other breast.
- After the skin over the breast area has stretched enough, the expander will be removed in a second operation and either flap reconstruction or a permanent implant will be inserted.
- The nipple and the dark skin surrounding it, called the areola, are reconstructed in a subsequent procedure.
John Hopkins Medicine - Tissue Expanders

Expanders could be in for up to a year or more if chemotherapy and radiation are done after surgery. Implants are placed 3-6 weeks after chemotherapy is complete or 6 months after radiation.

Common Side Effects:
- Pain and Stiffness
- Often numb at fill site
- Difficult to lie on side
- Postural changes

Tissue Flap Surgery

Information and pictures from *National Cancer Institute* unless otherwise specified

Quick Summary of Section

Tissue Flap Surgery:

- In tissue flap surgery, a reconstructive plastic surgeon builds a new breast-like shape from muscle, fat, and skin taken from other parts of your body (usually your belly, back, or buttock).

Autologous Tissue:

- Different sites in the body can provide flaps for breast reconstruction. Pedicled flap vs free flap.

Reconstruction with Autologous Tissue:

- Surgery and recovery; Possible complications

Abdomen: TRAM flap:

- Tissue comes from the lower abdomen as in a DIEP flap but includes muscle. It can be either pedicled or free.

Abdomen: DIEP flap:

- Tissue comes from the abdomen and contains only skin, blood vessels and fat, without the underlying muscle. This type of flap is a free flap.

Abdomen: SIEA flap:

- Tissue comes from the abdomen as in a DIEP flap but includes a different set of blood vessels. It also does not involve cutting of the abdominal muscle and is a free flap.

Back: Latissimus dorsi flap (LAT flap):

- Tissue comes from the middle and side of the back. This type of flap is pedicled when used for breast reconstruction.

Buttock (gluteal) flap:

- A gluteal flap is a free flap procedure that takes tissue from your buttocks and transplants it to your chest area.

Thigh flaps (TUG) and (IGAP):

- Transverse upper gracilis (TUG) flap, uses muscle and fatty tissue from the bottom of the buttocks to the inner thigh.

Nipple Reconstruction:

- After the chest heals from reconstruction surgery and the position of the breast mound on the chest wall has had time to stabilize, a surgeon can reconstruct the nipple and areola.

References

Tissue Flap Surgery *(Also see below)*	In tissue flap surgery, a reconstructive plastic surgeon builds a new breast-like shape from muscle, fat, and skin taken from other parts of your body (usually your belly, back, or buttock). • This new breast-like shape should last the rest of your life. • Women who are very thin or obese, smoke, or have serious health problems often cannot have tissue flap surgery. • Healing after tissue flap surgery often takes longer than healing after breast implant surgery. • You may have other problems, as well. For example, if you have a muscle removed, you might lose strength in the area from which it was taken. • You may get an infection or have trouble healing. • Tissue flap surgery is best done by a reconstructive plastic surgeon who has special training in this type of surgery and has done it many times before. *NIH NCI (10)*
Autologous Tissue	In autologous tissue reconstruction, a piece of tissue containing skin, fat, blood vessels, and sometimes muscle is taken from elsewhere in a woman's body and used to rebuild the breast. This piece of tissue is called a flap. • Different sites in the body can provide flaps for breast reconstruction. • Flaps used for breast reconstruction most often come from the abdomen or back. However, they can also be taken from the thigh or buttocks. Depending on their source, flaps can be pedicled or free. • With a pedicled flap, the tissue and attached blood vessels are moved together through the body to the breast area. Because the blood supply to the tissue used for reconstruction is left intact, blood vessels do not need to be reconnected once the tissue is moved. • With free flaps, the tissue is cut free from its blood supply. It must be attached to new blood vessels in the breast area, using a technique called microsurgery. This gives the reconstructed breast a blood supply. • Flaps taken from the thigh or buttocks are used for women who have had previous major abdominal surgery or who don't have enough abdominal tissue to reconstruct a breast. These types of flaps are free flaps. With these flaps an implant is often used as well to provide sufficient breast volume. • In some cases, an implant and autologous tissue are used together. For example, autologous tissue may be used to cover an implant when there isn't enough skin and muscle left after mastectomy to allow for expansion and use of an implant. *NIH NCI (10)*

Reconstruction with Autologous Tissue	• **Surgery and recovery**
	  ○ Longer surgical procedure than for implants
	  ○ The initial recovery period may be longer than for implants
	  ○ Pedicled flap reconstruction is usually a shorter operation than free flap reconstruction and usually requires a shorter hospitalization
	  ○ Free flap reconstruction is a longer, highly technical operation compared with pedicled flap reconstruction that requires a surgeon who has experience with microsurgery to re-attach blood vessels
	
	• **Possible complications**
	  ○ Necrosis (death) of the transferred tissue
	  ○ Blood clots may be more frequent with some flap sources
	  ○ Pain and weakness at the site from which the donor tissue was taken
	  ○ Obesity, diabetes, and smoking may increase the rate of complication.
	
	• **Other considerations**
	  ○ May provide a more natural breast shape than implants
	  ○ May feel softer and more natural to the touch than implants
	  ○ Leaves a scar at the site from which the donor tissue was taken
	  ○ Can be used to replace tissue that has been damaged by radiation therapy
	
	• All women who undergo mastectomy for breast cancer experience varying degrees of breast numbness and loss of sensation (feeling) because nerves that provide sensation to the breast are cut when breast tissue is removed during surgery.
	  ○ However, a woman may regain some sensation as the severed nerves grow and regenerate, and breast surgeons continue to make technical advances that can spare or repair damage to nerves.
	
	• Any type of breast reconstruction can fail if healing does not occur properly. In these cases, the implant or flap will have to be removed. If an implant reconstruction fails, a woman can usually have a second reconstruction using an alternative approach.
	  NIH NCI (9)

Abdomen: **TRAM flap**	Tissue comes from the lower abdomen as in a DIEP flap but includes muscle. It can be either pedicled or free. *NIH NCI (9)* • Your surgeon removes tissue — including muscle — from your abdomen in a procedure known as a transverse rectus abdominis muscle (TRAM) flap. • The TRAM flap can be transferred as a free flap or a pedicled flap. • A pedicled TRAM flap uses your whole rectus muscle — one of the four major muscles in your abdomen. • For a muscle-sparing free TRAM flap, your surgeon takes only a portion of your rectus abdominis muscle, which may help you retain abdominal strength after surgery. *Mayo Clinic - Breast reconstruction with flap surgery*

Pedicled Tram Flap (top) and Free TRAM Flap (bottom) – *Pictures from Mayo Clinic*

Rectus abdominis muscle

© MAYO FOUNDATION FOR MEDICAL EDUCATION AND RESEARCH. ALL RIGHTS RESERVED.

© MAYO FOUNDATION FOR MEDICAL EDUCATION AND RESEARCH. ALL RIGHTS RESERVED.

Mayo Clinic - https://www.mayoclinic.org/tests-procedures/breast-reconstruction-flap/about/pac-20384937

Abdomen: **DIEP flap**	Tissue comes from the abdomen and contains only skin, blood vessels, and fat, without the underlying muscle. This type of flap is a free flap. *NIH NCI (11)* • A newer procedure, deep inferior epigastric perforator (DIEP) flap, is similar to a TRAM flap, but only skin and fat are removed. • Most of the abdominal muscle is left in place and minimal muscle tissue is taken to form the new breast mound. • Reattaching blood vessels requires expertise in surgery through a microscope (microsurgery). • An advantage to this type of breast reconstruction is that you'll retain more strength in your abdomen. If your surgeon can't perform a DIEP flap procedure for anatomical reasons, he or she might opt for the TRAM procedure instead. *Mayo Clinic - Breast reconstruction with flap surgery*

DIEP flap – *Pictures from Mayo Clinic*

© MAYO FOUNDATION FOR MEDICAL EDUCATION AND RESEARCH. ALL RIGHTS RESERVED.

Mayo Clinic - https://www.mayoclinic.org/tests-procedures/breast-reconstruction-flap/about/pac-20384937

Abdomen: **SIEA flap** **(also called SIEP** **flap)**	Tissue comes from the abdomen as in a DIEP flap but includes a different set of blood vessels. It also does not involve cutting of the abdominal muscle and is a free flap. This type of flap is not an option for many women, as the necessary blood vessels are not adequate or do not exist. *NIH NCI (9)* • A variation of the DIEP flap, the superficial inferior epigastric artery (SIEA) flap uses the same abdominal tissue but relies on blood vessels that aren't as deep within the abdomen. • This provides a less invasive option, but not all women's SIEA blood vessels are adequate for this type of flap surgery. *Mayo Clinic - Breast reconstruction with flap surgery*

Back: **Latissimus dorsi** **flap (LAT flap)**	Tissue comes from the middle and side of the back. This type of flap is pedicled when used for breast reconstruction. (LD flaps can be used for other types of reconstruction as well.) *NIH NCI (9)* • This surgical technique takes skin, fat and muscle from your upper back, tunneling it under your skin to your chest. • Because the amount of skin and other tissue is generally less than in a TRAM flap surgery, this approach may be used for small and medium-sized breasts or for creating a pocket for a breast implant. • Although uncommon, some women experience muscle weakness in the back, shoulder or arm after this surgery. *Mayo Clinic - Breast reconstruction with flap surgery*

Latissimus dorsi (LD) flap

Latissimus
dorsi muscle

© MAYO FOUNDATION FOR MEDICAL EDUCATION AND RESEARCH. ALL RIGHTS RESERVED

Mayo Clinic - https://www.mayoclinic.org/tests-procedures/breast-reconstruction-flap/about/pac-20384937

Buttock (gluteal) **flap**	A gluteal flap is a free flap procedure that takes tissue from your buttocks and transplants it to your chest area. A gluteal flap may be an option for women who prefer tissue reconstruction but who don't have enough extra tissue in their backs or abdomens. *Mayo Clinic.org* • PAP flap: Tissue, without muscle, that comes from the upper inner thigh. • SGAP flap: Tissue comes from the buttocks as in an IGAP flap, but includes a different set of blood vessels and contains only skin, blood vessels, and fat. *NIH NCI (9)*
Thigh flaps **(TUG) and** **(IGAP)** *NIH NCI (11)*	Inner thigh (TUG). Another newer option, the transverse upper gracilis (TUG) flap, uses muscle and fatty tissue from the bottom of the buttocks to the inner thigh. TUG flap surgery, which isn't available everywhere, may be an option for women whose thighs touch and who have small to medium-sized breasts. *Mayo Clinic.org* • IGAP flap: Tissue comes from the buttocks and contains only skin, blood vessels, and fat. • TUG flap: Tissue, including muscle that comes from the upper inner thigh. *NIH NCI (9)*

Nipple Reconstruction	After the chest heals from reconstruction surgery and the position of the breast mound on the chest wall has had time to stabilize, a surgeon can reconstruct the nipple and areola. • Usually, the new nipple is created by cutting and moving small pieces of skin from the reconstructed breast to the nipple site and shaping them into a new nipple. A few months after nipple reconstruction, the surgeon can re-create the areola, usually using tattoo ink. However, in some cases, skin grafts may be taken from the groin or abdomen and attached to the breast to create an areola at the time of the nipple reconstruction. • Some women who do not have surgical nipple reconstruction may consider getting a realistic picture of a nipple created on the reconstructed breast from a tattoo artist who specializes in 3-D nipple tattooing. • A mastectomy that preserves a woman's own nipple and areola, called nipple-sparing mastectomy, may be an option for some women, depending on the size and location of the breast cancer and the shape and size of the breasts. *NIH NCI (9)*

Nipple Reconstruction

Mayo Clinic - https://www.mayoclinic.org/tests-procedures/breast-reconstruction-flap/about/pac-20384937

John Hopkins Medicine – Tissue Expander *YouTube Video https://www.youtube.com/watch?v=J9B23xnIoTw*

John Hopkins Medicine - Tissue Expanders
https://www.hopkinsmedicine.org/breast_center/treatments_services/reconstructive_breast_surgery/tissue_expanders.html

Mayo Clinic - Breast reconstruction with flap surgery - *https://www.mayoclinic.org/tests-procedures/breast-reconstruction-flap/about/pac-20384937*

NIH NCI (10) https://www.cancer.gov/types/breast/surgery-choices

NIH NCI (11) https://www.cancer.gov/types/breast/reconstruction-fact-sheet

Risks After Breast Surgery

Information and pictures from *National Cancer Institute* unless otherwise specified

Quick Summary of Section

Axillary Web Syndrome (Cording):

- Axillary Web Syndrome (AWS), also known as lymphatic cording, refers to a condition in which a rope-like soft-tissue density develops in the axilla, which may develop as a result of breast cancer treatment.

What causes AWS?

- The etiology of cording is not fully understood. The condition may be related to abnormalities in either the axillary vasculature or the lymphatics.

Who is at Risk for AWS?

- The incidence of cording after axillary lymph node dissection (ALND) has been reported as high as 72%, compared to 20% after sentinel lymph node biopsy (SLNB).

AWS: Pink Ribbon Program®

- Axillary web syndrome is a self-limiting and frequently overlooked cause of significant morbidity in the early post-operative period after breast cancer axillary surgery.

Managing AWS by Breastcancer.org (*Axillary Web Syndrome (Cording)*:

- If you have symptoms of AWS, ask your doctor to refer you to a physical therapist or other medical professional (such as a nurse or physician) who specializes in breast cancer rehabilitation.

Scar Tissue / Adhesions / Myofascial Release:

- Breast and axillary surgery, and radiotherapy in breast cancer   patients cause scar tissue formation, fibrosis and adhesions at all levels of soft tissues of the upper body.
- Postural restoration through myofascial release (medical massage) is needed by most people, but especially those having significant scarring on the front of the body.

Seroma / Compression:

- A serous fluid collection that develops under the skin flaps during mastectomy or in the axillary dead space.

Resources

CORDING OR AXILLARY WEB SYNDROME (AWS)

Axillary Web Syndrome (Cording)	Axillary Web Syndrome (AWS), also known as lymphatic cording, refers to a condition in which a rope-like soft-tissue density develops in the axilla, which may develop as a result of breast cancer treatment. It usually appears in the 5 to 8 week period following breast cancer surgery and can lead to shoulder pain and restricted motion. *NCBI: PMC: Atypical presentation of axillary web syndrome*
	
	Cords are palpable bands of tissue which can occur in the axilla, across the antecubital fossa into the forearm and wrist, and in the breast or abdominal wall. The incidence of cording following breast cancer treatment ranges from 6 – 72%, and the condition can cause pain and limited range of motion in the upper extremity. *NCBI: PMC: Cording Following Treatment for Breast Cancer*
	
	When does it happen:
	• Typically, 3-4 weeks post – op.
	• Less often 2-4 weeks
	• Less often over 4 weeks
	   Klose: Breast Cancer Rehabilitation
	
	Mondor disease is a rare condition that is characterized by scarring and inflammation of the veins located just beneath the skin of the chest. The affected veins are initially red and tender and subsequently become a painless, tough, fibrous band that is accompanied by tension and retraction of the nearby skin.
	• In most cases, the condition is benign and resolves on its own; however, Mondor disease can rarely be associated with breast cancer. Although the condition most commonly affects the chest, Mondor disease of other body parts (including the penis, groin, and abdomen) has been described, as well.
	• Mondor disease is thought to occur when pressure or trauma on the veins causes blood to stagnate. In most cases, the condition arises after recent breast surgery, but it can also be associated with physical strain and/or tight-fitting clothing (i.e. bras).
	• Treatments are available to help relieve symptoms until the condition resolves.
	   NIH: NCATS: Mondor Disease

What causes AWS	The etiology of cording is not fully understood. The condition may be related to abnormalities in either the axillary vasculature or the lymphatics.
	• Anatomic studies of resected cords reveal that these structures may represent dilated and thrombosed lymphatics and/or thrombosed superficial veins.
	• The condition is considered to be a variation of (Mondor's disease (*See below*), a rare thrombophlebitis of the subcutaneous veins caused by trauma such as surgery.
	   NCBI: PMC: Cording Following Treatment for Breast Cancer
	
	• AWS: may be attributed to lymph venous injury during axillary lymph node dissection due to either tissue retraction and/or patient positioning.
	• Another theory is that because of the interruption in axillary flow, lymphatic vessels are dilating and scalloping to the skin.
	   Summit Education: Oncology Rehab Dec 12, 2019

Who is at Risk?	The incidence of cording after axillary lymph node dissection (ALND) has been reported as high as 72%, compared to 20% after sentinel lymph node biopsy (SLNB). • Younger age, lower BMI, and being African-American have also been implicated as potential risk factors. • While cording has been reported to cause limited range of motion, the extent to which this translates into dysfunction performing daily functional reaching activities has yet to be reported. • Little data exists on whether cording is associated with an increased risk of developing upper extremity lymphedema. *NCBI: PMC: Cording Following Treatment for Breast Cancer* **Body habitus:** • Pt's that have AWS were found to be more often of lower weight with a BMI between 23-25. • Pt's that were obese with a BMI between 26-28.9, unlike with lymphedema, tend to have a lower incidence of cording. *Klose: Breast Cancer Rehabilitation.*
Axillary Web Syndrome by *Pink Ribbon Program*®	Axillary web syndrome is a self-limiting and frequently overlooked cause of significant morbidity in the early post-operative period after breast cancer axillary surgery, which is characterized by axillary pain that runs down the medial arm, limited shoulder range of motion affecting mainly shoulder abduction, and cords of subcutaneous tissue extending from axilla into the medial arm, made visible or palpable and painful by shoulder abduction. • In addition, soft tissue may give a cordlike appearance due to increased tension between the skin of the upper arm and adherence of an axillary scar to underlying fascia. • Lymphatic cording is associated with pain and limitation of shoulder movement, and it is common to find shoulder abduction restricted to less than 90°. • Exercise interventions should typically include supine exercises involving assisted shoulder flexion, active abduction, horizontal abduction, and a trunk rotational stretch with shoulder abduction, stretching exercises for levator scapulae, upper trapezius, pectoralis major, and medial and lateral rotators muscles of the shoulder. *Pink Ribbon Program*®

Managing AWS by *Breastcancer.org:* *Axillary Web* *Syndrome* *(Cording)*	If you have symptoms of AWS, ask your doctor to refer you to a physical therapist or other medical professional (such as a nurse or physician) *who specializes in breast cancer rehabilitation.* It's not a good idea to wait and see if the condition will resolve on its own. Your natural reaction to the pain of cording will be to avoid moving the arm and shoulder, which can lead to more tightness in the shoulder and chest area. Over time, this may cause more serious problems with function and mobility. Moving and stretching under the guidance of an experienced therapist are the best ways to resolve the condition and stop the pain. Together, you and your therapist can develop a treatment plan that's right for you. Your plan may include: • **Stretching and flexibility exercises**: Your therapist can work with you to help you learn exercises that gently stretch the cords and improve your pain-free range of motion. He or she can teach you exercises to do at home and advise you on how often to do them. • **Manual therapy**: Your therapist also may gently massage the cord tissue. Using manual therapy, your therapist would gently pull the tissue on your outstretched arm, starting in the upper arm and moving down into the forearm. This sometimes causes the cord to snap or break, and you may even hear a popping sound when that happens. It's usually not painful, and it often brings relief by extending your arm's pain-free range of motion. • **Moist heat**: Your therapist may apply warm, moist pads directly to the cords as part of therapy. However, it's important that he or she use caution when doing this. Prolonged heat can increase the production of lymph, which can lead to the fluid overload known as lymphedema. If your therapist recommends moist heat, just be sure he or she is experienced in its use for cording. • **Pain medication**: You may need to take some form of pain medication, such as an NSAID (non-steroidal anti-inflammatory drug, such as Motrin or aspirin), if you experience pain that prevents you from stretching the arm. But remember that the best treatment for the pain is doing the stretching exercises that help the condition get better. • **Low-level laser therapy**: Some therapists use a small, hand-held device to apply low- level laser beams directly to the skin. Laser therapy can help break down the hardened scar tissue. • With the exception of pain medication, all of these treatments focus on releasing the tight scar tissue that makes up the cord(s). o You may notice that releasing the cord in certain parts of the arm can magnify the tightness in other areas — not because the cording is getting worse, but because the scar tissue is still "stuck" in those other areas. For example, releasing the cord in the upper arm and elbow will reduce pain and improve range of motion, but the wrist and forearm may feel tighter at first. o "I describe the cord to my patients as being like a fishing line that is stuck in several places along the fishing rod," says Nicole Stout, MPT, CLT-LANA, physical therapist and lymphedema specialist, the Breast Care Center, National Naval Medical Center. "You can release a few of the stuck spots, but it then magnifies the tightness in the other areas that are still stuck." Fortunately, cording usually resolves for most people after a few therapy sessions, or at least within a few months. • It's possible to have limited range of motion for many months or even longer, but that's not typical. For some people, cording may get better and then come back later, but usually cording is a one-time event that doesn't become a persistent problem. • Experts still aren't exactly sure what happens to the cords after they break down. Some experts believe that they simply get reabsorbed by the body, but other experts say that we simply don't yet know what happens to the cords. *Breastcancer.org Axillary Web Syndrome (Cording)*

SCAR TISSUE / ADHESIONS / MYOFASCIAL RELEASE

Scar Tissue / Adhesions	An adhesion is a band of scar tissue that binds 2 parts of your tissue that are not normally joined together. Adhesions may appear as thin sheets of tissue similar to plastic wrap or as thick fibrous bands. The tissue develops when the body's repair mechanisms respond to any tissue disturbance, such as surgery, infection, trauma, or radiation. *Web MD: Adhesions, General and After Surgery* Breast and axillary surgery, and radiotherapy in breast cancer patients cause scar tissue formation, fibrosis and adhesions at all levels of soft tissues of the upper body. • The occurrence or persistence of upper limb impairments after breast cancer treatment can partially be explained by the presence of myofascial dysfunctions (*fascia surrounding and separating muscle tissue*). • Myofascial dysfunctions are expressed as myofascial trigger points and adhesions or restrictions of the myofascial tissues. • The latter are impairments of gliding of the myofascial tissues relative to each other. • Muscle manipulation during surgery, scar tissue formation, soft tissue adhesions and adaptive postures following surgery or fibrosis from radiotherapy can cause myofascial adhesions. *NCBI: An evaluation tool for Myofascial Adhesions* **According to *Klose (K) and BreastCancer.org (B)*, tissue adhesion can cause:** • Pain *(K)* • Postural changes *(K)* • Impaired shoulder function *(K)* • Movement compensations *(K)* • Nerve pain or numbness if scar tissue forms around nerves. *(B)* • A lump of scar tissue forms in the hole left after breast tissue is removed. If scar tissue forms around a stitch from surgery it's called a suture granuloma and also feels like a lump. *(B)* • Changes in breast appearance. Scar tissue and fluid retention can make breast tissue appear a little firmer or rounder than before surgery and/or radiation. *(B)* *Klose: Breast Cancer Rehabilitation (K)* and *BreastCancer.org: Scar Tissue Formation (B)*
Myofascial Release	Postural restoration through myofascial release (medical massage) is needed by most people, but especially those having significant scarring on the front of the body. • These scars draw the shoulders forward causing the head and neck to also pull forward. This leads to neck and shoulder aches and pains. • The body is meant to be in alignment. When we live and move in non-optimal alignment, serious orthopedic injuries can occur. • Most commonly, I have seen breast cancer survivors develop neck and shoulder impingement. Neck and shoulder impingement can cause shooting pain down the arm and lead to another surgery. Impingement syndromes start with achiness in the neck and shoulders. • Myofascial release is a type of medical massage that is NOT painful. Focus is placed on gently releasing tension along thickenings of fascia and scar tissue. Releasing this tension restores posture and alignment. It also relieves knots and painful areas in all parts of the body. *Breast Cancer Resource Center: Benefits of Myofascial Release Therapy after Mastectomy & Lumpectomy*

SEROMA / COMPRESSION

Seroma	A serous fluid collection that develops under the skin flaps during mastectomy or in the axillary dead space after axillary dissection.
	• Incidence of seroma formation after breast surgery varies between 2.5% and 51%.
	• Although seroma is not life threatening, it can lead to significant morbidity:
	o Flap necrosis
	o Wound dehiscence
	o Predisposes to sepsis
	o Prolonged recovery period
	o Multiple physician visits
	o May delay adjuvant therapy.
	• Fluid collection is ideally managed by repeated needle aspiration to seal the skin flaps against the chest wall.
	• Several factors have been investigated as the cause of seroma formation these include
	o Duration of wound drainage
	o Use of pressure garment
	o Postoperative arm activity
	o Preoperative chemotherapy
	o Use of electrocautery
	NCBI: Seroma formation after surgery for breast cancer
Compression	**Acute Management with Compression:**
	• Compression with pads and elastic garments
	• Apply immediate compression after aspiration, when possible
	Seroma Management Body Shapers:
	• Avoid shelf bras
	• Look for wide straps and good trunk coverage
	• Breast cup vs. flat fabric design (depending on surgery)
	• Ensure coverage into the axilla
	• Nighttime use if large breasted: daytime use if supportive enough to be used as a bra
	• If currently on radiation, consult radiation oncologist
	Klose: Breast Cancer Rehabilitation

Breast Cancer Resource Center: Benefits of Myofascial Release Therapy after Mastectomy & Lumpectomy
https://bcrc.org/benefits-myofascial-release-therapy-mastectomy-lumpectomy/

Breastcancer.org Axillary Web Syndrome (Cording) https://www.breastcancer.org/treatment/side_effects/aws

BreastCancer.org: Scar Tissue Formation https://www.breastcancer.org/treatment/side_effects/scar_tissue

Klose: Breast Cancer Rehabilitation

NCBI: Seroma formation after surgery for breast cancer https://www.ncbi.nlm.nih.gov/pmc/articles/PMC543447/

NCBI: An evaluation tool for Myofascial Adhesions in Patients after Breast Cancer
https://www.ncbi.nlm.nih.gov/pmc/articles/PMC5844553/#:~:text=Breast%20and%20axillary%20surgery%20and,
level%20and%20deeper%20myofascial%20structures.

NCBI: PMC: Atypical presentation of axillary web syndrome (AWS)
https://www.ncbi.nlm.nih.gov/pmc/articles/PMC5178020/

NCBI: PMC: Cording Following Treatment for Breast Cancer
https://www.ncbi.nlm.nih.gov/pmc/articles/PMC3786257/

NIH: NCATS: Mondor Disease: https://rarediseases.info.nih.gov/diseases/7054/mondor-disease

Pink Ribbon Program®

Summit Education: Oncology Rehab Dec 12, 2019

Web MD: Adhesions, General and After Surgery https://www.webmd.com/a-to-z-guides/adhesion-general-post-surgery#1

Breast Surgery Exercise & Contraindications / Precautions
Information and pictures from *National Cancer Institute* unless otherwise specified

Quick Summary this Section

Exercise Contraindications / Precautions After Breast Surgery
- TRAM Flap Reconstruction
- Latissimus Dorsi Flap Reconstruction
- DIEP Flap Reconstruction
- Tissue Expander
- Lymphedema and Exercise
- Axillary node dissection
- Peripheral Neuropathy
- Nerves that may be Damaged during Surgery

Things to Avoid, Post Op Healing & Mastectomy:
- Avoid 2 - weeks Post op
- Post op healing concerns
- Recommendations post mastectomy

Exercise Examples - Post Mastectomy:
- Examples of Exercises
- Stretches or Edema Control after Mastectomy

Home Exercise Guide Breast and / or Lymphedema:
- Home Exercise Guide For Post Surgery and / or Lymphedema

References

EXERCISE CONTRAINDICATIONS / PRECAUTIONS AFTER BREAST SURGERY

TRAM Flap Reconstruction	TRAM stands for the transverse rectus abdominis muscle, which is located in the lower abdomen, between the waist and the pubic bone. A TRAM flap uses a part of this muscle, its blood vessels, and some belly fat to rebuild the breast. • After TRAM flap surgery, you can start walking the next day, though it will probably hurt because of the incision in your abdomen. • For the first two days, many physical therapists recommend women do calf exercises and deep breathing exercises to help prevent blood clots. • You can start arm rehabilitation exercises 3 or 4 days after surgery. • Once the drains are removed, you can start stretching your chest, shoulders, and arms. It's also a good idea to walk regularly as you recover. • Don't do any abdominal ("abs") exercises until about 6 weeks after surgery or whenever your surgeon says it's OK to start. Start slowly and gently while continuing your stretching exercises and walking or other low-intensity aerobic exercise. • Those with a unilateral TRAM Flap may need minor assistance in lowering themselves back onto the floor. • Bi-lateral Tram Flap, will not be able to roll backwards or subsequently roll back to an upright position without assistance. *BreastCancer.org* and *CETI (Pilates)*
Latissimus Dorsi Flap Reconstruction	The latissimus dorsi is the muscle below the shoulder and behind the armpit. A latissimus dorsi flap uses an oval section of this muscle, skin, and fat to rebuild the breast. • Because this type of reconstruction affects the shoulder muscle, you should wait to start any gentle shoulder stretching until about 2 weeks after surgery. • Wait until about 3 months after surgery to do any resistance/strength exercises. • If you have any shortness of breath, pain, or tightness in your chest, stop exercising immediately. Tell your doctor what happened and work with him or her to develop a plan of movements that are right for you. • LAT Flap - may have noticeable weakness and instability in the affected shoulder(s). • Retract the shoulders prior to initiating the movement. This will help to contract the rhomboids and other scapular stabilizers. • Keep in mind that if you had a LAT Flap that one, or both, of the latissimus muscles are now in their chest wall. Because they are still "attached," they may feel a contraction in their chest when back exercises are performed. *BreastCancer.org* and *CETI (Pilates)*
DIEP Flap Reconstruction	DIEP stands for deep inferior epigastric perforator. In a DIEP flap, fat, skin, and blood vessels, but no muscles, are cut from the wall of the lower belly and moved up to your chest to rebuild your breast. • After DIEP flap surgery, you can start walking the next day, though it will probably hurt because of the incision in your abdomen. • For the first 2 days, many physical therapists recommend women do calf exercises and deep breathing exercises to help prevent blood clots. • You can start arm rehabilitation exercises 3 or 4 days after surgery. • Once the drains are removed, you can start stretching your chest, shoulders, and arms. It's also a good idea to walk regularly as you recover. • Don't do any abdominal ("abs") exercises until about 6 weeks after surgery or whenever your surgeon says it's OK to start. *BreastCancer.org*

Tissue Expander	If you have a tissue expander in (a temporary inflatable implant that stretches the skin to make room for the final implant), you can usually start gentle shoulder stretching exercises about 2 weeks after surgery once your mastectomy scar has started to heal. • Many physical therapists recommend doing these stretches right after a warm shower because the muscles and skin are more flexible. • If you have expanders or breast implants, you will want to begin with limited ROM. It is rare, but possible, that the implants will move out of their "pocket," and need surgical correction. • ***No chest exercises when tissue expanders are in place.*** *BreastCancer.org* and *CETI (Pilates)*

Lymphedema and Exercise
 	
If you have lymphedema or are at risk, talk with a certified lymphedema therapist before beginning exercise.
 	
This includes anyone who has had lymph nodes removed or radiation.
 	
Increasing resistance too quickly can exacerbate condition.
 	
(See lymphedema section)
	Both light exercise and aerobic exercise (physical activity that causes the heart and lungs to work harder) help the lymph vessels move lymph out of the affected limb and decrease swelling.
	• **If you have lymphedema or are at risk, talk with a certified lymphedema therapist before beginning exercise. This includes *anyone* who has had lymph nodes removed or radiation.**
	    ○ Patients who have lymphedema or who are at risk for lymphedema should talk with a certified lymphedema therapist before beginning an exercise routine. Adding resistance
	        ▪ (*See the Lymphology Association of North America* (https://www.clt-lana.org/) *web site for a list of certified lymphedema therapists in the US*)
	• Wear a pressure garment if lymphedema has developed.
	    ○ Patients who have lymphedema should wear a well-fitting pressure garment during all exercise that uses the affected limb or body part.
	    ○ When it is not known for sure if a woman has lymphedema, upper-body exercise without a garment may be more helpful than no exercise at all.
	    ○ Patients who do not have lymphedema do not need to wear a pressure garment during exercise.
	• Avoid wrapping a band around your hand when using for resistance. This will put you at risk for increased edema by cutting off the circulation. Hold the band or use a band that has handles.
	• Breast cancer survivors should begin with light upper-body exercise and increase it slowly.
	    ○ Some studies with breast cancer survivors show that upper-body exercise is safe in women who have lymphedema or who are at risk for lymphedema.
	    ○ Weight-lifting that is slowly increased may keep lymphedema from getting worse.
	    ○ Exercise should start at a very low level, increase slowly over time, and *be overseen by the lymphedema therapist*.
	    ○ If exercise is stopped for a week or longer, it should be started again at a low level and increased slowly.
	    ○ If symptoms (such as swelling or heaviness in the limb) change or increase for a week or longer, talk with the lymphedema therapist.
	    ○ It is likely that exercising at a low level and slowly increasing it again over time is better for the affected limb than stopping the exercise completely.
	• More studies are needed to find out if weight-lifting is safe for cancer survivors with lymphedema in the legs. *NIH NCI (12)*

Axillary Node Dissection	• If you have undergone an axillary node dissection, or radiation/dissection to the nodes in the neck, you may struggle with scar tissue/adhesions in that area. • Gently ease into the stretch and only go as far as you can, with mild discomfort, but NO pain • Start with a few repetitions and gradually increase as tolerated (no swelling). *CETI (Pilates)* **Also see Lymphedema**
Peripheral Neuropathy	• Some cancer treatments cause peripheral neuropathy, a result of damage to the peripheral nerves. These nerves carry information from the brain to other parts of the body. • Feet or lower extremity – caution with standing on uneven surface, such as a Bosu ball or balance pads due to decreased sensation in feet. Increased risk of falling. • Hands – caution with holding dumbbells or grasping resistance bands.
Nerves that may be Damaged during Surgery	Several structures, including vessels and muscles with their nerve supply, are related to the breast and should be preserved during mastectomy or axillary node dissection. • The **lateral pectoral nerve** passes medially around the medial pectoralis minor, and the medial pectoral nerve passes laterally around the pectoralis minor. These nerves can be severed during surgery. ***This results in numbness, motor atrophy, decreased sweat production in armpit and arm.*** • The **medial pectoral nerve** innervates pectoralis minor and the lateral portion of the pectoralis major muscles. Preservation of this nerve is particularly important to prevent atrophy of the pectoral muscles if submuscular implant reconstruction is planned. • The **thoracodorsal nerve** is identifiable medial to the thoracodorsal vein. ***Injury may result in a weakening of the latissimus.*** • The **long thoracic nerve** of Bell is located more medially in the axilla. It runs just beneath the fascia of the serratus anterior, medial to the thoracodorsal complex. ***Injury to this nerve will result in weakness in the serratus and cause winging of the scapula.*** *Pink Ribbon Program©*

Neurogenic causes of scapular winging and the physical exam

	Medial winging	**Lateral winging**	
Injured nerve	Long thoracic	Spinal accessory	Dorsal scapular
Muscle palsy	Serratus anterior	Trapezius	Rhomboids
Physical exam	Arm flexion; push-up motion against a wall	Arm abduction; external rotation against resistance	Arm extension from full flexion
Position of the scapula compared to normal	Entire scapula displaced more medial and superior	Superior angle more laterally displaced	Inferior angle more laterally displaced

NCBI: Scapular winging: anatomical review, diagnosis, and treatments

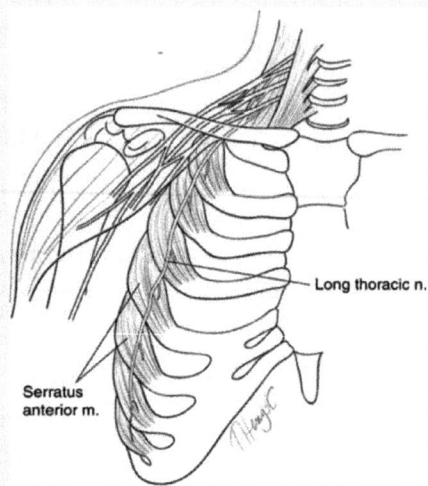

NCBI: Scapular winging: anatomical review, diagnosis, and treatments

| Latissimus dorsi | Pec Major | Pec Minor |

Scapular – normal   Scapular – winging

WikiMedia Commons: *https://commons.wikimedia.org/*

AVOID during the FIRST 2 WEEKS AFTER SURGERY
Cancer Research UK and *Dana Farber*

Your surgeon may suggest slightly different timings, so check if you are unsure.
- Don't lift your arm above the height of your shoulder or stretch behind your back.
- Don't lift anything heavier than a bag of sugar.

You might not realize that some everyday things can strain your muscles. Avoid doing any of the following with your arm on the side of your surgery. Avoiding these things helps your muscles to slowly stretch and heal.

- Pushing yourself up off the bed
- Pushing doors open
- Pulling things towards you, such as pulling washing out of the washing machine

IMPLANT
The implant has been placed under the muscle at the front of your chest. It stretches the chest muscle more than usual. By avoiding the movements listed above, the implant won't move and you won't overstretch the muscle or the wound, so it can all heal and settle down.
- When you are fastening your bra, do it up at the front, swivel it round, and put your arm on the side you had surgery in first. When you put your coat on, make sure you put the side you had surgery in the armhole first.
Cancer Research UK

If you have a lumpectomy or partial mastectomy with or without a sentinel lymph node biopsy:
- Avoid any activity that bounces or jostles the breast for two weeks after surgery (i.e.: running, jumping, using the elliptical machine).
- Perform shoulder range of motion as tolerated, beginning 1-2 days after surgery.
- If you have an axillary node dissection: You may want to use pillows to elevate your arm at night to decrease swelling during the first week. Putting a pillow between your arm and your side at night will prevent you from rolling on to the surgical site.
- You should avoid repetitive motions with the arm on the surgical side, such as vacuuming, for two weeks after surgery.
- Avoid heavy lifting for 4 weeks.

If you have a mastectomy without reconstruction:
- Perform shoulder range of motion as tolerated, even while the drains are in.
- You may return to low-impact exercises after surgery once your pain is controlled and you feel comfortable.

If you have breast reconstruction:
- You should not lift your arm above shoulder level until cleared by your plastic surgeon.
- You may return to low-impact exercises four weeks after surgery.

Walking is a great exercise to begin immediately to reduce bone loss, counter fatigue and nausea, and prevent muscle atrophy. After surgery, try to walk around for a few minutes 2-3 times per day.

If you've had a mastectomy do not lift your arm past shoulder level while the drains are in.

Dana Farber

POST OP HEALING CONCERNS
©Klose Training: Breast Cancer Rehabilitation

Not Enough Movement	• Tissue adhesions • Shoulder/rib/clavicle stiffness • Decreased lymphangiomotoricity
Not Enough Compression	• Axillary/mastectomy/flap site seroma • Breast edema
Too Much Movement	• Mastectomy skin flaps will not adhere > seroma • ALND > seroma • Lack of lymphatic regeneration > increased risk of lymphedema
Seroma and Lymph Edema Prevention	• To early and/or too aggressive exercise may be increasing the incidence of seroma and lymphedema • ***Avoid wall walks and ROM past shoulder height, at least for the initial 2-3 weeks post-surgery*** • Avoid extreme forward reaching
Post Op Movement Restrictions	• Limit shoulder flexion to 90 degrees for 7-14 days to avoid seroma formation and encourage lymphatic regeneration. • Range of motion in shoulder as far as possible, avoiding pain, after 14 days if no seroma, and per surgeon recommendations. • Encourage using the arm as normally as possible without pain, within surgeons guidelines.

Recommendations Post Mastectomy

3-7 Days
- Avoid lying on side or arm of mastectomy
- Elevate affected side above heart at about a 45 degree angle 2-3x a day to avoid swelling.
- Use your arm to brush hair or trying to reach

First 4 weeks
- Do not use resistance
- Do not do overhead laps in pool
- Do not do body weight exercises or certain yoga poses such as push-ups or downward dog
- Avoid sports, such as skiing, tennis, canoe or any other exercises that extreme stretching of the shoulder.
- Be aware of lymphedema symptoms
- Do stretches in a warm shower or after once cleared to take a shower.
- Do stretches until feeling a slight stretch, not pain.
- Try doing the exercises twice a day 5-7 each.
- You do not have to start with every exercise listed – start with the ones lying down, then move to seated, and then standing.

After 4 – 6 weeks progress as tolerated and/or instructed by MD or physical therapy to include resistance.

Follow MD orders

Examples of Exercises, Stretches or Edema Control after Mastectomy			
1-2 WEEKS POST-OP	**Exercise or Stretch**	**Section**	**Number**
	DIAPHRAGMATIC BREATHING 6x a day for 5-10 repetitions	Duration, Frequency, Intensity	Pg 158
	OPEN AND CLOSE YOUR FIST CLENCH	NA	--
	SHOUDER SHRUGS	Upper Extremity	87
	SHOULDER ROLLS	Upper Extremity	89
	NECK ROTATION and SIDE BENDS	Flexibility	47
	SHOULER RAISE / ELBOW CIRCLES	NA	--
	PENDULUM SHOULDER FORWARD/BACK	Upper Extremity	29
	PENDULUM SHOULDER – SIDE TO SIDE	Upper Extremity	30
	PENDULUM SHOULDER CIRCLES	Upper Extremity	31
	BODY TURNS (rotations)	NA	--
	ELBOW FLEXION EXTENSION – SUPINE Bicep curl without weight on affected side to prevent edema	Upper Extremity	1
	BICEPS CURLS – SEATED Bicep curl without weight on affected side to prevent edema	Upper Extremity	3

3-4 WEEKS POST-OP	Exercise or Stretch	Section	Number
	V RAISE	Upper Extremity	45
	FLEXION – SUPINE - SINGLE OR BILATERAL	Upper Extremity	35
	FLEXION – SUPINE - DOWEL	Upper Extremity	37
	FLEXION - TABLE SLIDE	Flexibility	67
	FLEXION - TABLE SLIDE - BALL	Flexibility	68
	WALL WALK	Flexibility	66
	WALL WALK – Lateral	NA	--
	TRUNK ROTATION – SEATED	Flexibility	61
	CHEST STRETCH – SEATED or STANDING	Flexibility	71
	CHEST STRETCH – SUPINE	NA	--
	SCAPULAR RETRACTIONS - BILATERAL	Upper Extremity	92

4-6 WEEKS POST-OP Or Per MD order	Exercise or Stretch	Section	Number
	SHOULDER EXTENSION - STANDING	Upper Extremity	51
	SHOULDER EXTENSION – BILATERAL Standing dowel without weight	Upper Extremity	53
	LYING DOWN EXTENSION - TABLE or BED	Flexibility	77
	SHOULDER EXTENSION – DOWEL - STANDING	Flexibility	78
	EXTERNAL ROTATION - SUPINE – DOWEL *INTERNAL ROTATION ON OPPOSITE ARM*	Flexibility	69
	EXTERNAL ROTATION - 90-90 – DOWEL	Flexibility	70
	EXTERNAL ROTATION – SEATED – DOWEL *INTERNAL ROTATION ON OPPOSITE ARM*	Flexibility	71
	SCAPULAR PROTRACTION - SUPINE – BILATERAL	Upper Extremity	9
	ABDUCTION - TABLE SLIDE – BALL	Flexibility	75
	ABDUCTION WITH DOWEL	Flexibility	76
	CHEST STRETCH - STEP THROUGH	Flexibility	80

HOME EXERCISE GUIDE FOR POST SURGERY AND/OR LYMPHEDEMA

Breathing Patterns

Diaphragmatic Breathing

Lie either on your back with your knees bent or sit up

Inhale through your nose; as you do so, allow your stomach to rise. Limit movement in your chest. Attempt to push your bottom ribs out to the side as you breathe in.

Exhale through your mouth; as you do so, allow your stomach to fall. Limit movement in your chest.

Diaphragmatic breathing 6x a day for 5-10 repetitions

Purse Lip Breathing – Shortness of Breath

(PLB) is a breathing technique that consists of inhaling through the nose with the mouth closed and then exhaling through tightly pressed (pursed) lips. This technique is frequently in those with cardiac or respiratory issues. "*Smell the Roses then Blow Out the Candle*".

Breathing with Exercise

Exhale on the exertion. For example exhale when you are lying on your back and pushing a weight up or when bending your arm doing a bicep curl,. Inhale as you bring the weight slowly to your chest or when you straighten your arm with a bicep curl..

1-2 WEEKS POST OP or PER MD ORDERS

Description	Pictures
Other information at beginning of book. UE = Upper Extremity Section Flex = Flexibility Section	See UE or Flex section of book for other pictures
FIST CLENCH *Lymphedema control and circulation* Hands on thighs, open and close hand	
FIST CLENCH *Lymphedema control and circulation* Open and close your hand 15-20x with arm elevated above heart to prevent edema	
FIST CLENCH *Lymphedema control and circulation* Open and close your hand 15-20x with arm elevated above heart to prevent edema **NOT OVERHEAD first 1-2 weeks and/or until drains are out**	
SHRUGS UE 87 Raise your shoulders upward towards your ears as shown. Shrug both shoulders at the same time. Inhale up/exhale down	

Description	Pictures
Other information at beginning of book. UE = Upper Extremity Section Flex = Flexibility Section	See UE or Flex section of book for other pictures
SHOULDER ROLLS - Backwards UE 89 Move your shoulders in a circular pattern so that you are moving in an up, back and down direction. Perform small circles if needed for comfort.	
NECK ROTATION and SIDE BENDS Flex 47 SIDE BENDS: (*Top*) Tilt your head as if you are trying to touch your ear to your shoulder. ROTATION: (*Bottom*) Turn you head to the side as if looking over your shoulder.	
NECK FLEXION AND EXTENSION Flex 48 EXTENSION: Look up as if you are looking at the sky moving your neck only. FLEXION: Look down as if you are looking at the floor. For an extra stretch gently put both hands behind your head to move chin towards the chest and hold.	
SHOULDER RAISE / ELBOW CIRCLES Place your fingertips onto your shoulders. Slowly raise the elbow up to the side, then move it forwards, gently circling your arm. You are aiming to get your elbow level with your shoulder. Try to increase the height each time you do the exercises until you get level with your shoulder.	
ISOMETRIC CHEST PRESS Place the palms of your hands together with your elbows bent and arms at shoulder level or below. Exhale while pushing hands together and inhale and relax. 5-10x.	

Description	Pictures
Other information at beginning of book. UE = Upper Extremity Section Flex = Flexibility Section	See UE or Flex section of book for other pictures

PENDULUM SHOULDER FORWARD/BACK
UE 29

Start in a standing position and lean forward as allowed by MD – First picture

Shift your body weight forward then back to allow your injured arm to swing forward and back freely. Your affected arm should be fully relaxed.

PENDULUM SHOULDER – SIDE TO SIDE
UE 30

Start in a standing position and lean forward as allowed by MD as above

Shift your body weight side to side to allow your injured arm to swing side to side freely. Your affected arm should be fully relaxed.

PENDULUM SHOULDER CIRCLES
UE 31

Start in a standing position and lean forward as allowed by MD as above

Shift your body weight in circles to allow your injured arm to swing in circles freely. Your injured arm should be fully relaxed.

REVERSE PENDULUM SHOULDER CIRCLES
Shift your body weight in reverse circles to allow your injured arm to swing in circles freely. Your injured arm should be fully relaxed.

Description	Pictures
Description Other information at beginning of book. UE = Upper Extremity Section Flex = Flexibility Section	**Pictures** See UE or Flex section of book for other pictures
BODY TURNS / ROTATIONS Cross your arms across your body so that your hands are placed lightly on your elbows. Slowly turn to look to the left and then to the right.	
ELBOW FLEXION EXTENSION – SUPINE UE 1 Lie on your back and rest your elbow on a small rolled up towel. Bend at your elbow and then lower back down.	 Extension Flexion
BICEPS CURLS UE 3 Bend your elbow and move your forearm upwards and lower back down. Bicep curl without weight on affected side to prevent edema	

3-4 WEEKS POST OP or PER MD ORDERS

Description	Pictures
Other information at beginning of book. UE = Upper Extremity Section Flex = Flexibility Section	See UE or Flex section of book for other pictures

V RAISE UE 45 Start with your arms down by your side, palms facing inward, thumbs up and your elbows straight. Raise up your arms in the form of a V to shoulder height as shown keeping elbows straight then return to starting position	
FLEXION – SUPINE - SINGLE OR BILATERAL UE 35 Lie on your back with your arm at your side. Slowly raise arm up and forward towards overhead until you feel a stretch – not pain. Can bend your knees for comfort. **NOT OVERHEAD first 2 weeks and/or until drains are out**	
FLEXION – SUPINE - DOWEL UE 37 Can use a broom handle, cane etc. Lie on your back holding dowel with both hands. Slowly raise up and forward towards overhead until you feel a stretch. Your unaffected arm will help lift the wand higher. Hold for 5 seconds, then gently lower arms. Return to starting position. Repeat. **NOT OVERHEAD first 2 weeks and/or until drains are out**	

Description	Pictures
Other information at beginning of book. UE = Upper Extremity Section Flex = Flexibility Section	See UE or Flex section of book for other pictures

Description	Pictures
FLEXION - TABLE SLIDE Shoulder blade stretch Flex 67 Stand rest your affected / target arm on a table either palm down or on side and gently slide it forward and then back. You should feel your shoulder blade move as you do this	
FLEXION - TABLE SLIDE - BALL Flex 68 Stand and rest your target arm on top of a ball on a table. Gently roll the ball forward and then back. You should feel your shoulder blade move as you do this	
WALL WALK - Front Flex 66 Place your target hand on the wall with the palm facing the wall. Walk your fingers up the wall towards overhead. Slide or walk your hand back down the wall to the starting position. You may feel tight, but it shouldn't be painful. If it is very painful, tell your specialist physiotherapist or breast care nurse. **NOT OVERHEAD first 2 weeks and/or until drains are out**	
WALL WALK – Lateral Walk your fingers up the wall sideways – Stand with the side you had the operation next to the wall. Walk your fingers up the wall so that the palm of your hand is facing the wall. **NOT OVERHEAD first 2 weeks and/or until drains are out**	

Description	Pictures
Other information at beginning of book. UE = Upper Extremity Section Flex = Flexibility Section	See UE or Flex section of book for other pictures

TRUNK ROTATION – SEATED Flex 61 Sit up as tall with erect posture. Rotate in one direction, using your hand to press against the opposite thigh to aide in further rotation. Exhale to increase the rotation and stretch. Return to the starting position, maintain an upright posture -repeat in the opposite direction.	
CHEST STRETCH – SEATED or STANDING Flex 71 TOP: Bend arms at a 90-degree angle. Move elbows back until feeling a stretch in front of shoulders/chest. BOTTOM: Clasp hands in back of head. Move elbows back until feeling a stretch in front of shoulders/chest.	
CHEST STRETCH – SUPINE Lie on your back. Put your fingers lightly on your ears or behind your head, with your elbows pointing up towards the ceiling. Slowly let your elbows fall back towards the floor/bed to feel a stretch in the chest and front of the shoulders. Should feel a stretch – not pain.	

Description	Pictures
Other information at beginning of book. UE = Upper Extremity Section Flex = Flexibility Section	See UE or Flex section of book for other pictures

SCAPULAR RETRACTIONS - Bilateral UE 92 Draw your shoulder blades back and down. Squeeze your shoulder blades together, bringing your elbows behind you toward your spine. Elbows will move with you, but don't force the motion with your elbows. Keep your shoulders level as you do this. Do not lift your shoulders up toward your ears. Return to the starting position and repeat 5 to 7 times. CHEST STRETCH Stand up, keeping your arms relaxed and straight by your side. Then slowly take your arms behind you, as if you are trying to touch your hands together at the back. UK **CAREFUL WITH CHEST EXPANDER OR NEW IMPLANTS**	

OTHER EXERCISES PER PHYSICAL THERAPY, CERTFIED CANCER EXERCISE SPECIALIST or OTHER TRAINED SPECIALIST

Description	Pictures
Other information at beginning of book. UE = Upper Extremity Section Flex = Flexibility Section	See UE or Flex section of book for other pictures
SHOULDER EXTENSION - STANDING UE 51 Start with arms by your side. Draw your arm back behind your waist. Keep your elbows straight.	
SHOULDER EXTENSION - STANDING UE 53 Hold a dowel or cane behind your back with both arms. Draw your arms back.	
LYING DOWN EXTENSION - TABLE or BED Flex 77 Lie on your back and gently let target arm drop off table or bed. May want to have someone there to guard or have strap and hold with the other hand.	

Description	Pictures
Description Other information at beginning of book. UE = Upper Extremity Section Flex = Flexibility Section	**Pictures** See UE or Flex section of book for other pictures
SHOULDER EXTENSION – DOWEL - STANDING Flex 78 Stand and hold a dowel/cane. Use the unaffected arm to help push the target arm back to a stretch, not pain. The elbow should remain straight the entire time. Can cup affected arm in back of dowel if unable to grasp *(see 2nd picture)*	
EXTERNAL ROTATION - SUPINE – DOWEL *INTERNAL ROTATION ON OPPOSITE ARM* Flex 69 Lie on your back holding a dowel/cane with both hands. On the target side, maintain approx. 90-degree bend at the elbow with your arm approximately 30-45 degrees away from your side. Use your other arm to push the dowel/cane to rotate the affected arm back into a stretch, not pain. Hold and then return to the starting position.	
EXTERNAL ROTATION - 90-90 – DOWEL Flex 70 Lie on your back and hold a dowel with your elbows out to the side and rested down. Roll your arms back towards overhead until a stretch is felt, not pain. Keep elbows bent at a 90-degree angle.	

Description	Pictures
Description Other information at beginning of book. UE = Upper Extremity Section Flex = Flexibility Section	**Pictures** See UE or Flex section of book for other pictures
EXTERNAL ROTATION – SEATED – DOWEL *INTERNAL ROTATION ON OPPOSITE ARM* Flex 71 Using the unaffected arm, push the dowel into the hand of the target arm. Keep the arm at a 90-degree angle and push until a stretch is felt, not pain. Hold and repeat. If needed, use towel under arm for positioning *(see 2nd picture)*	
SCAPULAR PROTRACTION - SUPINE SINGLE OR BILATERAL UE 9 Lie on your back with your arms extended out in front of your body and towards the ceiling. While keeping your elbows straight, protract your shoulders reaching forward towards the ceiling. Keep your elbows straight the entire time.	
ABDUCTION - TABLE SLIDE – BALL Flex 75 Stand and rest your target arm on top of a ball on a table and gently roll it to the side and back.	

Description	Pictures
Other information at beginning of book. UE = Upper Extremity Section Flex = Flexibility Section	See UE or Flex section of book for other pictures

| ABDUCTION WITH DOWEL
Flex 76

Hold a dowel/cane in front. Slowly push the dowel of the unaffected arm towards the target arm upward and to the side until a stretch is felt, not pain. | |
| CHEST STRETCH - STEP THROUGH
Flex 80

Stand with arms in doorway at a 90-degree angle. Step through until you feel a stretch through the chest and hold.
No pain should be felt.
 Keep shoulders down and back. Take another step to increase stretch.

Can modify starting with arms lower and bring up as tolerated. | |

NCBI: Scapular winging: anatomical review, diagnosis, and treatments:
https://www.ncbi.nlm.nih.gov/pmc/articles/PMC2684151/

CETI: Pilates https*: //www.thecancerspecialist.com/*

Dana Farber - *https://www.dana-farber.org/*

Klose Training ©: Breast Cancer Rehabilitation - *https://klosetraining.com/*

American Cancer Society - Physical Activity and the Cancer Patient - *https://www.cancer.org/treatment/survivorship-during-and-after-treatment/staying-active/physical-activity-and-the-cancer-patient.html*

Cancer Research UK - Exercise guidelines for Cancer Patients
https://www.cancerresearchuk.org/about-cancer/coping/physically/exercise-guidelines Clinical Exercise Physiology, pg. 440

NIH NCI (12) https://www.cancer.gov/about-cancer/treatment/side-effects/lymphedema/lymphedema-pdq

Pink Ribbon Program© - *https://www.pinkribbonprogram.com/*

Cancer Therapies
Information and pictures from *National Cancer Institute* unless otherwise specified

Quick Summary this Section

Chemotherapy:
- Chemotherapy works by stopping or slowing the growth of cancer cells, which grow and divide quickly.

Radiation:
- Radiation therapy (also called radiotherapy) is a cancer treatment that uses high doses of radiation to kill cancer cells and shrink tumors.

Hormone Therapy:
- Hormone therapy is a cancer treatment that removes hormones or blocks their action and stops cancer cells from growing. Hormones are substances made by glands in the body and circulated in the bloodstream.

Targeted Therapy:
- Targeted therapy is a type of treatment that uses drugs or other substances to identify and attack specific cancer cells without harming normal cells

Immunotherapy:
- Immunotherapy is a type of cancer treatment that helps your immune system fight cancer. The immune system helps your body fight infections and other diseases.
- It is made up of white blood cells and organs and tissues of the lymph system.

Stem Cell Therapy / Transplant:
- Stem cell transplants are procedures that restore blood-forming stem cells in people who have had theirs destroyed by the high doses of chemotherapy or radiation therapy that are used to treat certain cancers.

Other Therapies / Treatments:
- Ablation, Active surveillance, Biological, Bisphosphonate therapy, Chemoprevention, Chimeric antigen receptor, Electrocautery, Embolization therapy, Endoscopic stent placement, High-intensity–focused ultrasound therapy and more.

Side Effects and Late Side Effects:
- Side Effects and Late Side Effects of therapies and surgeries

Eating Hints: Before, during, and after Cancer Treatment:
- Clear Liquids, Full Liquid Diet, Foods and Drinks that Are Easy on the Stomach
- Low Fiber, High Fiber, High Protein, Foods and Drinks that Are Easy to Chew and Swallow

CHEMOTHERAPY
Information and pictures from *National Cancer Institute* unless otherwise specified

Quick Summary of Section

How Chemotherapy Works against Cancer and Who Receives It:

- Chemotherapy works by stopping or slowing the growth of cancer cells, which grow and divide quickly.

How Your Doctor Decides Which Chemotherapy Drugs to Give You:

- There are many different chemotherapy drugs.

How Chemotherapy Is Used with Other Cancer Treatments:

- When used with other treatments

How Often You Receive Chemotherapy

- Treatment schedules for chemotherapy vary widely. You may receive chemotherapy in cycles.
- A cycle is a period of chemotherapy treatment followed by a period of rest.

Ways Chemotherapy May be Given:

- Oral, intravenous, intrathecal, intraperitoneal, intra-arterial, topical, catheter, port, pump

The Most Common Chemotherapy Drugs/ Examples for Breast Cancer *(Medical News Today)*

Side Effects and Exercise Precautions:

- Chemotherapy not only kills fast-growing cancer cells but also kills or slows the growth of healthy cells that grow and divide quickly.

How Chemotherapy Works against Cancer and Who Receives it	Chemotherapy is used to treat many types of cancer. For some people, chemotherapy may be the only treatment you receive. But most often, you will have chemotherapy and other cancer treatments. • The types of treatment that you need depends on the type of cancer you have, if it has spread and where, and if you have other health problems. *NIH NCI (14)* Chemotherapy is used to: • Treat cancer: Chemotherapy can be used to cure cancer, lessen the chance it will return, or stop or slow its growth. • Ease cancer symptoms: Chemotherapy can be used to shrink tumors that are causing pain and other problems. *NIH NCI (14)* Chemotherapy is a drug treatment that works by stopping or slowing the growth of cancer cells, which grow and divide quickly. But it can also harm healthy cells that divide quickly, such as those that line your mouth and intestines or cause your hair to grow. • Damage to healthy cells may cause side effects. Often, side effects get better or go away after chemotherapy is over. *Cancer.gov publication – Chemotherapy and You*

How Your Doctor Decides Which Chemotherapy Drugs to Give You	There are many different chemotherapy drugs. Which ones are included in your treatment plan depends mostly on: • The type of cancer you have and how advanced it is • Whether you have had chemotherapy before • Whether you have other health problems, such as diabetes or heart disease *NIH NCI (14)*
How Chemotherapy Is Used with Other Cancer Treatments	When used with other treatments, chemotherapy can: • Make a tumor smaller before surgery or radiation therapy. This is called neoadjuvant chemotherapy. • Destroy cancer cells that may remain after treatment with surgery or radiation therapy. This is called adjuvant chemotherapy. • Help other treatments work better. • Kill cancer cells that have returned or spread to other parts of your body. *NIH NCI (14)*

How Often You Receive Chemotherapy	Treatment schedules for chemotherapy vary widely. How often and how long you get chemotherapy depends on:
	• Your type of cancer and how advanced it is
	• Whether chemotherapy is used to:
	    ○ Cure your cancer
	    ○ Control its growth
	    ○ Ease symptoms
	• The type of chemotherapy you are getting
	• How your body responds to chemotherapy
	
	You may receive chemotherapy in cycles. A cycle is a period of chemotherapy treatment followed by a period of rest.
	• For instance, you might receive chemotherapy every day for 1 week followed by 3 weeks with no chemotherapy. These 4 weeks make up one cycle.
	• The rest period gives your body a chance to recover and build new healthy cells.
	NIH NCI (14)

Ways Chemotherapy May be Given	**Oral**
	    The chemotherapy comes in pills, capsules, or liquids that you swallow
	Intravenous (IV)
	    The chemotherapy goes directly into a vein
	Injection
	    Chemotherapy is given by a shot in a muscle in your arm, thigh, or hip, or right under the skin in the fatty part of your arm, leg, or belly
	Intrathecal
	    Chemotherapy is injected into the space between the layers of tissue that cover the brain and spinal cord
	Intraperitoneal (IP)
	    Chemotherapy goes directly into the peritoneal cavity, which is the area in your body that contains organs such as your intestines, stomach, and liver
	Intra-arterial (IA)
	    Chemotherapy is injected directly into the artery that leads to the cancer
	Topical
	    The chemotherapy comes in a cream that you rub onto your skin
	
	Chemotherapy is often given through a thin needle that is placed in a vein on your hand or lower arm. Your nurse will put the needle in at the start of each treatment and remove it when the treatment is over.
	IV chemotherapy may also be given through catheters or ports, sometimes with the help of a pump.
	
	Catheter
	    • A catheter is a thin, soft tube. A doctor or nurse places one end of the catheter in a large vein, often in your chest area. The other end of the catheter stays outside your body.
	    • Most catheters stay in place until you have finished your chemotherapy treatments.
	    • Catheters can also be used to give you other drugs and to draw blood. Be sure to watch for signs of infection around your catheter.
	
	Port
	    • A port is a small, round disc that is placed under your skin during minor surgery. A surgeon puts it in place before you begin your course of treatment, and it remains there until you have finished. A catheter connects the port to a large vein, most often in your chest.
	    • Your nurse can insert a needle into your port to give you chemotherapy or draw blood.
	    • This needle can be left in place for chemotherapy treatments that are given for longer than one day.
	    • Be sure to watch for signs of infection around your port.
	
	Pump
	    • Pumps are often attached to catheters or ports. They control how much and how fast chemotherapy goes into a catheter or port, allowing you to receive your chemotherapy outside of the hospital.
	    • Pumps can be internal or external. External pumps remain outside your body.
	    • Internal pumps are placed under your skin during surgery.
	      NIH NCI (14)

Types of Chemotherapy Drugs and Examples

Medical News Today

There are several main types of chemotherapy drugs that doctors use to target different types of cancer. The sections below look at these in more detail.

Alkylating agents

These were some of the earliest cancer treatments, and they are still common. They work by disrupting the DNA inside cells, which prevents them from dividing. They can help treat many types of cancer, but they are most effective against slow-growing cancers.

Some *examples* of alkylating agents include:
- altretamine
- busulfan
- carboplatin
- carmustine
- cisplatin
- cyclophosphamide
- dacarbazine
- ifosfamide
- lomustine
- melphalan
- temozolomide
- trabectedin

Antimetabolites

These drugs work by pretending to be nutrients that cells need to grow. The cell eventually starves to death after consuming them. These medications only work at specific stages in a cell's growth cycle.

Some *examples* of antimetabolites include:
- 5-fluorouracil
- 6-mercaptopurine
- azacitidine
- capecitabine
- clofarabine
- cytarabine
- floxuridine
- fludarabine
- gemcitabine
- methotrexate
- pemetrexed
- pentostatin
- pralatrexate
- trifluridine and tipiracil, which is a combination drug that comes in the form of a pill

Types of Chemotherapy Drugs and Examples *and* **The Most Common Chemotherapies for Breast Cancer** *Continued* *Medical News Today*	**Plant alkaloids** Plant alkaloids are plant-based substances that prevent cancerous cells from dividing and growing into more cells. They can work throughout a cell's growth cycle, but they are most effective during certain phases. Some *examples* of plant alkaloids include: • vincristine • vinblastine • vinorelbine • paclitaxel • docetaxel • etoposide • teniposide • irinotecan • topotecan **Anti-tumor antibiotics** These drugs differ from antibiotics for treating infections. They work by causing DNA strands to unravel, which prevents the cell from dividing. Some *examples* of anti-tumor antibiotics include: • daunorubicin • doxorubicin • doxorubicin liposomal • epirubicin • idarubicin • valrubicin **The Most Common Chemotherapies for Breast Cancer** Doctors administer chemotherapy in cycles of treatment and recovery. These cycles are generally 2–3 weeks long and may repeat for 3–6 months. Most people receive chemotherapy drugs through an injection or infusion. The following sections look at some common chemotherapy medications for breast cancer. **Breast cancer** For breast cancer, a variety of chemotherapy drugs may be necessary, including: • anthracyclines, such as doxorubicin • cyclophosphamide • epirubicin • fluorouracil • methotrexate • taxanes, such as paclitaxel • docetaxel

Side Effects (See *Side Effects* and *Late Effects* for more information)	**Possible Side Effects:** • Chemotherapy not only kills fast-growing cancer cells but also kills or slows the growth of healthy cells that grow and divide quickly. • Examples are cells that line your mouth and intestines and those that cause your hair to grow. • Damage to healthy cells may cause side effects, such as mouth sores, nausea, and hair loss. Side effects often get better or go away after you have finished chemotherapy. Cancer treatments can cause side effects—problems that occur when treatment affects healthy tissues or organs. Ask your health care team what side-effects you are likely to have. • Anemia • Appetite Loss • Bleeding and Bruising (Thrombocytopenia) • Constipation • Delirium • Diarrhea • Edema (Swelling) • Fatigue • Fertility Issues in Boys and Men • Fertility Issues in Girls and Women • Hair Loss (Alopecia) • Infection and Neutropenia • Lymphedema • Memory or Concentration Problems • Mouth and Throat Problems • Nausea and Vomiting • Nerve Problems (Peripheral Neuropathy) • Pain • Sexual Health Issues in Men • Sexual Health Issues in Women • Skin and Nail Changes • Sleep Problems • Urinary and Bladder Problems The most common side effect is fatigue, which is feeling exhausted and worn out. You can prepare for fatigue by: • Asking someone to drive you to and from chemotherapy • Planning time to rest on the day of and day after chemotherapy • Asking for help with meals and childcare on the day of and at least one day after chemotherapy *NIH NCI (14)*

Exercise Precautions or per MD Recommendations **CETI**	**CETI – Exercise Precautions:** • **IV Chemotherapy** – No exercise for 24 hours • **Hematocrit** less than 25% - No Exercise • **Hemoglobin** less than 24% 8g/dl due to anemia – No Exercise • **White blood** cell counts *less than 300 mm3* – No Exercise • **White blood** cell counts – Avoid public gyms unless blood cell count is *above 500 mm3* • **Platelet count** *less than 5000 mm3* – No resistance training – risk of internal bleeding/hemorrhage • **Platelet count** *less than 30,000 mm3* – Gentle Active Range of Motion • **Adriamycin use (doxorubicin)** – No exercise on the day of chemotherapy. May cause heart to bear irregularly for 24 hours, so only low impact exercise for 24- 48 post treatment – no more than 15-20 beats over resting heart rate.
References	Cancer.gov publication – Chemotherapy and *You* *https://www.cancer.gov/publications/patient-education/chemotherapy-and-you.pdf* CETI: Cancer Exercise Training Institute https*://www.thecancerspecialist.com/* Medical News Today – Types of Chemotherapy Drugs: *https://www.medicalnewstoday.com/articles/most-common-chemo-drugs#types-of-chemotherapy-drugs* NIH NCI (14) *Chemotherapy https://www.cancer.gov/about-cancer/treatment/types/chemotherapy* **List of Cancer Drugs and Side Effects A-Z** National Cancer Institute - *https://www.cancer.gov/about-cancer/treatment/drugs*

RADIATION
Information and pictures from *National Cancer Institute* unless otherwise specified

Quick Summary of Section

What is Radiation?

- Radiation therapy (also called radiotherapy) is a cancer treatment that uses high doses of radiation to kill cancer cells and shrink tumors.

How Radiation Works against Cancer:

- At high doses, radiation therapy kills cancer cells or slows their growth by damaging their DNA.

Types of Radiation Therapy:

- There are two main types of radiation therapy, external beam and internal.

How Often will I have External Beam Radiation Therapy?

- Most people have external beam radiation therapy once a day, five days a week, Monday through Friday.
- Treatment lasts anywhere from 2 to 10 weeks, depending on the type of cancer you have and the goal of your treatment.

Positioning for Breast Cancer:

- Must have adequate shoulder range of motion lying on your back
- Pillows and supports are used to keep your arm out of the treatment field.

Side Effects *(also see Side Effects)*:

- Fatigue
- Hair loss in the radiation field
- Swelling / Edema (*also see lymphedema*)
- Tenderness
- Skin changes

Late Effects:

- Late Effects are not common, but may include Inflammation in the lung or lymphedema
- In breast cancer, possibility of cancer in the opposite breast.

Treatment Areas And Possible Side Effects

- Other radiation therapy side effects you may have depend on the part of the body that is treated.

What is Radiation	Radiation therapy (also called radiotherapy) is a cancer treatment that uses high doses of radiation to kill cancer cells and shrink tumors. • At low doses, radiation is used in x-rays to see inside your body, as with x-rays of your teeth or broken bones. *NIH NCI (15)*

How Radiation Works against Cancer	• At high doses, radiation therapy kills cancer cells or slows their growth by damaging their DNA. • Cancer cells whose DNA is damaged beyond repair stop dividing or die. When the damaged cells die, they are broken down and removed by the body. • Radiation therapy does not kill cancer cells right away. It takes days or weeks of treatment before DNA is damaged enough for cancer cells to die. Then, cancer cells keep dying for weeks or months after radiation therapy ends. *NIH NCI (15)*
Types of Radiation Therapy	There are two main types of radiation therapy, external beam and internal. **External Beam Radiation Therapy** • External beam radiation therapy comes from a machine that aims radiation at your cancer. The machine is large and may be noisy. It does not touch you, but can move around you, sending radiation to a part of your body from many directions. • External beam radiation therapy is a local treatment, which means it treats a specific part of your body. For example, if you have cancer in your breast, you will have radiation only to your chest/breast, not to your whole body. **Internal Radiation Therapy** • Internal radiation therapy is a treatment in which a source of radiation is put inside your body. The radiation source can be solid or liquid. • Internal radiation therapy with a solid source is called brachytherapy. • In this type of treatment, seeds, ribbons, or capsules that contain a radiation source are placed in your body, in or near the tumor. • Like external beam radiation therapy, brachytherapy is a local treatment and treats only a specific part of your body. • With brachytherapy, the radiation source in your body will give off radiation for a while. *NIH NCI (15)*
How Often Will I Have External Beam Radiation Therapy?	• Most people have external beam radiation therapy once a day, five days a week, Monday through Friday. • Treatment lasts anywhere from 2 to 10 weeks, depending on the type of cancer you have and the goal of your treatment. • This span of time is called a course of treatment. Radiation therapy may also be given on other schedules. These schedules include: • Accelerated fractionation, which is treatment given in larger daily or weekly doses to reduce the number of weeks of treatment • Hyperfractionation, which is smaller doses of radiation given more than once a day • Hypofractionation, which is larger doses given once a day (or less often) to reduce the number of treatments Your doctor may prescribe one of these treatment schedules if he or she feels that it will work better for you. *NIH NCI (16)*

Positioning *(Breast Cancer)*	• Must have adequate shoulder range of motion lying on your back • Pillows and supports are used to keep your arm out of the treatment field.
Skin Changes	Radiation therapy can cause skin changes in your treatment area. Here are some common skin changes: • Redness. Your skin in the treatment area may look as if you have a mild to severe sunburn or tan. • Severe itching. The skin in your treatment area may itch very badly. It is important to avoid scratching, which can cause skin breakdown and infection. Skin breakdown is a problem that happens when the skin in the treatment area peels off faster than it can grow back. • Dry and peeling skin. The skin in your treatment area can get very dry. It may get so dry that it starts to peel, as if you have had a bad sunburn. If it peels off faster than it can grow back, you may develop sores or ulcers. • Moist reaction. The skin in your treatment area can become wet, sore, and infected. This problem is more common where you have skin folds, such as your buttocks, behind your ears, and under your breasts. It may also occur where your skin is very thin, such as your neck. • Swollen skin. The skin in your treatment area may be swollen and puffy. **Why they occur:** Radiation kills healthy skin cells in the treatment area. When people get radiation therapy almost every day, their skin cells do not have enough time to grow back between treatments. Skin changes can happen anywhere on the body that gets radiation. **How long they last:** • Skin changes may start a few weeks after you begin radiation therapy. Many of these changes go away a few weeks after treatment is over. But even after radiation therapy ends, some skin changes may remain. • Skin in the treatment area may always look darker and blotchy. • It may feel very dry or thicker than before. • You will always burn quickly and be sensitive to the sun.

Skin Changes
 	
Continued
	Ways to manage
	• Skin care. Take extra good care of your skin during radiation therapy. Be gentle and do not rub, scrub, or scratch in the treatment area. Use creams that your doctor or nurse suggests.
	• Do not put anything on your skin that is very hot or cold. Do not use heating pads, ice packs, or other hot or cold items on the treatment area.
	• Be gentle when you shower or take a bath. You can take a lukewarm shower every day. If you prefer to take a lukewarm bath, do so only every other day and don't soak for too long. Whether you take a shower or bath, make sure to use a mild soap. Dry yourself with a soft towel by patting, not rubbing, your skin. Be careful not to wash off the ink markings that you need for radiation therapy.
	• Use only those lotions and skin products that your doctor or nurse suggests. If you are using a prescribed cream for a skin problem or acne, tell your doctor or nurse before you begin radiation treatment.
	• Check with your doctor or nurse before using any of the following skin products: *Bubble bath * Cornstarch * Cream * Deodorant * Hair removers * Makeup * Oil *
	Ointment * Perfume * Powder * Soap * Sunscreen
	• Cool, humid places. Your skin may feel much better when you are in cool, humid places. You can make rooms more humid by putting a bowl of water on the radiator or using a humidifier. If you use a humidifier, be sure to follow the directions about cleaning it to prevent bacteria.
	• Soft fabrics. Wear clothes and use bed sheets that are made of very soft fabrics.
	• Do not wear clothes in your treatment area that are tight and do not breathe, such as girdles, body shapers, and pantyhose.
	• Protect your skin from the sun every day. The sun can burn you even on cloudy days or when you are outside for just a few minutes.
	     o Do not go to the beach or sunbathe.
	     o Wear a broad-brimmed hat, long-sleeved shirt, and long pants when you are outside.
	     o Talk with your doctor or nurse about sunscreen lotions. He or she may suggest that you use a sunscreen with an SPF of 30 or higher. You will need to protect your skin from the sun even after radiation therapy is over. Do not use tanning beds. Tanning beds expose you to the same harmful effects as the sun.
	• Adhesive tape. Do not put adhesive bandages or other types of sticky tape on your skin in the treatment area. Talk with your doctor or nurse about ways to bandage without tape.
	• Shaving. Ask your doctor or nurse if you can shave the treatment area. If you can shave use an electric razor, but do not use a pre-shave liquid.
	• Talk with your doctor or nurse. Some skin changes can be very serious. Your treatment team will check for skin changes each time you have radiation therapy. Make sure to report any skin changes that you notice.
	• Medicine. Medicines can help with some skin changes. These include lotions for dry or itchy skin, antibiotics to treat infection, and drugs to reduce swelling or itching.
	NIH NCI (16)

Side Effects (Also see *Side Effects* and *Late Side Effects*)	• Fatigue • Hair loss in the radiation field • Swelling / Edema (also see lymphedema) • Tenderness • Skin changes *(see below)*

Late Effects (Also see *Side Effects* and *Late Side Effects*)	Late Effects are not common, but may include: • Inflammation of the lung after radiation therapy to the breast, especially when chemotherapy is given at the same time. • Arm lymphedema, especially when radiation therapy is given after lymph node dissection. • In women younger than 45 years who receive radiation therapy to the chest wall after mastectomy, there may be a higher risk of developing breast cancer in the other breast. *NIH NCI (15)*
Treatment Areas and Possible Side Effects	Other radiation therapy side effects you may have depend on the part of the body that is treated. See more information in the *Side Effects* section. Treatment areas and possible side effects: **Breast** • Fatigue • Hair loss • Skin changes • Swelling (edema) • Tenderness **Chest** • Fatigue • Hair loss • Skin changes • Throat problems, such as trouble swallowing • Cough • Shortness of breath **Head and Neck** • Fatigue • Hair loss • Mouth problems • Skin changes • Taste changes • Throat problems, such as trouble swallowing • Less active thyroid gland
References	NCI – National Cancer Institute – Radiation Therapy Side Effects: *https://www.cancer.gov/about-cancer/treatment/types/radiation-therapy/side-effects* NIH NCI (15) Radiation *https://www.cancer.gov/about-cancer/treatment/types/radiation-therapy* *NIH NCI (16)* Radiation Therapy and You. *https://www.cancer.gov/publications/patient- education/radiationttherapy.pdf*

HORMONE THERAPY
Information and pictures from *National Cancer Institute* unless otherwise specified

Quick Summary of Section

Hormone Therapy:

Hormone therapy is a cancer treatment that removes hormones or blocks their action and stops cancer cells from growing. Hormones are substances made by glands in the body and circulated in the bloodstream.

Breast Cancer & Drugs Used *(Pink Ribbon Program®)*

- Tamoxifen
- Arimidex
- Herceptin

Hormone Therapy	Hormone therapy is a cancer treatment that removes hormones or blocks their action and stops cancer cells from growing. Hormones are substances made by glands in the body and circulated in the bloodstream.

- Some hormones can cause certain cancers to grow. If tests show that the cancer cells have places where hormones can attach (receptors), drugs, surgery, or radiation therapy is used to reduce the production of hormones or block them from working.

Hormone therapy is used to

- Treat cancer. Hormone therapy can lessen the chance that cancer will return or stop or slow its growth.
- Ease cancer symptoms. Hormone therapy may be used to reduce or prevent symptoms in men with prostate cancer who are not able to have surgery or radiation therapy.

Types of hormone therapy

- Hormone therapy falls into two broad groups, those that block the body's ability to produce hormones and those that interfere with how hormones behave in the body.

Who receives hormone therapy?

- Hormone therapy is used to treat prostate and breast cancers that use hormones to grow. Hormone therapy is most often used along with other cancer treatments.
- The types of treatment that you need depend on the type of cancer, if it has spread and how far, if it uses hormones to grow, and if you have other health problems.

How hormone therapy is used with other cancer treatments

- Range of scores for the Decipher test showing low, intermediate, and high risk of prostate cancer metastasis
- Genetic Test May Help Predict Whether Prostate Cancer Will Spread
- The test may help determine whether to treat with hormone therapy.

Hormone Therapy *Continued*	**When used with other treatments, hormone therapy can** • Make a tumor smaller before surgery or radiation therapy. This is called neoadjuvant therapy. • Lower the risk that cancer will come back after the main treatment. This is called adjuvant therapy. • Destroy cancer cells that have returned or spread to other parts of your body. *(Hormone Therapy to Treat Cancer – NCI)*
Hormone Therapy **Breast Cancer** See also References *National Cancer Institute* **List of Cancer Drugs and Side Effects A-Z**	• The hormone estrogen, which makes some breast cancers grow, is made mainly by the ovaries. Treatment to stop the ovaries from making estrogen is called ovarian ablation. • Hormone therapy with tamoxifen is often given to patients with early localized breast cancer that can be removed by surgery and those with metastatic breast cancer (cancer that has spread to other parts of the body). Hormone therapy with tamoxifen or estrogens can act on cells all over the body and may increase the chance of developing endometrial cancer. Women taking tamoxifen should have a pelvic exam every year to look for any signs of cancer. Any vaginal bleeding, other than menstrual bleeding, should be reported to a doctor as soon as possible. • Hormone therapy with a luteinizing hormone-releasing hormone (LHRH) agonist is given to some premenopausal women who have just been diagnosed with hormone receptor positive breast cancer. LHRH agonists decrease the body's estrogen and progesterone. • Hormone therapy with an aromatase inhibitor is given to some postmenopausal women who have hormone receptor positive breast cancer. Aromatase inhibitors decrease the body's estrogen by blocking an enzyme called aromatase from turning androgen into estrogen. Anastrozole, letrozole, and exemestane are types of aromatase inhibitors. • For the treatment of early localized breast cancer that can be removed by surgery, certain aromatase inhibitors may be used as adjuvant therapy instead of tamoxifen or after 2 to 3 years of tamoxifen use. For the treatment of metastatic breast cancer, aromatase inhibitors are being tested in clinical trials to compare them to hormone therapy with tamoxifen. • In women with hormone receptor positive breast cancer, at least 5 years of adjuvant hormone therapy reduces the risk that the cancer will recur (come back). • Other types of hormone therapy include megestrol acetate or anti-estrogen therapy such as fulvestrant. *NIH NCI (17)*

Tamoxifen **Arimidex** **Herceptin** *Pink Ribbon* *Program®*	**Tamoxifen** was approved for treating breast cancer more than two decades ago. The standard treatment used to last 5 years, but researchers have found that taking tamoxifen for 10 years produced more reductions in breast cancer recurrence and death than taking tamoxifen for 5 years. • Tamoxifen: slows cancer growth by blocking estrogen-positive receptor sites. Some breast cancers are spread through estrogen. These are classified as estrogen-positive cancers. • By blocking the estrogen receptors, the drug slows or stops the growth of cancer cells that are already present in the body. Needs to be taken for 5 years after surgery/treatment. **Side effects:** • Menopause • Fatigue • Weight Gain • Hot Flashes • Depression • Osteoporosis due to menopause • Endometrial Cancer (cancer of the lining of the uterus) • Uterine sarcoma (cancer of the connective tissue of the uterus • Pulmonary embolism (blood clot in the lung) • Deep vein thrombosis (blood clot in a major vein) **Arimidex** is an aromatase inhibitor, which reduces the body's production of estrogen. An aromatase inhibitor is a drug that blocks aromatase, an enzyme needed to make estrogen. • Prescribed for post-menopausal women only • Prescribed after Tamoxifen • Has fewer side effects • Joint pain is a significant side effect **Herceptin:** Some breast cancers make excessive amounts of a protein called human growth factor receptor 2 (HER2), which helps breast cancer cells grow and survive. • Trastuzumab is a biological class of drugs known as monoclonal antibodies. It blocks HER2 and cause the cancer cells to die. • For women with HER2-positive breast cancers, the drug Herceptin has been shown to dramatically reduce the risk of recurrence. • It has now become standard treatment to give Herceptin along with adjuvant (after-surgery) chemotherapy in those with metastatic breast cancer. • Herceptin has far fewer immediate side effects than chemotherapy -- for example, there is usually no nausea or hair loss. • However, it causes muscle weakness and there is a small but real risk of heart damage (cardiac dysfunction) and possible lung damage. • Some other adverse effects have been reported as anaphylaxis and severe dyspnea, allergic or hypersensitivity reactions, hematological toxicity hepatic and renal toxicity, diarrhea and an increased risk of infections. *Pink Ribbon Program®*

References	NIH NCI (17) *https://www.cancer.gov/types/breast/patient/breast-treatment-pdq#_185*
	National Cancer Institute – NCI - Hormone Therapy to Treat Cancer: *https://www.cancer.gov/about- cancer/treatment/types/hormone-therapy*
	National Cancer Institute – NCI - Hormone Therapy for Prostate Cancer: *https://www.cancer.gov/types/prostate/prostate-hormone-therapy-fact-sheet*
	Pink Ribbon Program® *https://www.pinkribbonprogram.com/*
	List of Cancer Drugs and Side Effects A-Z National Cancer Institute - *https://www.cancer.gov/about-cancer/treatment/drugs*

TARGETED THERAPY
Information and pictures from *National Cancer Institute* unless otherwise specified

Quick Summary of Section

Targeted Therapy:
- Targeted therapy is a type of treatment that uses drugs or other substances to identify and attack specific cancer cells without harming normal cells.

Drugs Used in Targeted Therapy *(Breast Cancer)*:
- Monoclonal antibody therapy
- Tyrosine kinase inhibitors are targeted therapy drugs that block signals needed for tumors to grow.
- Cyclin-dependent kinase inhibitors are targeted therapy drugs that block proteins called cyclin-dependent kinases, which cause the growth of cancer cells.

Targeted Therapy	**What is targeted therapy?**
	Targeted therapy is a type of cancer treatment that targets proteins that control how cancer cells grow, divide, and spread. It is the foundation of precision medicine. As researchers learn more about the DNA changes and proteins that drive cancer, they are better able to design treatments that target these proteins. Targeted therapy is a type of treatment that uses drugs or other substances to identify and attack specific cancer cells without harming normal cells.
	  • Monoclonal antibodies, tyrosine kinase inhibitors, cyclin-dependent kinase inhibitors, mammalian target of rapamycin (mTOR) inhibitors, and PARP inhibitors are types of targeted therapies used in the treatment of breast cancer.
	  • Monoclonal antibody therapy is a cancer treatment that uses antibodies made in the laboratory, from a single type of immune system cell.
	
	What are the types of targeted therapy?
	  • Most targeted therapies are either small-molecule drugs or monoclonal antibodies.
	  • Small-molecule drugs are small enough to enter cells easily, so they are used for targets that are inside cells.
	  • Monoclonal antibodies, also known as therapeutic antibodies, are proteins produced in the lab. These proteins are designed to attach to specific targets found on cancer cells. Some monoclonal antibodies mark cancer cells so that they will be better seen and destroyed by the immune system. Other monoclonal antibodies directly stop cancer cells from growing or cause them to self-destruct. Still others carry toxins to cancer cells.
	
	Who is treated with targeted therapy?
	  • For some types of cancer, most patients with that cancer will have a target for a certain drug, so they can be treated with that drug. Most of the time, the tumor will need to be tested to see if it contains targets for which we have drugs.
	  • Testing your cancer for targets that could help you and your doctor choose your treatment is called biomarker testing.
	  • You may need to have a biopsy for biomarker testing. A biopsy is a procedure in which your doctor removes a piece of the tumor for testing. There are some risks to having a biopsy. These risks vary depending on the size of the tumor and where it is located. Your doctor will explain the risks of having a biopsy for your type of tumor.

Targeted Therapy *Continued*	**How does targeted therapy work against cancer?** Most types of targeted therapy help treat cancer by interfering with specific proteins that help tumors grow and spread throughout the body. They treat cancer in many ways. They can: • Help the immune system destroy cancer cells. One reason that cancer cells thrive is because they can hide from your immune system. Certain targeted therapies can mark cancer cells, so it is easier for the immune system to find and destroy them. Other targeted therapies help boost your immune system to work better against cancer. • Stop cancer cells from growing. Healthy cells in your body usually divide to make new cells only when they receive strong signals to do so. These signals bind to proteins on the cell surface, telling the cells to divide. This process helps new cells form only as your body needs them. Some cancer cells have changes in the proteins on their surface that tell them to divide whether or not signals are present. Some targeted therapies interfere with these proteins, preventing them from telling the cells to divide. This process helps slow cancer's uncontrolled growth. • Stop signals that help form blood vessels. Tumors need to form new blood vessels to grow beyond a certain size. In a process called angiogenesis, these new blood vessels form in response to signals from the tumor. Some targeted therapies called angiogenesis inhibitors are designed to interfere with these signals to prevent a blood supply from forming. Without a blood supply, tumors stay small. Or, if a tumor already has a blood supply, these treatments can cause blood vessels to die, which causes the tumor to shrink. Learn more about Angiogenesis Inhibitors. • Deliver cell-killing substances to cancer cells. Some monoclonal antibodies are combined with toxins, chemotherapy drugs, and radiation. Once these monoclonal antibodies attach to targets on the surface of cancer cells, the cells take up the cell-killing substances, causing them to die. Cells that don't have the target will not be harmed. • Cause cancer cell death. Healthy cells die in an orderly manner when they become damaged or are no longer needed, but cancer cells have ways of avoiding this dying process. Some targeted therapies can cause cancer cells to go through this process of cell death. • Starve cancer of the hormones it needs to grow. Some breast and prostate cancers require certain hormones to grow. Hormone therapies are a type of targeted therapy that can work in two ways. Some hormone therapies prevent your body from making specific hormones. Others prevent the hormones from acting on your cells, including cancer cells. **Are there drawbacks to targeted therapy?** • Targeted therapy does have some drawbacks. These include: • Cancer cells can become resistant to targeted therapy. For this reason, they may work best when used with other types of targeted therapy or with other cancer treatments, such as chemotherapy and radiation. • Drugs for some targets are hard to develop. Reasons include the target's structure, the target's function in the cell, or both.

Targeted Therapy *Continued*	**What are the side effects of targeted therapy?** • Targeted therapy can cause side effects. The side effects you may have depend on the type of targeted therapy you receive and how your body reacts to the therapy. • The most common side effects of targeted therapy include diarrhea and liver problems. Other side effects might include problems with blood clotting and wound healing, high blood pressure, fatigue, mouth sores, nail changes, the loss of hair color, and skin problems. Skin problems might include rash or dry skin. Very rarely, a hole might form through the wall of the esophagus, stomach, small intestine, large bowel, rectum, or gallbladder. • There are medicines for many of these side effects. These medicines may prevent the side effects from happening or treat them once they occur. • Most side effects of targeted therapy go away after treatment ends. *(Targeted Therapy to Treat Cancer)*

Drugs used in Targeted Therapy For Breast Cancer
 	
See also References
National Cancer Institute
List of Cancer Drugs and Side Effects A-Z
	Types of monoclonal antibody therapy include the following:
	
	• ***Trastuzumab*** is a monoclonal antibody that blocks the effects of the growth factor protein HER2, which sends growth signals to breast cancer cells. It may be used with other therapies to treat HER2 positive breast cancer.
	
	• ***Pertuzumab*** is a monoclonal antibody that may be combined with trastuzumab and chemotherapy to treat breast cancer. It may be used to treat certain patients with HER2 positive breast cancer that has metastasized (spread to other parts of the body). It may also be used as neoadjuvant therapy in certain patients with early stage HER2 positive breast cancer.
	
	• ***Ado-trastuzumab emtansine*** is a monoclonal antibody linked to an anticancer drug. This is called an antibody-drug conjugate. It is used to treat HER2 positive breast cancer that has spread to other parts of the body or recurred (come back).
	
	• ***Sacituzumab govitecan*** is a monoclonal antibody that carries an anticancer drug to the tumor. This is called an antibody-drug conjugate. It is being studied to treat women with triple-negative breast cancer who have received at least two previous chemotherapy regimens.
	
	Tyrosine kinase inhibitors are targeted therapy drugs that block signals needed for tumors to grow. Tyrosine kinase inhibitors may be used with other anticancer drugs as adjuvant therapy. Tyrosine kinase inhibitors include the following:
	
	• **Lapatinib** is a tyrosine kinase inhibitor that blocks the effects of the HER2 protein and other proteins inside tumor cells. It may be used with other drugs to treat patients with HER2 positive breast cancer that has progressed after treatment with trastuzumab.
	
	• **Neratinib** is a tyrosine kinase inhibitor that blocks the effects of the HER2 protein and other proteins inside tumor cells. It may be used to treat patients with early stage HER2 positive breast cancer after treatment with trastuzumab.
	
	Cyclin-dependent kinase inhibitors are targeted therapy drugs that block proteins called cyclin- dependent kinases, which cause the growth of cancer cells. Cyclin-dependent kinase inhibitors include the following:
	
	• **Palbociclib** is a cyclin-dependent kinase inhibitor used with the drug letrozole to treat breast cancer that is estrogen receptor positive and HER2 negative and has spread to other parts of the body.
	    ○ It is used in postmenopausal women whose cancer has not been treated with hormone therapy.
	    ○ Palbociclib may also be used with fulvestrant in women whose disease has gotten worse after treatment with hormone therapy.

Drugs used in Targeted Therapy For Breast Cancer
 	
Continued
	• ***Ribociclib** is a cyclin-dependent kinase inhibitor* used with letrozole to treat breast cancer that is hormone receptor positive and HER2 negative and has come back or spread to other parts of the body.
	   ○ It is used in postmenopausal women whose cancer has not been treated with hormone therapy.
	   ○ It is also used with fulvestrant in postmenopausal women with hormone receptor positive and HER2 negative breast cancer that has spread to other parts of the body or has recurred.
	   ○ It is also used in premenopausal women with hormone receptor positive and HER2 negative breast cancer that has spread to other parts of the body or has recurred..
	• ***Abemaciclib** is a cyclin-dependent kinase inhibitor* used to treat hormone receptor positive and HER2 negative breast cancer that is advanced or has spread to other parts of the body. It may be used alone or with other drugs to treat breast cancer that has gotten worse after other treatment.
	• ***Alpelisib** is a cyclin-dependent kinase inhibitor* used with the drug fulvestrant to treat hormone receptor positive and HER2 negative breast cancer that has a certain gene change and is advanced or has spread to other parts of the body.
	   ○ It is used in postmenopausal women whose breast cancer has gotten worse during or after treatment with hormone therapy.
	
	Mammalian target of rapamycin (mTOR) inhibitors block a protein called mTOR, which may keep cancer cells from growing and prevent the growth of new blood vessels that tumors need to grow. mTOR inhibitors include the following:
	• **Everolimus** is an mTOR inhibitor used in postmenopausal women with advanced hormone receptor positive breast cancer that is also HER2 negative and has not gotten better with other treatment.
	
	PARP inhibitors are a type of targeted therapy that block DNA repair and may cause cancer cells to die. PARP inhibitors include the following:
	• **Olaparib** is a PARP inhibitor used to treat patients with mutations in the BRCA1 or BRCA2 gene and HER2 negative breast cancer that has spread to other parts of the body. PARP inhibitor therapy is being studied for the treatment of patients with triple-negative breast cancer.
	• **Talazoparib** is a PARP inhibitor used to treat patients with mutations in the BRCA1 or BRCA2 genes and HER2 negative breast cancer that is locally advanced or has spread to other parts of the body.
	NIH NCI (17)

References	*NIH NCI (17) https://www.cancer.gov/types/breast/patient/breast-treatment-pdq#_185* National Cancer Institute – NCI - Targeted Therapy to Treat Cancer: *https://www.cancer.gov/about- cancer/treatment/types/targeted-therapies* **List of Cancer Drugs and Side Effects A-Z** National Cancer Institute - *https://www.cancer.gov/about-cancer/treatment/drugs*

IMMUNOTHERAPY

Information and pictures from *National Cancer Institute* unless otherwise specified

Quick Summary of Section

Immunotherapy:

Immunotherapy is a type of treatment that helps your immune system fight against cancer.

- The immune system helps your body fight infections and other diseases. It is made up of white blood cells and organs and tissues of the lymph system.

Types:

Several types of immunotherapies are used to treat cancer.

- These treatments can either help the immune system attack the cancer directly or stimulate the immune system in a more general way.

Side Effects:

- The most common side effects are skin reactions at the needle site.
- You may also have flu-like symptoms.

Description	Immunotherapy is a type of cancer treatment that helps your immune system fight cancer. The immune system helps your body fight infections and other diseases. It is made up of white blood cells and organs and tissues of the lymph system. • Immunotherapy is a type of biological therapy. Biological therapy is a type of treatment that uses substances made from living organisms to treat cancer. • One reason that cancer cells thrive is because they are able to hide from your immune system. Certain immunotherapies can mark cancer cells so it is easier for the immune system to find and destroy them. • Other immunotherapies boost your immune system to work better against cancer. Different forms of immunotherapy may be given in different ways. These include: • **Intravenous (IV)** - The immunotherapy goes directly into a vein. • **Oral** - The immunotherapy comes in pills or capsules that you swallow. • **Topical** - The immunotherapy comes in a cream that you rub onto your skin. This type of immunotherapy can be used for very early skin cancer. • **Intravesical** - The immunotherapy goes directly into the bladder.
Types	Several types of immunotherapies are used to treat cancer. These treatments can either help the immune system attack the cancer directly or stimulate the immune system in a more general way. Types of immunotherapies that help the immune system act directly against the cancer include: • **Checkpoint inhibitors**, which are drugs that help the immune system respond more strongly to a tumor. These drugs work by releasing "brakes" that keep T cells (a type of white blood cell and part of the immune system) from killing cancer cells. These drugs do not target the tumor directly. Instead, they interfere with the ability of cancer cells to avoid immune system attack. • **Adoptive cell transfer**, which is a treatment that attempts to boost the natural ability of your T cells to fight cancer. In this treatment, T cells are taken from your tumor. Then those that are most active against your cancer are grown in large batches in the lab.

Types *Continued*	• **Monoclonal antibodies,** also known as therapeutic antibodies, which are immune system proteins created in the lab. These antibodies are designed to attach to specific targets found on cancer cells. o Some monoclonal antibodies mark cancer cells so that they will be better seen and destroyed by the immune system. o Other monoclonal antibodies directly stop cancer cells from growing or cause them to self-destruct. o Still others carry toxins to cancer cells. o Because therapeutic monoclonal antibodies recognize specific proteins on cancer cells, they are also considered *targeted* therapies. • *Treatment vaccines,* which work against cancer by boosting your immune system's response to cancer cells. Treatment vaccines are different from the ones that help prevent disease. Types of immunotherapies that enhance the body's immune response to fight the cancer include: • **Cytokines,** which are proteins made by your body's cells. They play important roles in the body's normal immune responses and also in the immune system's ability to respond to cancer. The two main types of cytokines used to treat cancer are called interferons and interleukins. • **BCG,** which stands for Bacillus Calmette-Guérin, is an immunotherapy that is used to treat bladder cancer. It is a weakened form of the bacteria that causes tuberculosis. When inserted directly into the bladder with a catheter, BCG causes an immune response against cancer cells.
Side Effects	The most common side effects are skin reactions at the needle site. These side effects include: • Pain, Soreness • Swelling • Redness, Itchiness, Rash You may have flu-like symptoms, which include: • Fever, Chills • Weakness, Dizziness • Nausea or vomiting • Muscle or joint aches • Fatigue • Headache • Trouble breathing • Low or high blood pressure Other side effects might include: • Swelling and weight gain from retaining fluid • Heart palpitations • Sinus congestion • Diarrhea • Risk of infection • *White blood cell counts – Avoid public gyms unless blood cell count is above 500 mm3* (CETI: Cancer Exercise Training Institute *https: //www.thecancerspecialist.com/*) *Immunotherapy rarely causes severe or even fatal allergic reactions.*

STEM CELL THERAPY / Transplant
Information and pictures from *National Cancer Institute* unless otherwise specified

Quick Summary of Section

Stem Cell Therapy / Transplant

- Stem cell transplants are procedures that restore blood-forming stem cells in people who have had theirs destroyed by the high doses of chemotherapy or radiation therapy that are used to treat certain cancers.

Types:

- The blood-forming stem cells that are used in transplants can come from the bone marrow, bloodstream, or umbilical cord.

How Stem Cell Transplants Work Against Cancer:

- Stem cell transplants do not usually work against cancer directly. Instead, they help you recover your body's ability to produce stem cells after treatment with very high doses of radiation therapy, chemotherapy, or both.

Side Effects:

- The high doses of cancer treatment that you have before a stem cell transplant can cause problems such as bleeding and an increased risk of infection.

Description	Stem cell transplants are procedures that restore blood-forming stem cells in people who have had theirs destroyed by the high doses of chemotherapy or radiation therapy that are used to treat certain cancers. Blood-forming stem cells are important because they grow into different types of blood cells. The main types of blood cells are: • white blood cells, which are part of your immune system and help your body fight infection • red blood cells, which carry oxygen throughout your body • platelets, which help the blood clot o You need all three types of blood cells to be healthy.
Types	In a stem cell transplant, you receive healthy blood-forming stem cells through a needle in your vein. Once they enter your bloodstream, the stem cells travel to the bone marrow, where they take the place of the cells that were destroyed by treatment. The blood-forming stem cells that are used in transplants can come from the bone marrow, bloodstream, or umbilical cord. Transplants can be: • **Autologous**, which means the stem cells come from you, the patient • **Allogeneic**, which means the stem cells come from someone else. The donor may be a blood relative but can also be someone who is not related. • **Syngeneic**, which means the stem cells come from your identical twin, if you have one To reduce possible side effects and improve the chances that an allogeneic transplant will work, the donor's blood-forming stem cells must match yours in certain ways.

How Stem Cell Transplants Work Against Cancer	Stem cell transplants do not usually work against cancer directly. Instead, they help you recover your body's ability to produce stem cells after treatment with very high doses of radiation therapy, chemotherapy, or both.. • However, in multiple myeloma and some types of leukemia, the stem cell transplant may work against cancer directly. This happens because of an effect called graft-versus-tumor that can occur after allogeneic transplants. • *Graft-versus-tumor* occurs when white blood cells from your donor (the graft) attack any cancer cells that remain in your body (the tumor) after high-dose treatments. This effect improves the success of the treatments. **Who receives stem cell transplants?** Stem cell transplants are most often used to help people with leukemia and lymphoma. • They may also be used for neuroblastoma and multiple myeloma.
Side Effects	The high doses of cancer treatment that you have before a stem cell transplant can cause problems such as bleeding and an increased risk of infection. Talk with your doctor or nurse about other side effects that you might have and how serious they might be. If you have an allogeneic transplant, you might develop a serious problem called graft-versus-host disease. • **Graft-versus-host disease** can occur when white blood cells from your donor (the graft) recognize cells in your body (the host) as foreign and attack them. • This problem can cause damage to your skin, liver, intestines, and many other organs. • It can occur a few weeks after the transplant or much later. • Graft-versus-host disease can be treated with steroids or other drugs that suppress your immune system. The closer your donor's blood-forming stem cells match yours, the less likely you are to have graft-versus-host disease. • Your doctor may also try to prevent it by giving you drugs to suppress your immune system.
References	National Cancer Institute - NCI - Stem Cell Transplants in Cancer Treatment: *https://www.cancer.gov/about-cancer/treatment/types/stem-cell-transplant*

OTHER THERAPIES / TREATMENTS
Information and pictures from National Cancer Institute unless otherwise specified

Ablation therapy	Ablation therapy removes or destroys tissue. Different types of ablation therapy are used for liver cancer: **Radiofrequency ablation:** - The use of special needles that are inserted directly through the skin or through an incision in the abdomen to reach the tumor. High-energy radio waves heat the needles and tumor which kills cancer cells. **Microwave therapy:** - A type of treatment in which the tumor is exposed to high temperatures created by microwaves. This can damage and kill cancer cells or make them more sensitive to the effects of radiation and certain anticancer drugs. **Percutaneous ethanol injection:** - A cancer treatment in which a small needle is used to inject ethanol (pure alcohol) directly into a tumor to kill cancer cells. Several treatments may be needed. Usually local anesthesia is used, but if the patient has many tumors in the liver, general anesthesia may be used. **Cryoablation:** - A treatment that uses an instrument to freeze and destroy cancer cells. This type of treatment is also called cryotherapy and cryosurgery. The doctor may use ultrasound to guide the instrument. **Electroporation therapy:** - A treatment that sends electrical pulses through an electrode placed in a tumor to kill cancer cells. Electroporation therapy is being studied in clinical trials.
Active surveillance	Active surveillance is closely following a patient's condition without giving any treatment unless there are changes in test results. It is used to find early signs that the condition is getting worse. • In active surveillance, patients are given certain exams and tests, including digital rectal exam, PSA test, transrectal ultrasound, and transrectal needle biopsy, to check if the cancer is growing. • When the cancer begins to grow, treatment is given to cure the cancer.
Biologic therapy	Biologic therapy is a treatment that uses the patient's immune system to fight cancer. Substances made by the body or made in a laboratory are used to boost, direct, or restore the body's natural defenses against cancer. This type of cancer treatment is also called biotherapy or immunotherapy. The following types of biologic therapy are being used or studied in the treatment of renal cell cancer: • **Nivolumab:** Nivolumab is a monoclonal antibody that boosts the body's immune response against renal cell cancer cells. • **Interferon:** Interferon affects the division of cancer cells and can slow tumor growth. Interleukin-2 (IL-2): IL-2 boosts the growth and activity of many immune cells, especially lymphocytes (a type of white blood cell)
Bisphosphonate therapy	Bisphosphonate drugs, such as clodronate or zoledronate, reduce bone disease when cancer has spread to the bone. • Men who are treated with antiandrogen therapy or orchiectomy are at an increased risk of bone loss. In these men, bisphosphonate drugs lessen the risk of bone fracture (breaks). • The use of bisphosphonate drugs to prevent or slow the growth of bone metastases is being studied in clinical trials.
Chemoprevention	Chemoprevention is the use of drugs, vitamins, or other substances to reduce the risk of cancer or to reduce the risk cancer will recur (come back).

Chimeric antigen receptor (CAR) T-cell therapy	CAR T-cell therapy is a type of immunotherapy that changes the patient's T cells (a type of immune system cell) so they will attack certain proteins on the surface of cancer cells. T cells are taken from the patient and special receptors are added to their surface in the laboratory. The changed cells are called chimeric antigen receptor (CAR) T cells. • The CAR T cells are grown in the laboratory and given to the patient by infusion. The CAR T cells multiply in the patient's blood and attack cancer cells. CAR T-cell therapy is being studied in the treatment of adult ALL that has recurred (come back).
Electrocautery	Electrocautery is a treatment that uses a probe or needle heated by an electric current to destroy abnormal tissue. For tumors in the airways, electrocautery is done through an endoscope.
Embolization therapy **AKA** **Chemoembolization**	Embolization therapy is the use of substances to block or decrease the flow of blood through the hepatic artery to the tumor. When the tumor does not get the oxygen and nutrients it needs, it will not continue to grow. Embolization therapy is used for patients who cannot have surgery to remove the tumor or ablation therapy and whose tumor has not spread outside the liver. *The liver receives blood from the hepatic portal vein and the hepatic artery. Blood that comes into the liver from the hepatic portal vein usually goes to the healthy liver tissue. Blood that comes from the hepatic artery usually goes to the tumor. When the hepatic artery is blocked during embolization therapy, the healthy liver tissue continues to receive blood from the hepatic portal vein.* There are two main types of embolization therapy: • **Transarterial embolization (TAE):** A small incision (cut) is made in the inner thigh and a catheter (thin, flexible tube) is inserted and threaded up into the hepatic artery. Once the catheter is in place, a substance that blocks the hepatic artery and stops blood flow to the tumor is injected. • **Transarterial chemoembolization (TACE):** This procedure is like TAE except an anticancer drug is also given. The procedure can be done by attaching the anticancer drug to small beads that are injected into the hepatic artery or by injecting the anticancer drug through the catheter into the hepatic artery and then injecting the substance to block the hepatic artery. Most of the anticancer drug is trapped near the tumor and only a small amount of the drug reaches other parts of the body. This type of treatment is also called *chemoembolization.*
Endoscopic stent placement	An endoscope is a thin, tube-like instrument used to look at tissues inside the body. An endoscope has a light and a lens for viewing and may be used to place a stent in a body structure to keep the structure open. An endoscopic stent can be used to open an airway blocked by abnormal tissue.
High-intensity–focused ultrasound therapy	High-intensity–focused ultrasound therapy is a treatment that uses ultrasound (high-energy sound waves) to destroy cancer cells. To treat prostate cancer, an endorectal probe is used to make sound waves.
Monoclonal antibody therapy	Monoclonal antibody therapy is a cancer treatment that uses antibodies made in the laboratory, from a single type of immune system cell. These antibodies can identify substances on cancer cells or normal substances that may help cancer cells grow. • The antibodies attach to the substances and kill the cancer cells, block their growth, or keep them from spreading. Monoclonal antibodies are given by infusion. They may be used alone or to carry drugs, toxins, or radioactive material directly to cancer cells.

Proton beam radiation therapy	Proton beam radiation therapy is a type of high-energy, external radiation therapy that targets tumors with streams of protons (small, positively charged particles). • This type of radiation therapy is being studied in the treatment of prostate cancer.
Radioactive iodine	A radioactive form of iodine, often used for imaging tests or to treat an overactive thyroid, thyroid cancer, and certain other cancers. For imaging tests, the patient takes a small dose of radioactive iodine that collects in thyroid cells and certain kinds of tumors and can be detected by a scanner. • To treat thyroid cancer, the patient takes a large dose of radioactive iodine, which kills thyroid cells. • Radioactive iodine is also used in internal radiation therapy for prostate cancer, intraocular (eye) melanoma, and carcinoid tumors. • Radioactive iodine is given by mouth as a liquid or in capsules, by infusion, or sealed in seeds, which are placed in or near the tumor to kill cancer cells.
Radiofrequency ablation	Radiofrequency ablation is the use of a special probe with tiny electrodes that kill cancer cells. • Sometimes the probe is inserted directly through the skin and only local anesthesia is needed. • In other cases, the probe is inserted through an incision in the abdomen. • This is done in the hospital with general anesthesia.
Radiopharmaceutical therapy	Radiopharmaceutical therapy uses a radioactive substance to treat cancer. Radiopharmaceutical therapy includes the following: • Alpha emitter radiation therapy uses a radioactive substance to treat prostate cancer that has spread to the bone. • A radioactive substance called radium-223 is injected into a vein and travels through the bloodstream. The radium-223 collects in areas of bone with cancer and kills the cancer cells.
Radiosensitizers	Radiosensitizers are substances that make tumor cells easier to kill with radiation therapy. The combination of chemotherapy and radiation therapy given with a radiosensitizer is being studied in the treatment of non-small cell lung cancer.
Steroid therapy	Steroids are hormones made naturally in the body by the adrenal glands and by reproductive organs. Some types of steroids are made in a laboratory. • Certain steroid drugs have been found to help chemotherapy work better and help stop the growth of cancer cells. • Steroids can also help the lungs of the fetus develop faster than normal. This is important when delivery is induced early.
Vaccine therapy	Vaccine therapy uses a substance or group of substances meant to cause the immune system to respond to a tumor and kill it. Vaccine therapy is being studied in the treatment of stage III melanoma that can be removed by surgery.
Watchful waiting	Watchful waiting is closely monitoring a patient's condition without giving any treatment until signs or symptoms appear or change. This is also called observation. • During this time, problems caused by the disease, such as infection, are treated.

SIDE EFFECTS and LATE SIDE EFFECTS
Information and pictures from *National Cancer Institute* unless otherwise specified

Quick Summary of Section	SIDE EFFECTS
NIH (NCI) *https://www.cancer.gov/about-cancer/treatment/side-effects*	<ul><li>Anemia</li><li>Appetite Loss</li><li>Bleeding & Bruising (Thrombocytopenia)</li><li>Constipation</li><li>Delirium</li><li>Diarrhea</li><li>Edema (Swelling)</li><li>Fatigue</li><li>Fertility Issues in Girls and Women</li><li>Hair Loss (Alopecia)</li><li>Infection and Neutropenia</li><li>Memory or Concentration Issues</li><li>Mouth and Throat Problems</li><li>Nausea and Vomiting</li><li>Nerve Problems (Peripheral Neuropathy)</li><li>Pain</li><li>Skin and Nail Changes</li><li>Sleep Problems</li><li>Urinary and Bladder Problems</li><li>Bone Loss</li><li>Brain Changes</li></ul> **LATE EFFECTS** <ul><li>Eye Problems</li><li>Hearing Loss</li><li>Heart Problems</li><li>Hot Flashes and Night Sweats</li><li>Joint Changes</li><li>Lung Problems</li><li>Mouth Changes</li><li>Joint Changes</li></ul>

SIDE EFFECT AND POSSIBLE CAUSE	DESCRIPTION	WAYS TO MANAGE
Anemia *Chemotherapy *Radiation therapy	• Anemia is a condition that can make you feel very tired, short of breath, and lightheaded. • Other signs of anemia may include feeling dizzy or faint, headaches, a fast heartbeat, and/or pale skin. • Cancer treatments, such as chemotherapy and radiation therapy can cause anemia. • When you are anemic, your body does not have enough red blood cells. Red blood cells are the cells that that carry oxygen from the lungs throughout your body to help it work properly. • You will have blood tests to check for anemia. Treatment for anemia is also based on your symptoms and on what is causing the anemia.	**Save your energy and ask for help.** Choose the most important things to do each day. When people offer to help, let them do so. They can take you to the doctor, make meals, or do other things you are too tired to do. **Balance rest with activity.** Take short naps during the day, but keep in mind that too much bed rest can make you feel weak. You may feel better if you take short walks or exercise a little every day. **Eat and drink well. Talk** with your doctor, nurse, or a registered dietitian to learn what foods and drinks are best for you. You may need to eat foods that are high in protein or iron.
Appetite Loss *Chemotherapy *Radiation therapy	• Cancer treatments may lower your appetite or change the way food tastes or smells. • Side effects such as mouth and throat problems, or nausea and vomiting can also make eating difficult. • Cancer-related fatigue can also lower your appetite. • Talk with your health care team if you are not hungry or if your find it difficult to eat. Don't wait until you feel weak, have lost too much weight, or are dehydrated, to talk with your doctor or nurse. It's important to eat well, especially during treatment for cancer.	**Drink plenty of liquids.** Drinking plenty of liquids is important, especially if you have less of an appetite. Losing fluid can lead to dehydration, a dangerous condition. You may become weak or dizzy and have dark yellow urine if you are not drinking enough liquids. **Choose healthy and high-nutrient foods.** Eat a little, even if you are not hungry. It may help to have five or six small meals throughout the day instead of three large meals. Most people need to eat a variety of nutrient-dense foods that are high in protein and calories. **Be active.** Being active can actually increase your appetite. Your appetite may increase when you take a short walk each day.

SIDE EFFECT AND POSSIBLE CAUSE	DESCRIPTION	WAYS TO MANAGE

Bleeding & Bruising **(Thrombocytopenia)** *Chemotherapy *Targeted therapy	• Some cancer treatments, such as chemotherapy and targeted therapy, can increase your risk of bleeding and bruising.
	 • These treatments can lower the number of platelets in the blood. Platelets are the cells that help your blood to clot and stop bleeding. When your platelet count is low, you may bruise or bleed a lot or very easily and have tiny purple or red spots on your skin. This condition is called thrombocytopenia.
	 • It is important to tell your doctor or nurse if you notice any of these changes.
	 • Call your doctor or nurse if you have more serious problems, such as:
	    o Bleeding that doesn't stop after a few minutes; bleeding from your mouth, nose, or when you vomit; bleeding from your vagina when you are not having your period (menstruation); urine that is red or pink; stools that are black or bloody; or bleeding during your period that is heavier or lasts longer than normal.
	    o Head or vision changes such as bad headaches or changes in how well you see, or if you feel confused or very sleepy.
		Avoid certain medicines. Many over-the-counter medicines contain aspirin or ibuprofen, which can increase your risk of bleeding. When in doubt, be sure to check the label. Get a list of medicines and products from your health care team that you should avoid taking. You may also be advised to limit or avoid alcohol if your platelet count is low.
		
		 Take extra care to prevent bleeding. Brush your teeth gently, with a very soft toothbrush. Wear shoes, even when you are inside. Be extra careful when using sharp objects. Use an electric shaver, not a razor. Use lotion and a lip balm to prevent dry, chapped skin and lips. Tell your doctor or nurse if you are constipated or notice bleeding from your rectum.
		
		 Care for bleeding or bruising. If you start to bleed, press down firmly on the area with a clean cloth. Keep pressing until the bleeding stops. If you bruise, put ice on the area.

SIDE EFFECT AND POSSIBLE CAUSE	DESCRIPTION	WAYS TO MANAGE
Constipation *Chemotherapy *Pain medications	• Constipation is when you have infrequent bowel movements and stool that may be hard, dry, and difficult to pass. • You may also have stomach cramps, bloating, and nausea when you are constipated. • Cancer treatments such as chemotherapy can cause constipation. • Certain medicines (such as pain medicines), changes in diet, not drinking enough fluids, and being less active may also cause constipation. • It is easier to prevent constipation than to treat its complications which may include fecal impaction or bowel obstruction.	**Eat high-fiber foods.** Adding bran to foods such as cereals or smoothies is an easy way to get more fiber in your diet. Ask your health care team how many grams of fiber you should have each day. If you have had an intestinal obstruction or intestinal surgery, you should not eat a high-fiber diet. **Drink plenty of liquids.** Most people need to drink at least 8 cups of liquid each day. You may need more based on your treatment, medications you are taking, or other health factors. Drinking warm or hot liquids may also help. **Try to be active every day.** Ask your health care team about exercises that you can do. Most people can do light exercise, even in a bed or chair. Other people choose to walk or ride an exercise bike for 15 to 30 minutes each day. **Learn about medicine.** Use only medicines and treatments for constipation that are prescribed by your doctor, since some may lead to bleeding, infection, or other harmful side effects in people being treated for cancer. Keep a record of your bowel movements to share with your doctor or nurse.

SIDE EFFECT AND POSSIBLE CAUSE	DESCRIPTION	WAYS TO MANAGE
Delirium Causes may include: *Advanced cancer *Older age *Dehydration *Infection *Taking certain medicines, such as high doses of opioids *Withdrawal from or stopping certain medicines *Early monitoring of someone with these risk factors for delirium may prevent it or allow it to be treated more quickly.*	• Delirium is a confused mental state that includes changes in awareness, thinking, judgment, sleeping patterns, as well as behavior. • Although delirium can happen at the end of life, many episodes of delirium are caused by medicine or dehydration and are reversible. • The symptoms of delirium usually occur suddenly (within hours or days) over a short period of time and may come and go. • Although delirium may be mistaken for depression or dementia, these conditions are different and have different treatments. Types of Delirium: • *Hypoactive delirium:* The patient seems sleepy, tired, or depressed • *Hyperactive delirium:* The patient is restless, anxious, or suddenly agitated and uncooperative • *Mixed delirium:* The patient changes back and forth between hypoactive delirium and hyperactive delirium Changes caused by delirium can be upsetting for family members and dangerous to the person with cancer, especially if judgment is affected. People with delirium may be more likely to fall, unable to control their bladder and/or bowels, and more likely to become dehydrated. Their confused state may make it difficult to talk with others about their needs and make decisions about care.	**Treat the causes of delirium**: If medicines are causing delirium, then reducing the dose or stopping them may treat delirium. If conditions such as dehydration, poor nutrition, and infections are causing the delirium, then treating these may help. **Control surroundings:** If the symptoms of delirium are mild, it may help to keep the room quiet and well lit, with a clock or calendar and familiar possessions. Having family members around and keeping the same caregivers, as much as possible, may also help. **Consider medicines:** Medicines are sometimes given to treat the symptoms of delirium. However, these medicines have serious side effects and patients receiving them require careful observation by a doctor. **Sometimes sedation may help**: After discussion with family members, sedation is sometimes used for delirium at the end of life, if it does not get better with other treatments. The doctor will discuss the decisions involved in using sedation to treat delirium with the family.

SIDE EFFECT AND POSSIBLE CAUSE	DESCRIPTION	WAYS TO MANAGE
Diarrhea *Treatments for cancer *Medications *Infections *Stress *Certain Cancers	• Diarrhea means having bowel movements that are soft, loose, or watery more often than normal. • If diarrhea is severe or lasts a long time, the body does not absorb enough water and nutrients. This can cause you to become dehydrated or malnourished. • Cancer treatments, or the cancer itself, may cause diarrhea or make it worse. • Some medicines, infections, and stress can also cause diarrhea. • Tell your health care team if you have diarrhea. • Diarrhea that leads to dehydration (the loss of too much fluid from the body) and low levels of salt and potassium (important minerals needed by the body) can be life threatening. • Call your health care team if you feel dizzy or light headed, have dark yellow urine or are not urinating, or have a fever of 100.5 °F (38 °C) or higher.	**Drink plenty of fluid each day.** Most people need to drink 8 to 12 cups of fluid each day. Ask your doctor or nurse how much fluid you should drink each day. For severe diarrhea, only clear liquids or IV (intravenous) fluids may be advised for a short period. **Eat small meals that are easy on your stomach.** Eat six to eight small meals throughout the day, instead of three large meals. Foods high in potassium and sodium (minerals you lose when you have diarrhea) are good food choices, for most people. Limit or avoid foods and drinks that can make your diarrhea worse. **Check before taking medicine.** Check with your doctor or nurse before taking medicine for diarrhea. Your doctor will prescribe the correct medicine for you. **Keep your anal area clean and dry.** Try using warm water and wipes to stay clean. It may help to take warm, shallow baths. These are called sitz baths.
Edema (Swelling) *Chemotherapy *Radiation *Certain Cancers *Unrelated conditions	Edema, a condition in which fluid builds up in your body's tissues, may be caused by some types of chemotherapy, certain cancers, and conditions not related to cancer. Signs of edema may include: • Swelling in your feet, ankles, and legs • Swelling in your hands and arms • Swelling in your face or abdomen • Skin that is puffy, shiny, or looks slightly dented after being pressed • Shortness of breath, a cough, or irregular heartbeat Tell your health care team if you notice swelling. Your doctor or nurse will determine what is causing your symptoms, advise you on steps to take, and may prescribe medicine. Some problems related to edema are serious. Call your doctor or nurse if you feel short of breath, have a heartbeat that seems different or is not regular, have sudden swelling or swelling that is getting worse or is moving up your arms or legs, you gain weight quickly, or you don't urinate at all or urinate only a little.	**Get comfortable**. Wear loose clothing and shoes that are not too tight. When you sit or lie down, raise your feet with a stool or pillows. Avoid crossing your legs when you sit. Talk with your health care team about wearing special stockings, sleeves, or gloves that help with circulation if your swelling is severe. **Exercise.** Moving the part of your body with edema can help. Your doctor may give you specific exercises, including walking, to improve circulation. However, you may be advised not to stand or walk too much at one time. **Limit salt (sodium) in your diet.** Avoid foods such as chips, bacon, ham, and canned soup. Check food labels for the sodium content. Don't add salt or soy sauce to your food. **Take your medicine.** If your doctor prescribes a medicine called a diuretic, take it exactly as instructed. The medicine will help move the extra fluid and salt out of your body.

SIDE EFFECT AND POSSIBLE CAUSE	DESCRIPTION	WAYS TO MANAGE
Fatigue *Chemotherapy *Immunotherapy *Radiation therapy *Bone marrow transplant *Surgery *Anemia *Pain *Medications *Emotions	• Fatigue is a common side effect of many cancer treatments, including chemotherapy, immunotherapy, radiation therapy, bone marrow transplants, and surgery. • Conditions such as anemia, as well as pain, medications, and emotions, can also cause or worsen fatigue. • People often describe cancer-related fatigue as feeling extremely tired, weak, heavy, run down, and having no energy. • Resting does not always help with cancer-related fatigue. Cancer-related fatigue is one of the most difficult side effects for many people to cope with. • Tell your health care team if you feel extremely tired and are not able to do your normal activities or are very tired even after resting or sleeping. • There are many causes of fatigue. Keeping track of your levels of energy throughout the day will help your doctor to assess your fatigue. Write down how fatigue affects your daily activities and what makes the fatigue better or worse.	**Make a plan that balances rest and activity.** Choose activities that are relaxing for you. Many people choose to listen to music, read, meditate, practice guided imagery, or spend time with people they enjoy. Relaxing can help you save your energy and lower stress. Light exercise may also be advised by your doctor to give you more energy and help you feel better. **Plan time to rest.** If you are tired, take short naps of less than 1 hour during the day. However, too much sleep during the day can make it difficult to sleep at night. Choose the activities that are most important to you and do them when you have the most energy. Ask for help with important tasks such as making meals or driving. **Eat and drink well.** Meet with a registered dietitian to learn about foods and drinks that can increase your level of energy. Foods high in protein and calories will help you keep up your strength. Some people find it easier to eat many small meals throughout the day instead of three big meals. Stay well hydrated. Limit your intake of caffeine and alcohol. **Meet with a specialist.** It may help to meet with a counselor, psychologist, or psychiatrist. These experts help people to cope with difficult thoughts and feelings. Lowering stress may give you more energy. Since pain that is not controlled can also be major source of fatigue, it may help to meet with a pain or palliative care specialist.

SIDE EFFECT AND POSSIBLE CAUSE	DESCRIPTION	CANCER TREATMENTS MAY AFFECT YOUR FERTILITY
Fertility Issues in Boys and Men **Possible Cause:** See 2nd column *Cancer Treatments May Affect Your Fertility*	Many cancer treatments can affect a boy's or a man's fertility. Most likely, your doctor will talk with you about whether or not cancer treatment may lower fertility or cause infertility. However, not all doctors bring up this topic. Sometimes you, a family member, or parents of a child being treated for cancer may need to initiate this conversation. Whether or not your fertility is affected depends on factors such as: <ul><li>Your baseline fertility</li><li>Your age at the time of treatment</li><li>The type of cancer and treatment(s)</li><li>The amount (dose) of treatment</li><li>he length (duration) of treatment</li><li>The amount of time that has passed since treatment</li><li>Other personal health factors</li></ul>*Emotional Considerations and Support for Fertility Issues* For some men, infertility can be one of the most difficult and upsetting long-term effects of cancer treatment. Although it might feel overwhelming to think about your fertility right now, most people benefit from having talked with their doctor (or their child's doctor, when a child is being treated for cancer) about how treatment may affect their fertility and learning about options to preserve their fertility. Although most people want to have children at some point in their life, families can come together in many ways. For extra support during this time, reach out to your health care team with questions or concerns, as well as to professionally led support groups.	Cancer treatments are important for your future health, but they may harm reproductive organs and glands that control fertility. Changes to your fertility may be temporary or permanent. Talk with your healthcare team to learn what to expect based on your treatment(s): **Chemotherapy** (especially alkylating drugs) can damage sperm in men and sperm-forming cells (germ cells) in young boys. **Hormone therapy** (also called endocrine therapy) can decrease the production of sperm. **Radiation therapy** to the reproductive organs as well as radiation near the abdomen, pelvis, or spine may lower sperm counts and testosterone levels, causing infertility. <ul><li>Radiation may also destroy sperm cells and the stem cells that make sperm. Radiation therapy to the brain can damage the pituitary gland and decrease the production of testosterone and sperm.</li><li>For some types of cancers, the testicles can be protected from radiation through a procedure called testicular shielding.</li></ul>**Surgery** for cancers of the reproductive organs and for pelvic cancers (such as bladder, colon, prostate, and rectal cancer) can damage these organs and/or nearby nerves or lymph nodes in the pelvis, leading to infertility. **Stem cell transplants** such as bone marrow transplants and peripheral blood stem cell transplants, involve receiving high doses of chemotherapy and/or radiation. These treatments can damage sperm and sperm-forming cells. **Other treatments:** Talk with your doctor to learn whether other types of treatment, such as immunotherapy and targeted cancer therapy, may affect your fertility.

SIDE EFFECT AND POSSIBLE CAUSE	DESCRIPTION	CANCER TREATMENTS MAY AFFECT YOUR FERTILITY
Fertility Issues in Girls and Women **Possible Cause:** See 2nd column *Cancer Treatments May Affect Your Fertility*	Many cancer treatments can affect a girl's or woman's fertility. Most likely, your doctor will talk with you about whether or not cancer treatment may increase the risk of, or cause, infertility. However, not all doctors bring up this topic. Sometimes you, a family member, or parents of a child being treated for cancer may need to initiate this conversation. Whether or not your fertility is affected depends on factors such as: • Your baseline fertility • Your age at the time of treatment • The type of cancer and treatment(s) • The amount (dose) of treatment • The length (duration) of treatment • The amount of time that has passed since treatment • Other personal health factors ***Emotional Considerations and Support for Fertility Issues*** For some women, infertility can be one of the most difficult and upsetting long-term effects of cancer treatment. While it might feel overwhelming to think about your fertility right now, most people benefit from having talked with their doctor (or their child's doctor, when a child is being treated for cancer) about how treatment may affect their fertility and about options to preserve fertility.	Cancer treatments are important for your future health, but they may harm reproductive organs and glands that control fertility. Changes to your fertility may be temporary or permanent. Talk with your health care team to learn what to expect, based on your treatment(s): **Chemotherapy** (especially alkylating agents) can affect the ovaries, causing them to stop releasing eggs and estrogen. This is called primary ovarian insufficiency (POI). • Sometimes POI is temporary, and your menstrual periods and fertility return after treatment. Other times, damage to your ovaries is permanent and fertility doesn't return. • You may have hot flashes, night sweats, irritability, vaginal dryness, and irregular or no menstrual periods. • Chemotherapy can also lower the number of healthy eggs in the ovaries. • Women who are closer to the age of natural menopause may have a greater risk of infertility. • The National Institute for Child Health and Human Development (NICHD) has more information about primary ovarian insufficiency. **Hormone therapy** (also called endocrine therapy) used to treat cancer can disrupt the menstrual cycle, which may affect your fertility. Side effects depend on the specific hormones used and may include hot flashes, night sweats, and vaginal dryness. **Bone marrow transplants, peripheral blood stem cell transplants,** and other stem cell transplants involve receiving high doses of chemotherapy and/or radiation. These treatments can damage the ovaries and may cause infertility. **Other treatments:** Talk with your doctor to learn whether or not other types of treatment such as immunotherapy and targeted cancer therapy may affect your fertility.

SIDE EFFECT AND POSSIBLE CAUSE	DESCRIPTION	WAYS TO MANAGE
Hair Loss (Alopecia) *Chemotherapy *Radiation (Localized)	• Some types of chemotherapy cause the hair on your head and other parts of your body to fall out. • Radiation therapy can also cause hair loss on the part of the body that is being treated. • Hair loss is called alopecia. ***Ways to Care for Your Hair When It Grows Back*** **Be gentle**. When your hair starts to grow back, you will want to be gentle with it. Avoid too much brushing, curling, and blow-drying. You may not want to wash your hair as frequently. **After chemotherapy.** Hair often grows back in 2 to 3 months after treatment has ended. Your hair will be very fine when it starts to grow back. Sometimes your new hair can be curlier or straighter—or even a different color. In time, it may go back to how it was before treatment. **After radiation therapy.** Hair often grows back in 3 to 6 months after treatment has ended. If you received a very high dose of radiation your hair may grow back thinner or not at all on the part of your body that received radiation.	***Ways to Manage Hair Loss*** Talk with your health care team about ways to manage before and after hair loss: **Treat your hair gently.** You may want to use a hairbrush with soft bristles or a wide-tooth comb. Do not use hair dryers, irons, or products such as gels or clips that may hurt your scalp. Wash your hair with a mild shampoo. Wash it less often and be very gentle. Pat it dry with a soft towel. **You have choices.** Some people choose to cut their hair short to make it easier to deal with when it starts to fall out. Others choose to shave their head. If you choose to shave your head, use an electric shaver so you won't cut yourself. If you plan to buy a wig, get one while you still have hair so you can match it to the color of your hair. If you find wigs to be itchy and hot, try wearing a comfortable scarf or turban. **Protect and care for your scalp.** Use sunscreen or wear a hat when you are outside. Choose a comfortable scarf or hat that you enjoy and that keeps your head warm. If your scalp itches or feels tender, using lotions and conditioners can help it feel better. **Talk about your feelings.** Many people feel angry, depressed, or embarrassed about hair loss. It can help to share these feelings with someone who understands. Some people find it helpful to talk with other people who have lost their hair during cancer treatment. Talking openly and honestly with your children and close family members can also help you all. Tell them that you expect to lose your hair during treatment.

SIDE EFFECT AND POSSIBLE CAUSE	DESCRIPTION	WAYS TO MANAGE

Infection and Neutropenia
 	
*Surgery
*Chemotherapy
	• An infection is the invasion and growth of germs in the body, such as bacteria, viruses, yeast, or other fungi.
	• An infection can begin anywhere in the body, may spread throughout the body, and can cause one or more of these signs:
	  o Fever of 100.5 °F (38 °C) or higher or chills
	  o Cough or sore throat
	  o Diarrhea
	  o Ear pain, headache or sinus pain, or a stiff or sore neck
	  o skin rash
	  o Sores or white coating in your mouth or on your tongue
	  o Swelling or redness, especially where a catheter enters your body
	  o Urine that is bloody or cloudy, or pain when you urinate
	• Call your health care team if you have signs of an infection.
	• Infections during cancer treatment can be life threatening and require urgent medical attention.
	• Be sure to talk with your doctor or nurse before taking medicine—even aspirin, acetaminophen (such as Tylenol®), or ibuprofen (such as Advil®) for a fever. These medicines can lower a fever but may also mask or hide signs of a more serious problem.
	• Some types of cancer and treatments such as chemotherapy may increase your risk of infection. This is because they lower the number of white blood cells, the cells that help your body to fight infection. During chemotherapy, there will be times in your treatment cycle when the number of white blood cells (called neutrophils) is particularly low, and you are at increased risk of infection.
	• Stress, poor nutrition, and not enough sleep can also weaken the immune system, making infection more likely.
		Ways to Prevent Infection
		
		Your health care team will talk with you about these and other ways to prevent infection:
		
		Wash your hands often and well. Use soap and warm water to wash your hands well, especially before eating. Have people around you wash their hands well too.
		
		Stay extra clean. If you have a catheter, keep the area around it clean and dry. Clean your teeth well and check your mouth for sores or other signs of an infection each day. If you get a scrape or cut, clean it well. Let your doctor or nurse know if your bottom is sore or bleeds, as this could increase your risk of infection.
		
		Avoid germs. Stay away from people who are sick or have a cold. Avoid crowds and people who have just had a live vaccine, such as one for chicken pox, polio, or measles. Follow food safety guidelines; make sure the meat, fish, and eggs you eat are well cooked. Keep hot foods hot and cold foods cold. You may be advised to eat only fruits and vegetables that can be peeled, or to wash all raw fruits and vegetables very well.

SIDE EFFECT AND POSSIBLE CAUSE	DESCRIPTION	WAYS TO MANAGE
Memory or Concentration Issues *Chemotherapy *Immunotherapy *Radiation therapy (brain)	• Whether you have memory or concentration problems (sometimes described as a mental fog or chemo brain) depends on the type of treatment you receive, your age, and other health-related factors. • Cancer treatments such as chemotherapy may cause difficulty with thinking, concentrating, or remembering things. • So can some types of radiation therapy to the brain and immunotherapy. • These cognitive problems may start during or after cancer treatment. Some people notice very small changes, such as a bit more difficulty remembering things, whereas others have much greater memory or concentration problems. • Your doctor will assess your symptoms and advise you about ways to manage or treat these problems. Treating conditions such as poor nutrition, anxiety, depression, fatigue, and insomnia may also help.	It's important for you or a family member to tell your health care team if you have difficulty remembering things, thinking, or concentrating. Here are some steps you can take to manage minor memory or concentration problems: **Plan your day.** Do things that need the most concentration at the time of day when you feel best. Get extra rest and plenty of sleep at night. If you need to rest during the day, short naps of less than 1 hour are best. Long naps can make it more difficult to sleep at night. Keep a daily routine. **Exercise your body and mind.** Exercise can help to decrease stress and help you to feel more alert. Exercise releases endorphins, also known as "feel-good chemicals, "which give people a feeling of well-being. Ask what light physical exercises may be helpful for you. Mind–body practices such as meditation or mental exercises such as puzzles or games also help some people. **Get help to remember things.** Write down and keep a list handy of important information. Use a daily planner, recorder, or other electronic device to help you remember important activities. Make a list of important names and phone numbers. Keep it in one place so it's easy to find

SIDE EFFECT AND POSSIBLE CAUSE	DESCRIPTION	WAYS TO MANAGE

Mouth and Throat Problems
 	
*Chemotherapy
*Immunotherapy
*Radiation therapy (head & neck)
*Medications
 	
See Eating Hints
	• Cancer treatments may cause dental, mouth, and throat problems.
	• Radiation therapy to the head and neck may harm the salivary glands and tissues in your mouth and/or make it hard to chew and swallow safely.
	• Some types of chemotherapy and immunotherapy can also harm cells in your mouth, throat, and lips.
	• Drugs used to treat cancer and certain bone problems may also cause oral complications.
	Mouth and throat problems may include:
	   o Changes in taste or smell
	   o Dry mouth (xerostomia)
	   o Infections and mouth sores
	   o Pain or swelling in your mouth (oral mucositis)
	   o Sensitivity to hot or cold foods
	   o Swallowing problems (dysphagia)
	   o Tooth decay (cavities)
	
	Mouth problems are more serious if they interfere with eating and drinking because they can lead to dehydration and/or malnutrition.
	
	It's important to call your doctor or nurse if you have pain in your mouth, lips, or throat that makes it difficult to eat, drink, or sleep or if you have a fever of 100.5 °F (38 °C) or higher.
	
	Ways to Prevent Mouth and Dental Problems
	• Get a dental check-up before starting treatment.
	   o Before you start treatment, visit your dentist for a cleaning and check-up. Tell the dentist about your cancer treatment and try to get any dental work completed before starting treatment.
	• Check and clean your mouth daily.
	   o Check your mouth every day for sores or white spots.
	   o Rinse your mouth throughout the day with a solution of warm water, baking soda, and salt.
	   o Gently brush your teeth, gums, and tongue after each meal and before going to bed at night. Use a very soft toothbrush or cotton swabs.
	   o If you are at risk of bleeding, ask if you should floss.
		Your health care team may suggest that you take these and other steps to manage these problems:
		
		For a sore mouth or throat: Choose foods that are soft, wet, and easy to swallow. Soften dry foods with gravy, sauce, or other liquids. Use a blender to make milkshakes or blend your food to make it easier to swallow. Ask about pain medicine, such as lozenges or sprays that numb your mouth and make eating less painful. Avoid foods and drinks that can irritate your mouth; foods that are crunchy, salty, spicy, or sugary; and alcoholic drinks. Don't smoke or use tobacco.
		
		For a dry mouth: Drink plenty of liquids because a dry mouth can increase the risk of tooth decay and mouth infections. Keep water handy and sip it often to keep your mouth wet. Suck on ice chips or sugar-free hard candy, have frozen desserts, or chew sugar-free gum. Use a lip balm. Ask about medicines such as saliva substitutes that can coat, protect, and moisten your mouth and throat. Acupuncture may also help with dry mouth.
		
		For changes to your sense of taste: Foods may seem to have no taste or may not taste the way they used to or food may not have much taste at all. Radiation therapy may cause a change in sweet, sour, bitter, and salty tastes. Chemotherapy drugs may cause an unpleasant chemical or metallic taste in your mouth. If you have taste changes it may help to try different foods to find ones that taste best to you. Trying cold foods may also help. Here are some more tips to consider:
		• If food tastes bland, marinate foods to improve their flavor or add spices to foods.
		• If red meat tastes strange, switch to other high-protein foods such as chicken, eggs, fish, peanut butter.
		• If foods taste salty, bitter, or acidic, try sweetening them.
		• If foods taste metallic, switch to plastic utensils and non-metal cooking dishes.
		• If you have a bad taste in your mouth, try sugar-free lemon drops, gum, or mints.

SIDE EFFECT AND POSSIBLE CAUSE	DESCRIPTION	WAYS TO MANAGE
Nausea and Vomiting Cancer treatments, including, but not limited to chemotherapy	• Nausea is when you feel sick to your stomach, as if you are going to throw up. • Vomiting is when you throw up. • There are different types of nausea and vomiting caused by cancer treatment, including anticipatory, acute, and delayed nausea and vomiting. • Controlling nausea and vomiting will help you to feel better and prevent more serious problems such as malnutrition and dehydration. • Your doctor or nurse will determine what is causing your symptoms and advise you on ways to prevent them. • Medicines called anti-nausea drugs or antiemetics are effective in preventing or reducing many types of nausea and vomiting. The medicine is taken at specific times to prevent and/or control symptoms of nausea and vomiting. These foods and drinks may be easy on your stomach: SOUPS • Clear broth, such as chicken, beef, and vegetable DRINKS • Clear soda, such as ginger ale • Cranberry or grape juice • Oral rehydration drinks, such as Pedialyte® • Tea • Water MAIN MEAL AND SNACKS • Chicken—broiled or baked without the skin • Cream of wheat or rice cereal • Crackers or pretzels • Oatmeal • Pasta or noodles • Potatoes—boiled, without the skin • White rice • White toast FRIUITS and SWEETS • Bananas • Canned fruit such as applesauce, peaches, and pears • Gelatin (Jell-O®) • Popsicles and sherbet • Yogurt (plain or vanilla)	You may be advised to take these steps to feel better: **Take anti-nausea medicine.** Talk with your doctor or nurse to learn when to take your medicine. Most people need to take an anti-nausea medicine even on days when they feel well. Tell your doctor or nurse if the medicine doesn't help. There are different kinds of medicine, and one may work better than another for you. **Drink plenty of water and fluids.** Drinking will help to prevent dehydration, a serious problem that happens when your body loses too much fluid and you are not drinking enough. Try to sip on water, fruit juices, ginger ale, tea, and/or sports drinks throughout the day. **Have enough to eat and drink.** Take small sips of water during the day, if you find it hard to drink a full glass at one time. Eat 5 or 6 small meals during the day, instead of 3 big meals. **Avoid certain foods.** Don't eat greasy, fried, sweet, or spicy foods if you feel sick after eating them. If the smell of food bothers you, ask others to make your food. Try cold foods that do not have strong smells, or let food cool down before you eat it. **Try these tips on treatment days.** Some people find that it helps to eat a small snack before treatment. Others avoid eating or drinking right before or after treatment because it makes them feel sick. After treatment, wait at least 1 hour before you eat or drink. **Learn about complementary medicine practices that may help.** Acupuncture relieves nausea and/or vomiting caused by chemotherapy in some people. Deep breathing, guided imagery, hypnosis, and other relaxation techniques (such as listening to music, reading a book, or meditating) also help some people. *See Eating Hints*

SIDE EFFECT AND POSSIBLE CAUSE	DESCRIPTION	WAYS TO MANAGE
Nerve Problems (Peripheral Neuropathy)	• Some cancer treatments cause peripheral neuropathy, a result of damage to the peripheral nerves. These nerves carry information from the brain to other parts of the body. • Side effects depend on which peripheral nerves (sensory, motor, or autonomic) are affected. Damage to sensory nerves (nerves that help you feel pain, heat, cold, and pressure) can cause: • Tingling, numbness, or a pins-and-needles feeling in your feet and hands that may spread to your legs and arms • Inability to feel a hot or cold sensation, such as a hot stove • Inability to feel pain, such as from a cut or sore on your foot Damage to motor nerves (nerves that help your muscles to move) can cause: • Weak or achy muscles. You may lose your balance or trip easily. It may also be difficult to button shirts or open jars. • Muscles that twitch and cramp or muscle wasting (if you don't use your muscles regularly). • Swallowing or breathing difficulties (if your chest or throat muscles are affected) Damage to autonomic nerves (nerves that control functions such as blood pressure, digestion, heart rate, temperature, and urination) can cause: • Digestive changes such as constipation or diarrhea • Dizzy or faint feeling, due to low blood pressure • Sexual problems: men may be unable to get an erection and women may not reach orgasm • Sweating problems (either too much or too little sweating) • Urination problems, such as leaking urine or difficulty emptying your bladder	*Ways to Prevent or Manage Problems Related to Nerve Changes* You may be advised to take these steps: **Prevent falls.** Have someone help you prevent falls around the house. Move rugs out of your path so you will not trip on them. Put rails on the walls and in the bathroom, so you can hold on to them and balance yourself. Put bathmats in the shower or tub. Wear sturdy shoes with soft soles. Get up slowly after sitting or lying down, especially if you feel dizzy. **Take extra care in the kitchen and shower.** Use potholders in the kitchen to protect your hands from burns. Be careful when handling knives or sharp objects. Ask someone to check the water temperature, to make sure it's not too hot. **Protect your hands and feet**. Wear shoes, both inside and outside. Check your arms, legs, and feet for cuts or scratches every day. When it's cold, wear warm clothes to protect your hands and feet. **Ask for help and slow down.** Let people help you with difficult tasks. Slow down and give yourself more time to do things. **Ask about pain medicine and integrative medicine practices**. You may be prescribed pain medicine. Sometimes practices such as acupuncture, massage, physical therapy, yoga, and others may also be advised to lower pain. Talk with your health care team to learn what is advised for you.

SIDE EFFECT AND POSSIBLE CAUSE	DESCRIPTION	WAYS TO MANAGE
Pain See 1st Column *Different cancer treatments may cause specific types of pain.*	• Cancer itself and the side effects of cancer treatment can sometimes cause pain. • Pain is not something that you have to "put up with." Controlling pain is an important part of your cancer treatment plan. • Pain can suppress the immune system, increase the time it takes your body to heal, interfere with sleep, and affect your mood. Talk with your health care team about pain, especially if: • The pain isn't getting better or going away with pain medicine • the pain comes on quickly • The pain makes it hard to eat, sleep, or perform your normal activities • You feel new pain • You have side effects from the pain medicine such as sleepiness, nausea, or constipation ***Different cancer treatments may cause specific types of pain.*** Patients may have different types of pain depending on the treatments they receive, including: • **Spasms, stinging, and itching** caused by intravenous chemotherapy. • **Mucositis** (sores or inflammation in the mouth or other parts of the digestive system) caused by chemotherapy or targeted therapy. • **Skin pain, rash, or hand-foot syndrome** (redness, tingling, or burning in the palms of the hands and/or the soles of feet) caused by chemotherapy or targeted therapy. • **Pain in joints and muscles** throughout the body caused by paclitaxel or aromatase inhibitor therapy. • **Osteonecrosis** of the jaw caused by bisphosphonates given for cancer that has spread to the bone.	Here are some steps you can take, as you work with your health care team to prevent, treat, or lessen pain: **Keep track of your pain levels.** Each day, write about any pain you feel. Writing down answers to the questions below will help you describe the pain to your doctor or nurse. • What part of your body feels painful? • What does the pain feel like (is it sharp, burning, shooting, or throbbing) and where do you feel the pain? • When does the pain start? How long does the pain last? • What activities (such as eating, sleeping, or other activities) does pain interfere with? • What makes the pain feel better or worse? For example, do ice packs, heating pads, or exercises help? • Does pain medicine help? How much do you take? How often do you take it? • How bad is the pain, on a scale of 1 to 10, where "10" is the most pain and "1" is the least pain? **Take the prescribed pain medicine.** • Take the right amount of medicine at the right time. • Do not wait until your pain gets too bad before taking pain medicine. Waiting to take your medicine could make it take longer for the pain to go away or increase the amount of medicine needed to lower pain. • Do not stop taking the pain medicine unless your doctor advises you to. • Tell your doctor or nurse if the medicine no longer lowers the pain, or if you are in pain, but it's not yet time to take the pain medicine.

| Pain Continued | • **Pain syndromes caused by radiation,** including:
  o Pain from brachytherapy.
  o Pain from the position the patient stays in during radiation therapy.
  o Mucositis.
  o Inflammation of the mucous membranes in areas treated with radiation.
  o Dermatitis (inflammation of the skin in areas treated with radiation).
  o Pain flares (a temporary worsening of pain in the treated area). | **Meet with a pain specialist.** Specialists who treat pain often work together as part of a pain or palliative care team. These specialists may include a neurologist, surgeon, physiatrist, psychiatrist, psychologist, or pharmacist.
• Talk with your health care team to find a pain specialist.
• **Ask about integrative medicine.** Treatments such as acupuncture, biofeedback, hypnosis, massage therapy and physical therapy may also be used to treat pain.

Pain may affect quality of life after treatment ends.

• Pain that is severe or continues after cancer treatment ends increases the risk of anxiety and depression.
• Patients may be disabled by their pain, unable to work, or feel that they are losing support once their care moves from their oncology team back to their primary care team.
• Feelings of anxiety and depression can worsen pain and make it harder to control. |

SIDE EFFECT AND POSSIBLE CAUSE	DESCRIPTION	WAYS TO MANAGE
Skin and Nail Changes *Radiation therapy *Chemotherapy *Biological therapy *Targeted therapy	Cancer treatments may cause a range of skin and nail changes. Talk with your health care team to learn whether or not you will have these changes, based on the treatment you are receiving. **Radiation therapy** can cause the skin on the part of your body receiving radiation therapy to become dry and peel, itch (called pruritus), and turn red or darker. It may look sunburned or tan and be swollen or puffy. **Chemotherapy** • May damage fast growing skin and nail cells. This can cause problems such as skin that is dry, itchy, red, and/or that peels. • Some people may develop a rash or sun sensitivity, causing you to sunburn easily. • Nail changes may include dark, yellow, or cracked nails and/or cuticles that are red and hurt. • Chemotherapy in people who have received radiation therapy in the past can cause skin to become red, blister, peel, or hurt on the part of the body that received radiation therapy; this is called radiation recall. **Biological therapy** may cause itching (pruritus). **Targeted therapy** May cause a dry skin, a rash, and nail problems. These skin problems are more serious and need urgent medical attention: • Sudden or severe itching, a rash, or hives during chemotherapy. These may be signs of an allergic reaction. • Sores on the part of your body where you are receiving treatment that become painful, wet, and/or infected. This is called a moist reaction and may happen in areas where the skin folds, such as around your ears, breast, or bottom.	Depending on what treatment you are receiving, you may be advised to take these steps to protect your skin, prevent infection, and reduce itching: **Use only recommended skin products.** Use mild soaps that are gentle on your skin. Ask your nurse to recommend specific lotions and creams. Ask when and how often to use them. Ask what skin products to avoid. For example, you may be advised to not use powders or antiperspirants before radiation therapy. **Protect your skin.** Ask about lotions or antibiotics for dry, itchy, infected or swollen skin. Don't use heating pads, ice packs, or bandages on the area receiving radiation therapy. Shave less often and use an electric razor or stop shaving if your skin is sore. Wear sunscreen and lip balm or a loose-fitting long-sleeved shirt, pants, and a hat with a wide brim when outdoors. **Prevent or treat dry, itchy skin (pruritus).** Your doctor will work to assess the cause of pruritus. There are also steps you can take to feel better. Avoid products with alcohol or perfume, which can dry or irritate your skin. Take short showers or baths in lukewarm, not hot, water. Put on lotion after drying off from a shower, while your skin is still slightly damp. Keep your home cool and humid. Eat a healthy diet and drink plenty of fluids to help keep your skin moist and healthy. Applying a cool washcloth or ice to the affected area may also help. Acupuncture also helps some people. **Prevent or treat minor nail problems.** Keep your nails clean and cut short. Wear gloves when you wash the dishes, work in the garden, or clean the house. Check with your nurse about products that can help your nails. If your skin hurts in the area where you get treatment, tell your doctor or nurse. Your skin might have a moist reaction. Most often this happens in areas where the skin folds, such as behind the ears or under the breasts. It can lead to an infection if not properly treated. Ask your doctor or nurse how to care for these areas.

SIDE EFFECT AND POSSIBLE CAUSE	DESCRIPTION	WAYS TO MANAGE
Sleep Problems	• Sleeping well is important for your physical and mental health. A good night's sleep not only helps you to think clearly, it also lowers your blood pressure, helps your appetite, and strengthens your immune system. • Sleep problems such as being unable to fall asleep and/or stay asleep, also called insomnia, are common among people being treated for cancer. Studies show that as many as half of all patients have sleep-related problems. These problems may be caused by the side effects of treatment, medicine, long hospital stays, or stress. • Talk with your health care team if you have difficulty sleeping, so you can get the help you need. • Sleep problems that go on for a long time may increase the risk of anxiety or depression. • Your doctor will do an assessment, which may include a polysomnogram (recordings taken during sleep that show brain waves, breathing rate, and other activities such as heart rate) to correctly diagnose and treat sleep problems. Assessments may be repeated from time to time, since sleeping problems may change over time.	There are steps that you and your health care team can take to help you sleep well again. **Tell your doctor about problems that interfere with sleep.** Getting treatment to lower side effects such as pain or bladder or gastrointestinal problems may help you sleep better. **Cognitive behavioral therapy (CBT) and relaxation therapy** may help. Practicing these therapies can help you to relax. For example, a CBT therapist can help you learn to change negative thoughts and beliefs about sleep into positive ones. Strategies such as muscle relaxation, guided imagery, and self-hypnosis may also help you. **Set good bedtime habits.** Go to bed only when sleepy, in a quiet and dark room, and in a comfortable bed. If you do not fall asleep, get out of bed and return to bed when you are sleepy. Stop watching television or using other electrical devices for a couple of hours before going to bed. Don't drink or eat a lot before bedtime. While it's important to keep active during the day with regular exercise, exercising a few hours before bedtime may make sleep more difficult. **Sleep medicine may be prescribed.** Your doctor may prescribe sleep medicine for a short period if other strategies don't work. The sleep medicine prescribed will depend on your specific problem (such as trouble falling asleep or trouble staying asleep) as well as other medicines you are taking.

SIDE EFFECT AND POSSIBLE CAUSE	DESCRIPTION	WAYS TO MANAGE
Urinary and Bladder Problems *Radiation therapy *Chemotherapy *Immunotherapy *Surgery	***Symptoms of a Urinary Problem*** Some urinary or bladder changes may be normal, such as changes to the color or smell of your urine caused by some types of chemotherapy. Your health care team will determine what is causing your symptoms and will advise on steps to take to feel better. Irritation of the bladder lining (radiation cystitis): <ul><li>Pain or a burning feeling when you urinate</li><li>Blood in your urine</li><li>Trouble starting to urinate</li><li>Trouble emptying your bladder completely</li><li>Feeling that you need to urinate urgently or frequently</li><li>Leaking a little urine when you sneeze or cough</li><li>Bladder spasms, cramps, or discomfort in the pelvic area</li></ul>Urinary tract infection (UTI): <ul><li>Pain or a burning feeling when you urinate</li><li>Urine that is cloudy or red</li><li>Fever of 100.5 °F (38 °C) or higher, chills, and fatigue</li><li>Pain in your back or abdomen</li><li>Difficulty urinating or not being able to urinate</li></ul>In people being treated for cancer, a UTI can turn into a serious condition that needs immediate medical care. Antibiotics will be prescribed if you have a bacterial infection.	***Ways to Prevent or Manage*** Here are some steps you may be advised to take to feel better and to prevent problems: **Drink plenty of liquids.** Most people need to drink at least 8 cups of fluid each day, so that urine is light yellow or clear. You'll want to stay away from things that can make bladder problems worse. These include caffeine, drinks with alcohol, spicy foods, and tobacco products. **Prevent urinary tract infections.** Your doctor or nurse will talk with you about ways to lower your chances of getting a urinary tract infection. These may include going to the bathroom often, wearing cotton underwear and loose-fitting pants, learning about safe and sanitary practices for catheterization, taking showers instead of baths, and checking with your nurse before using products such as creams or lotions near your genital area. ***Drink more liquids*** <ul><li>Drink liquids such as water, soup, milkshakes, and cranberry juice. Add extra water to the juice.</li><li>Ask your doctor or nurse how many cups of liquid you should drink each day. Most people need to drink at least 8 cups a day.</li><li>Keep drinking liquids even if you have to go to the bathroom a lot. Liquids help your body to work well.</li></ul>Some liquids can make bladder problems worse. Talk with your doctor or nurse to learn what you should stop drinking or drink less of. These include: <ul><li>Drinks with caffeine, such as coffee, black tea, and soda.</li><li>Drinks with alcohol, such as beer, wine, mixed drinks, and liquor.</li></ul>

LATE SIDE EFFECT	DESCRIPTION	WAYS TO MANAGE
Bone Loss	<ul><li>Chemotherapy, steroid medicines, hormonal therapy, or radiation therapy may cause thinning of the bones.</li><li>With radiation therapy, bone loss will occur only in the part of the body that was treated.</li></ul>	After cancer treatment, you should have regular check-ups. During these visits, your doctor or nurse will do a physical exam and may order tests to check for bone loss. You can help lower your risk of bone loss by:<ul><li>Not smoking or using other tobacco products</li><li>Eating foods that are rich in calcium and vitamin D</li><li>Walking, jogging, or doing other weight-bearing exercise</li><li>Limiting how much alcohol you drink</li><li>If you had radiation to the head and neck, also see Mouth Changes for tips on managing bone loss in your jaw.</li></ul>
Brain Changes	Some chemotherapy drugs and radiation therapy to the brain can cause problems months or years after treatment ends. Late effects may include:<ul><li>Memory loss</li><li>Problems doing math</li><li>Problems concentrating</li><li>Slow processing of information</li><li>Personality changes</li><li>Movement problems</li></ul>Radiation to the brain can cause radiation necrosis. This problem may happen when an area of dead tissue forms at the site of the brain tumor. Radiation necrosis can cause movement problems, problems concentrating, slow processing of information, and headaches.	After cancer treatment, you should have regular check-ups. If you have symptoms of brain changes, you will have tests to see whether they are due to the cancer or are late side effects of your treatment. If you have late side effects, your doctor or nurse:<ul><li>Will talk with you about ways to manage late side effects</li><li>May refer you to a physical, occupational, or speech therapist who can help with problems caused by late side effects</li><li>May prescribe medicine or suggest surgery to help with the symptoms</li></ul>

LATE SIDE EFFECT	DESCRIPTION	WAYS TO MANAGE
Eye Problems	Chemotherapy, hormone therapy, immunotherapy, and steroid medicines may increase the risk of cataracts. Cataracts are a problem in which the lens of your eye becomes cloudy. Cataracts can cause: • Blurred, cloudy, or double vision • Sensitivity to light • Trouble seeing at night Some chemotherapy drugs can cause dry eye syndrome. This is a problem in which your eyes do not produce enough tears. • Symptoms include feeling as if your eyes are dry or have something in them.	If you are at risk for cataracts, you should have regular visits with an ophthalmologist (a medical doctor who treats eye problems). • If cataracts become serious, they can be treated with surgery. • In this type of surgery, an eye surgeon will remove the clouded lens and replace it with a plastic lens. You will usually have local anesthesia and be able to go home the same day. If you develop dry eye syndrome, your doctor may prescribe regular treatment with eye drops or ointments.
Hearing Loss	• Watch for signs of hearing loss. Let your doctor know right away if you notice changes in your hearing. • Treatment with certain chemotherapy drugs (in particular, cisplatin and high doses of carboplatin) and high doses of radiation to the brain can cause hearing loss.	• See an audiologist. An audiologist is a professional trained in hearing disorders. • If you had a cancer treatment that can cause hearing loss, you should have at least one visit with an audiologist after you have finished treatment. • Depending on the type and dose of cancer treatment that you received, you may need to see an audiologist more often.

LATE SIDE EFFECT	DESCRIPTION	WAYS TO MANAGE

Heart Problems	Certain cancer drugs, chemotherapy, and radiation therapy to the chest may cause heart problems. Examples of drugs that tend to cause heart problems include:
	• Trastuzumab
	• Doxorubicin
	• Daunorubicin (Cerubidine)
	• Epirubicin (Ellence)
	• Cyclophosphamide (Neosar)
	
	Heart problems caused by cancer treatment may include:
	• A weakening of the heart muscle, which is known as congestive heart failure.
	    o It can cause shortness of breath, dizziness, and swollen hands or feet.
	• Coronary artery disease, which occurs when the small blood vessels that supply blood and oxygen to the heart become narrow.
	    o It can cause chest pain or shortness of breath.
	    o This problem is more common in those who had high doses of radiation therapy to the chest.
		After cancer treatment, you should have regular check-ups. If you have heart problems, your doctor or nurse might suggest that you:
		
		Eat a heart-healthy diet: A heart-healthy diet includes a variety of fruits, vegetables, and whole grains. It also includes lean meats, poultry, fish, beans, and fat-free or low-fat milk or milk products. Your doctor will probably recommend that you follow a diet low in salt, because salt can cause extra fluid to build up in your body, making heart problems worse. *The American Heart Association* has many tips for heart-healthy eating.
		
		Watch fluid intake: Drinking too much fluid can worsen heart problems, so it's important for people who have heart failure to drink the correct amounts and types of fluid. Talk with your doctor about what amounts and types of fluid you should have each day. Let your doctor know right away if you have sudden weight gain. This could mean extra fluid is building up. Also, if you have heart failure, you shouldn't drink alcohol.
		
		Lose weight if you're overweight or obese: Carrying extra weight can put added strain on your heart. Work with your health care team to lose weight safely.
		
		Exercise: The right type and amount of exercise can help keep you and your heart healthy. Talk with your doctor about which activities you can safely do. Exercise can help you become more fit and stay as active as possible.
		
		Quit smoking and avoid using illegal drugs: Talk with your doctor about programs and products that can help you quit smoking. Also, try to avoid secondhand smoke. Smoking and drugs can make heart failure worse and harm your health.
		
		Get enough rest: *See Sleep Problems above under SIDE EFFECT AND POSSIBLE CAUSE.*
		
		Take medicines prescribed by your doctor: Your doctor may prescribe medicines based on the type of heart problem you have, how severe it is, and your response to certain medicines.

LATE SIDE EFFECT	DESCRIPTION	*NON-DRUG TREATMENT FOR HOT FLASHES AND NIGHT SWEATS IN PATIENTS WITH CANCER*	*DRUG TREATMENT FOR HOT FLASHES AND NIGHT SWEATS IN PATIENTS WITH CANCER*
Hot Flashes and Night Sweats	In patients with cancer, hot flashes and night sweats may be caused by the tumor, its treatment, or other conditions. Sweating happens with disease conditions such as fever and may occur without disease in warm climates, during exercise, and during hot flashes in menopause. Sweating helps balance body temperature by allowing heat to evaporate through the skin. Hot flashes and night sweats are common in patients with cancer and in cancer survivors. They are more common in women but can also occur in men. Many patients treated for breast cancer and prostate cancer have hot flashes. Menopause in women can have natural, surgical, or chemical causes. Chemical menopause in women with cancer is caused by certain types of chemotherapy, radiation, or hormone therapy with androgen (a male hormone).	**Treatments that help patients cope with stress and anxiety may help manage hot flashes.** Treatments that change how patients deal with stress, anxiety, and negative emotions may help manage hot flashes. These are called psychological interventions. Psychological interventions help patients gain a sense of control and develop coping skills to manage symptoms. Staying calm and managing stress may lower levels of a hormone called serotonin that can trigger hot flashes. Psychological interventions may help hot flashes and related problems when used together with drug treatment. **Hypnosis may help relieve hot flashes.** Hypnosis is a trance-like state that allows a person to be more aware, focused, and open to suggestion. Under hypnosis, the person can concentrate more clearly on a specific thought, feeling, or sensation without becoming distracted. In hypnosis, a therapist helps the patient to deeply relax and focus on cooling thoughts. This may lower stress levels, balance body temperature, and calm the heart rate and breathing rate. **Comfort measures may help relieve night sweats related to cancer.** Comfort measures may be used to treat night sweats related to cancer. Since body temperature goes up before a hot flash, doing the following may control body	**Hot flashes may be controlled with estrogen replacement therapy.** Hot flashes during natural or treatment-related menopause can be controlled with estrogen replacement therapy. However, many women are not able to take estrogen replacement (for example, women who have or had breast cancer). Hormone replacement therapy that combines estrogen with progestin may increase the risk of breast cancer or breast cancer recurrence. **Other drugs may be useful in some patients.** Studies of non-estrogen drugs to treat hot flashes in women with a history of breast cancer have reported that many of them do not work as well as estrogen replacement or have side effects. Megestrol (a drug like progesterone), certain antidepressants, anticonvulsants, and clonidine (a drug used to treat high blood pressure) are non-estrogen drugs used to control hot flashes. Some antidepressants may change how other drugs, work in the body.

Hot Flashes and Night Sweats
Continued

Treatment for breast cancer and prostate cancer can cause menopause or menopause-like effects, including severe hot flashes.

Certain types of drugs can cause night sweats. Drugs that may cause night sweats include the following:

- Tamoxifen.
- Aromatase inhibitors.
- Opioids.
- Tricyclic antidepressants
- Steroids.

temperature and help control symptoms:

- Wear loose-fitting clothes made of cotton.
- Use fans and open windows to keep air moving.
- Practice relaxation training and slow, deep breathing.

Herbs and dietary supplements should be used with caution.
Most studies of soy and black cohosh show they are no better than a placebo in reducing hot flashes. *Soy contains estrogen -like substances; the effect of soy on the risk of breast cancer growth or recurrence is not clear.* Studies of ground flaxseed to treat hot flashes have shown mixed results. Claims are made about several other plant-based and natural products as remedies for hot flashes. These include dong quai, milk thistle, red clover, licorice root extract, and chaste tree berry. Since little is known about how these products work or whether they affect the risk of breast cancer, women should be cautious about using them.

Acupuncture has been studied in the treatment of hot flashes.
Pilot studies of acupuncture and randomized clinical trials that compare true acupuncture and sham (inactive) treatment have been done in patients with hot flashes and results are mixed. A review of many studies combined showed that acupuncture had slight or no effects in breast cancer patients with hot flashes. (See the Vasomotor symptoms section in the PDQ health professional summary on Acupuncture for more information.)

Side effects of drug therapy may include the following:

- Antidepressants used to treat hot flashes over a short period of time may cause nausea, drowsiness, dry mouth, and changes in appetite.
- Anticonvulsants used to treat hot flashes may cause drowsiness, dizziness, and trouble concentrating.
- Clonidine may cause dry mouth, drowsiness, constipation, and insomnia.

Patients may respond in different ways to drug therapy. It is important that the patient's health care providers know about all medicines, dietary supplements, and herbs the patient is taking.

If one medicine does not improve symptoms, switching to another medicine may help.

LATE SIDE EFFECT	DESCRIPTION	WAYS TO MANAGE
Joint Changes	• Radiation therapy, some chemotherapy drugs, and steroids can cause scar tissue, weakness, and bone loss. • These problems can lead to loss of motion in joints, such as your jaw, shoulders, hips, or knees. • If you receive radiation therapy, these problems will occur only in the part of the body that was treated.	It is important to be aware of early signs of joint problems so these can be addressed before they worsen. These signs include: • Trouble opening your mouth wide • Pain when you make certain movements, such as reaching over your head or putting your hand in a back pocket Talk with your doctor or nurse. He or she may refer you to a physical therapist, which will assess your joint problems and give you exercises to do. Physical therapy exercises can decrease pain, increase strength, and improve movement.
Lung Problems	• Chemotherapy and radiation therapy to the chest may damage the lungs. • Cancer survivors who received both chemotherapy and radiation therapy to the chest may have a higher risk of lung damage. • Lung damage can cause shortness of breath, wheezing, fever, dry cough, congestion, and feeling tired. • Tell your doctor if you have any of these symptoms.	**Oxygen therapy:** If you have serious trouble breathing, your doctor may prescribe oxygen therapy. Oxygen is most often given through nasal prongs or a mask that fits over your mouth and nose. In some cases, you might receive oxygen through a ventilator. **Lose weight if you're overweight or obese:** Excess weight can make it hard to breathe. Work with your doctor and health care team to lose weight safely. **Exercise:** Talk with your doctor about which activities you can safely do. Exercise can help you become more fit and stay as active as possible. **Quit smoking and avoid using illegal drugs:** Talk with your doctor about programs and products that can help you quit smoking. Also, try to avoid secondhand smoke. Smoking and drugs can worsen lung problems and harm your health. For help to quit smoking, visit *Smokefree.gov* or call toll-free, 1-800-QUIT-NOW (1-800-784-8669). **Take medicines prescribed by your doctor:** Your doctor can prescribe medicines to help you relax when it is hard to breathe, relieve discomfort, and treat pain. **Some people with lung problems take steroid pills.** Steroids can interfere with the way the body uses specific nutrients, including calcium, potassium, sodium, protein, and vitamins C and D. If you take steroid pills for lung problems, it is very important to eat a balanced diet. A healthy diet that includes foods from each food group can make up for some of the effects of steroid therapy.

LATE SIDE EFFECT	DESCRIPTION	WAYS TO MANAGE
Mouth Changes	• Radiation therapy to your head or neck and some chemotherapy drugs can cause late side effects in your mouth. • Problems may include dry mouth, cavities, or bone loss in the jaw.	**Visit your dentist** You may be asked to have your teeth checked every 1 to 2 months for at least 6 months after radiation treatment ends. During this time, your dentist will look for changes in your mouth, teeth, and jaw. **Exercise your jaw** Your doctor or nurse may suggest that you open and close your mouth 20 times as far as you can without causing pain, three times a day, even if your jaw isn't stiff. **Stimulate saliva** Your doctor or nurse may suggest that you drink 8 to 10 cups of liquid per day. Keep a water bottle handy so you can sip throughout the day. You may also find sucking on sugarless candy or chewing gum helpful. **Take good care of your teeth and gums** Floss and use a mouthwash with fluoride every day. Brush your teeth after meals and before you go to bed. Also, avoid mouthwashes that contain alcohol. **Explore your treatment options** Ask your dentist to contact your radiation oncologist before you have dental or gum surgery. There may be other treatment options besides surgery. Also, do not have teeth pulled from the part of your mouth that received radiation.
Second Primary Cancer	• Cancer treatment can sometimes cause a new cancer many years after you have finished treatment. • When a new primary cancer occurs in a person with a history of cancer, it is known as a second primary cancer. • Second primary cancers do not occur very often, but they can happen.	• Talk with your doctor about the types of second cancers you may be at risk for. • Have regular check-ups for the rest of your life to check for cancer—the one you were treated for and any new cancer that may occur. Your doctor can suggest tests you may need to look for a new cancer and how often you should have them. • Tell your doctor if you have any new symptoms or problems.

NIH (NCI)
https://www.cancer.gov/about- cancer/treatment/side-effects

Eating Hints: Before, during, and after Cancer Treatment
by the *National Cancer Institute*

Clear Liquids
This list may help if you have appetite loss, constipation, diarrhea, or vomiting.

Soups	• Bouillon • Clear, fat-free broth • Consommé
Drinks	• Clear apple juice • Clear carbonated beverages • Fruit-flavored drinks; Fruit punch • Sports drinks • Water • Weak, caffeine-free tea
Sweets	• Fruit ices made without fruit pieces or milk • Gelatin • Honey • Jelly • Popsicles
Meal replacements and supplements	• Clear nutrition supplements (such as Resource® Breeze) and Carnation® Instant Breakfast® Juice

Full-Liquid Foods
This list may help if you have appetite loss, vomiting, or weight loss.

Cereals	• Refined hot cereals (such as Cream of Wheat®, Cream of Rice®, instant oatmeal, and grits)	
Soups	• Breakfast® Juice • Bouillon • Broth • Soup that has been strained or put through a blender	
Drinks	• Carbonated drinks • Coffee • Fruit drinks • Fruit punch • Milk, Milkshakes	• Smoothies • Sports drinks • Tea • Tomato juice, Vegetable juice • Water
Desserts and snacks	• Custard (soft or baked) • Frozen yogurt • Fruit purees that are watered down • Gelatin • Honey • Ice cream with no chunks (such as nuts or cookie pieces)	• Jelly • Pudding • Sherbet • Sorbet • Syrup • Yogurt (plain or vanilla) • Ice milk
Meal replacements and supplements	• Instant breakfast drinks (such as Carnation® Instant Breakfast®) • Liquid meal replacements (such as Ensure® and Boost®) • Clear nutrition supplements (such as Resource® Breeze, Carnation® Instant Breakfast®Juice, and Ensure®Clear)	

Foods and Drinks that Are Easy on the Stomach		
This list may help if you have nausea or once your vomiting is under control.		
Soups	• Clear broth (such as chicken, vegetable, or beef) • All kinds (strain or puree, if needed), except those made with foods that cause gas, such as dried beans and peas, broccoli, or cabbage	
Drinks	• Clear carbonated drinks that have lost their fizz • Cranberry or grape juice • Fruit-flavored drinks • Fruit punch • Milk • Sports drinks • Tea • Vegetable juices • Water	
Main meals and snacks	• Avocado • Beef, tender cuts only • Cheese, hard, mild types, such as American • Cheese, soft or semi-soft, such as cottage cheese or cream cheese • Chicken or turkey, broiled or baked without skin • Eggs • Fish, poached or broiled • Noodles • Pasta, plain • Peanut butter, creamy, and other nut butters	• Potatoes, without skins, boiled or baked • Pretzels • Refined cold cereals, such as corn flakes, Rice Krispies®, Rice Chex®, and Corn Chex® Refined hot cereals, such as Cream of Wheat® • Saltine crackers • Tortillas, white flour • Vegetables, tender, well-cooked • White bread • White rice • White toast
Desserts	• Angel food cake • Bananas • Canned fruit, such as applesauce, peaches, • and pears • Custard • Frozen yogurt • Gelatin • Ice cream; Ice milk • Lemon drop candy • Popsicles • Pudding • Sherbet; Sorbet • Yogurt (plain or vanilla)	
Meal replacements and supplements	• Instant breakfast drinks (such as Carnation® Instant Breakfast®) • Liquid meal replacements (such as Ensure®) • Clear nutrition supplements (such as Resource® Breeze, Carnation® Instant Breakfast® juice, and Ensure®Clear)	

	Low-Fiber Foods This list may help if you have diarrhea.
Main meals	• Chicken or turkey (skinless and baked, broiled, or grilled) • Cooked refined cereals (such as Cream of Rice®, instant oatmeal, and grits) • Eggs • Fish • Noodles • Potatoes, without skins (boiled or baked) • White bread • White rice
Fruits and vegetables	• Carrots, cooked • Canned fruit, such as peaches, pears, and applesauce • Fruit juice • Mushrooms • String beans, cooked • Vegetable juice
Sweets and snacks	• Angel food cake • Animal crackers • Custard • Gelatin • Ginger snaps • Graham crackers • Saltine crackers • Sherbet • Sorbet • Vanilla wafers • Yogurt (plain or vanilla)
Fats	• Oil • Salad dressing (without seeds) • Butter • Mayonnaise

High-Fiber Foods
This list may help if you have constipation or weight gain.

Main meals	• Bran muffins • Bran or whole-grain cereals • Cooked dried or canned peas and beans, such as lentils or pinto, black, red, or kidney beans • Peanut butter and other nut butters • Soups with vegetables and beans, such as lentil and split pea • Whole-grain cereals, such as oatmeal and shredded wheat • Whole-wheat bread; Whole-wheat pasta
Fruits and vegetables	• Apples • Berries, such as blueberries, blackberries, and strawberries • Broccoli • Brussels sprouts • Cabbage • Corn • Dried fruit, such as apricots, dates, prunes, and raisins • Green leafy vegetables, such as spinach, lettuce, kale, and collard greens • Peas • Potatoes with skins • Spinach • Sweet potatoes; Yams
Snacks	• Bran snack bars • Granola • Nuts • Popcorn • Seeds, such as pumpkin or sunflower • Trail mix

High Protein Foods
It is important to increase your protein to assist with energy and healing.

Drinks	• Whole Milk • Milkshakes • Smoothies made with Milk or Yogurt	
Main Meals and Snacks	• Bean Burger • Beans and Peas • Beef, Chicken, Fish, Turkey • Cheese, including cottage and cream • Custard and Pudding • Eggs • Hummus (chickpea spread)	• Nuts, seeds, wheat germ • Peanut butter and other nut butters • Soups with beans, lentils or peas • Soups, such as chicken or cream • Sour Cream • Yogurt, including frozen
Meal Replacement and Protein Supplements If requiring *Soy Free*, please read ingredients	• Liquid Meal Replacement, such as Ensure®, Boost® or other protein drinks • Use "instant breakfast powder" in milk drinks and desserts • Protein Powders - Mix with ice cream, milk, and fruit flavoring for a high-protein milkshake or smoothie • Powdered Milk – Add to foods, such as milkshakes, smoothies, scrambled eggs	

Foods and Drinks that Are Easy to Chew and Swallow

This list may help if you have dry mouth, sore mouth, sore throat, or trouble swallowing.

Main meals	<ul><li>Baby food</li><li>Casseroles</li><li>Chicken salad</li><li>Cooked refined cereals, such as Cream of Wheat®, Cream of Rice®, instant oatmeal, and grits</li><li>Cottage cheese</li><li>Eggs, soft boiled or scrambled</li><li>Egg salad</li><li>Macaroni and cheese</li><li>Mashed potatoes</li><li>Peanut butter, creamy</li><li>Pureed cooked foods</li><li>Soups</li><li>Stews</li><li>Tuna salad</li><li>Custard</li></ul>
Desserts and Snacks	<ul><li>Flan</li><li>Fruit, pureed or baby food</li><li>Gelatin</li><li>Ice cream</li><li>Milkshakes</li><li>Puddings</li><li>Sherbet</li><li>Smoothies</li><li>Soft fruits, such as bananas or applesauce</li><li>Sorbet</li><li>Yogurt, plain or vanilla</li></ul>
Meal replacements and supplements	<ul><li>Instant breakfast drinks, such as Carnation® Instant Breakfast®</li><li>Liquid meal replacements, such as Ensure®</li><li>Clear nutrition supplements, such as Resource® Breeze, Carnation® Instant Breakfast® juice, and Ensure® Clear</li></ul>

HOME EXERCISE GUIDE - TOC

Quick Summary this Section

Safety First

- Benefits / Before Starting a Routine
- Averages, Body Temperature
- Respiration, Blood Pressure, Heart Rate
- How to Monitor Intensity of Heart Rate
- Temperature – Heat and Cold
- Dehydration; Altitude

Components of a Conditioning Program

- Warm up/cool down
- Duration, Frequency, Intensity & Movement Patterns
- Breathing – Diaphragmatic, Pursed lip and with Exercise
- Equipment That May be Needed

Self-Tests:

- Prior to starting program

Exercise Worksheets:

- Exercises below with:
  - Exercise name and number for section
    - Reps, Sets, How many times a day and how long a stretch should be held (Ex. 20 seconds)

EXERCISE Flexibility (Stretching)	EXERCISE NUMBER	PAGE	REPS	SETS	X DAY	HOLD
PRAYER STRETCH and LATERAL	53					

Exercises:

- Myofascial release
- Flexibility / Stretches / ROM
- Core / Abdominal
- Strengthening - Upper and Lower Extremity
- Balance > Lower Extremity Standing Exercises
- Agility
- Endurance/Aerobic Capacity
- Calories
- Worksheet with room for notes under each section

EXERCISE Core / Stability / Balance	EXERCISE NUMBER	NOTES
PRONE BALL	27	

References

PHYSICAL AND PSYCHOLOGICAL BENEFITS OF KEEPING PHYSICALLY FIT

- Contributes positively to maintaining a healthy weight, building and maintaining healthy bone density, muscle strength, joint mobility, reducing surgical risks, and strengthening the immune system.
- Helps to prevent or treat serious and life-threatening chronic conditions such as high blood pressure, obesity, heart disease, Type 2 diabetes, insomnia, and depression.
- Endurance exercise before meals lowers blood glucose more than the same exercise after meals.
- It also improves mental health, helps prevent depression, helps to promote or maintain positive self-esteem, and can even augment an individual's sex appeal or body image.

(Physical Exercise - Wikipedia)

Before starting a routine here are some factors to consider

AGE	Men over 45 and women over 55 should have medical evaluation before starting a vigorous exercise program. If you will be participating in low to moderate exercise, it is suggested that those with, or have signs and symptoms of cardiopulmonary disease, set up a medical evaluation.
MEDICAL AND PHYSICAL CONDITION	It is very important for you to be aware of any medical or physical problems that may impede your performance. **If you have any of the following issues, please see a medical doctor and/or physical therapist to address issues before starting an exercise program:** • Cardiac issues • Pulmonary issues • Arthritis • Joint pain • Back pain • Diabetes • Acute or Chronic issues, such as, but not limited to, Parkinson's, Stroke, Autoimmune Diseases, Metabolic Disease or Orthopedic disorders/joint replacements.

VITAL SIGN AVERAGES

Adult (resting)

Body Temperature	98.6 Fahrenheit under tongue.
Respiration	12-20 breaths per minute

Blood Pressure
 	
Systolic/Diastolic
	120/80.
	Systolic is when the heart pumps blood to the body / Diastolic is blood that remains in arteries when the heart relaxes.
	Pre-hypertension: 120-139/80-89.
	Hypertension:
	    Stage I 140-159/90-99
	    Stage II over 160/100

Resting pulse	**Men**: 70 beats per minute. **Women:** 75 beats per minute.

HOW to MONITOR EXERCISE INTENSITY

Ways to monitor heart rate (HR):

Talk Test Method	This is a simple, subjective method for the beginner to determine your comfort zone while exercising. Are you able to breathe and talk comfortably throughout the workout without gasping for air? If not, reduce your activity level, catch your breath, and resume at a slower pace.
Heart Rate monitor or Watch	This is a device you wear on your wrist or chest, which allows you to measure your heart rate in real time. These devices range in price at about $50.00 for just a basic HR monitor or higher with other bells and whistles. Some of the popular manufacturers are Fitbit, Apple Watch, Garmin and Samsung Galaxy among others. (See *Target Heart Rate*)
Rate of Perceived Exertion	This method was designed by Dr. Gunnar Borg and is often called the Borg Scale (revised). It rates what you feel your level of exertion is from a scale of 1-10, one being at rest and ten at maximal exertion. A rate of 5-7 is recommended, somewhere between somewhat hard and very hard. Like the talk test method, this is subjective and should be used with HR monitoring.
Training Heart Rate	Measuring Heart Rate: Place your first and second finger over the pulse site and gently apply pressure. Palpate the number of beats for a full minute or 30 sec x 2, 15 sec x 4 or 6 sec x 10. If you have in irregular heartbeat, it is suggested counting the full 60 seconds. Do not use the thumb, as this has its own pulse.
	Take your pulse after you've been exercising for at least five minutes. An easy way to check your pulse without interrupting your workout too much is to take a quick 6-second count and then multiply that number by 10 to get your heart rate in beats per minute (BPM). Make sure your pulse is within your target heart rate zone (*see below*). You can then increase or decrease your intensity based on your heart rate. You can also wear a heart rate monitor.

Radial: Wrist following line from base of thumb.

Carotid: Side of larynx.

Target heart rate range (THR)	**Beginner or low fitness level**: 50-60%
	Intermediate or average fitness level: 60-70%
	Advanced or high fitness level: 75-85%
Percent of maximal heart rate	220 - Age = predicted maximum heart rate (HR). To get the desired exercise intensity, multiply the predicted maximal HR by the percentage. For example, a woman who is 40 years old of Intermediate fitness level would use the following equation at a 70% target heart rate: 220 – 40 (age) =180 predicted maximal HR. 180 x 0.70 (THR) = 126 BPM - desired exercise HR.
Karvonen Formula	Percentage of Heart-rate reserve. This formula factors in the resting HR as well, which will make the target heart rate higher than just the percentage of maximal heart rate. To figure this out, take the predicted maximal heart rate as above with a resting HR prior to exercise. Maximal HR – resting heart rate (RHR) = heart rate reserve; multiply by intensity + RHR + Target HR. See example under Percentage of maximal HR. Rest heart rate = 80. 220 – 40 (age) =180 (as above) – 80 (RHR) = 100 x 0.70 (THR) = 70 + 80 = 150 Target HR.

TEMPERATURE – HEAT and COLD

HEAT

Avoid exercise in the hottest part of the day, as well as in humid weather. People need to sweat to regulate internal body temperature and must evaporate to dissipate heat. During hot, humid weather, sweat cannot evaporate, and therefore cannot cool the body down. It is also important to drink plenty of cool water during exercise, about 7-10 oz. every 10-20 minutes during exercise (see *Dehydration*).

Heat cramps:	• Severe cramps that begin in hands, feet or calves • Hard, tense muscles
Heat exhaustion: Requires immediate medical attention, although not usually life threatening	• Fatigue • Nausea • Headache • Excessive thirst • Muscle aches and cramps • Confusion or anxiety • Weakness • Severe sweats that can be accompanied by cold, clammy skin • Slow heartbeat (decreased pulse rate) • Dizziness or fainting • Agitation
Heat Stroke: Can occur suddenly, with or without warning from heat exhaustion. Obtain immediate medical attention, as this can be *fatal*	• Nausea and vomiting • Headache • Increased body temperature, but DECREASED sweating. • Hot, flushed, DRY skin • Dizziness • Fatigue • Rapid heart rate • Shortness of breath • Decreased urination or may have blood in the urine. • Confusion or loss of consciousness • Convulsions

COLD

It is just as important to drink plenty of water when exercising in the cold weather secondary to increased urine production.   Be sure to dress in layers to help self-regulate body temperature. This simply involves taking off or putting back on clothing as dictated by the changing weather conditions. Choose clothing that will keep moisture out and away from the skin, such as Gortex® brand. Clothing that stays wet because of sweat will decrease your body temperature.

Hypothermia-Mild: A body temperature that is below normal. People with hypothermia are usually not aware of their condition due to confusion or being overly focused on their current activity. Hypothermia may or may not include shivering in the early stages	• Confusion • Lack of coordination • Fatigue • Nausea or vomiting • Dizziness
Hypothermia	• Shivering • Slurred speech • Mumbling • Clumsiness • Difficulty speaking • Stumbling • Poor decision making • Drowsiness • Weak pulse • Shallow breathing • Progressive loss of consciousness

DEHYDRATION

Excessive loss of body fluid (which can include water and solutes, usually sodium or electrolytes). It is also important to drink plenty of cool water during exercise, about 7-10 oz. every 10-20 minutes during exercise. During exercise, sports drinks may be necessary to keep an electrolyte balance as well.

Dehydration-Mild: About 2% of water depletion	• Thirst • Decreased urine volume • Abnormally dark urine • Unexplained tiredness • Irritability • Lack of tears when crying • Headache • Dry mouth • Dizziness when standing due to orthostatic hypotension • May cause insomnia.
Moderate: About 5% -6%of water depletion	• Grogginess or sleepiness • Headache • Nausea • May feel tingling in limbs (parenthesis)
Severe: About 10% -15% of water depletion	• Muscles may become spastic • Skin may shrivel and wrinkle (decreased skin turgor) • Vision may dim • Urination will be greatly reduced and may become painful • Delirium may begin.
Over 15% of water depletion	• Usually, fatal.

COMPONENTS OF A CONDITIONING PROGRAM

WARM UP and COOL DOWN

Warming up and cooling down are very important parts of the exercise routine. There are physical and psychological benefits to both these components that can be as simple as a slow walk before and after your exercise program.

Benefits of warming up	Benefits of cooling down
• Increases the temperature in the muscles, which increases the speed of contraction and relaxation. • Reduces premature lactic acid build up and fatigue during high level exercises. • Increases speed of nerve impulse conduction. • Increases elasticity of connective tissues • Increases muscle metabolism and oxygen consumption that enhances aerobic performance. • Alert for potential muscle injury that may arise during higher intensities. • Increases endorphins. • Allows the heart rate to get to a workable rate for beginning exercise. • Increases production of synovial fluid located between the joints to reduce friction. • Psychological warm up to mentally focus on training and competition.	• Prevents venous blood pooling at the extremities, which reduces chance of dizziness or fainting. • Reduces the potential for Delayed Onset Muscle Soreness (DOMS). • Aids in removing waste products in muscles, such as lactic acid. • Reduces the level of adrenaline and other exercise hormones in the blood to lower the chance of post-exercise disturbances in cardiac rhythm. • Allows the heart to return back safely to resting rate.

Start out every routine with a warmup first. Here are some suggestions

- Walking or outside
- Running up and down some stairs
- Jumping jacks
- Running in place
- Dynamic stretching

Equipment

- Treadmill
- Stationary or Recumbent bike
- Stair climber or Elliptical
- Mini trampoline

Duration, Frequency, Intensity and Movement Patterns

Intensity: How *much* mental and physical *effort* it takes to sustain an activity.	This can be done using the target heart rate range THR (optimum exercise intensity levels through beats per minute, talk test or rate of perceived exertion.
Duration: How *long* the training lasts.	The higher the intensity, the shorter the duration. The American College of Sports Medicine guidelines recommends all healthy adults aged 18–65 yr should participate in moderate intensity aerobic physical activity for a minimum of 30 min on five days per week, or vigorous intensity aerobic activity for a minimum of 20 min on three days per week.
Frequency: How *often* the training occurs,	Training should be performed at least every other day or three days a week. Cardiac/aerobic conditioning can be done daily, although you may want to vary exercises. Regarding strength training, it is important to give each muscle group 48 hours to recover. Alternate upper and lower body with isolated abdomen/core exercises every other day. For those working out several days a week, find a schedule that works for you as long as you give each muscle group 48 hours of recovery time.

Movement Patterns and Examples
 	
Basic movements that help to increase overall body strengthening
	• Bend and Lift: Squats, Dead Lifts and Leg presses
	  o Picking up item off floor
	• Single Leg: Step ups, Single leg stance, Lunges
	  o Walking up steps
	• Push: Shoulder press, Bench press, Push up
	  o Pushing Shopping cart or Lawn mower
	• Pull: Lat pull downs, Seated rows
	  o Vacuuming, Raking
	• Rotational
	  o Shoveling snow

Diaphragmatic Breathing

- Lie either on your back with your knees bent or sit up
- Inhale through your nose; as you do so, allow your stomach to rise. Limit movement in your chest. Attempt to push your bottom ribs out to the side as you breathe in.
- Exhale through your mouth; as you do so, allow your stomach to fall. Limit movement in your chest.
- Repeat for at least 10 cycles.

Pursed Lip Breathing

(PLB) is a breathing technique that consists of inhaling through the nose with the mouth closed and then exhaling through tightly pressed (pursed) lips. This technique is frequently in those with cardiac or respiratory issues.   *"Smell the Roses then Blow Out the Candle".*

Breathing with Exercise

Exhale on the exertion. For example, exhale when you are lying on your back and pushing a weight up or when bending your arm doing a bicep curl,. Inhale as you bring the weight slowly to your chest or when you straighten your arm with a bicep curl..

ANATOMY

ANATOMICAL POSITIONS and PLANES

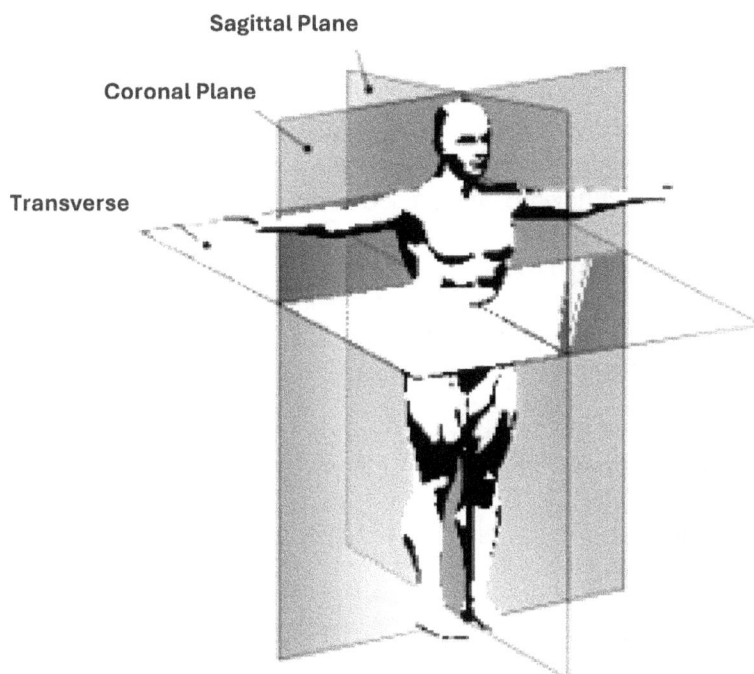

Anterior – Towards the front of the body.

Posterior – Towards the back of the body.

Distal – Away from the body or any point of reference, or from the point of attachment or origin.

Proximal – Closer to the body or any point of reference, or to the point of attachment or origin.

Medial – Situated towards the midline of the body.

Lateral – Position farther from the midline of the body.

Inferior – Away from the head or lower surface of a structure.

Superior – Towards the head or situated above.

Transverse /Axial / Horizontal plane is parallel to the ground, which separates the superior from the inferior or the head from the feet.

Coronal / Frontal/Frontal plane is perpendicular to the ground, which separates the anterior from the posterior or the front from the back

Sagittal / Lateral plane is a Y-Z plane, perpendicular to the ground, which separates left from right.

Upper Extremity (UE): Shoulders, Chest, Arms, Hands, etc

Lower Extremity (LE): Hips, Legs, Ankle Foot , etc

ANATOMICAL DIRECTIONS

Range of Motion (ROM): The distance and direction a joint can move between the flexed and extended position (*see flexion and extension below*). This can also be the act of attempting to increase the distance through therapeutic exercise and/or stretching for physiological gain.

Flexion - Bending movement that decreases the angle between two parts. Bending the knee or elbow are examples of flexion. Flexion of the hip or shoulder moves the limb forward (towards the front of the body).

Extension - The opposite of flexion; a straightening movement that increases the angle between body parts. The knees are extended when standing up. When straightening the arm, the elbow is extended. Extension of the hip or shoulder moves the limb backward (towards the back of the body).

Hyperextension – Extending the joint beyond extension.

Abduction - A lateral movement that pulls a structure or part away from the midline of the body. Raising the arms to the sides is an example of abduction.

Adduction - A medial movement that pulls a structure or part towards the midline of the body, or towards the midline of a limb. Dropping the arms to the sides, or bringing the knees together, are examples of adduction.

Internal rotation (or **medial rotation**). Inward rotary movement around the axis of the bone. Internal rotation of the shoulder or hip would point the toes or the flexed forearm inwards (towards the midline).

External rotation (or **lateral rotation**). External rotary movement around the axis of the bone. It would turn the toes or the flexed forearm outwards (away from the midline).

Elevation - Movement in a superior direction. Shrugging or bringing the shoulders up is an example of elevation.

Depression - Movement in an inferior direction, the opposite of elevation. Pushing the shoulders down is an example of depression.

Pronation - Internal rotation the hand or foot to face downward or posterior. Pronating the foot is a combination of eversion and abduction.

Supination - External rotation of the hand or foot to face upward or anterior. Raising the inside or medial margin of the foot.

Dorsiflexion – Movement at the ankle of the foot superiorly towards the shin. The up position of tapping the foot.

Plantarflexion – Movement at the ankle of the foot inferiorly away from the shin. Pointing the foot downward.

Eversion – Moving the sole of the foot away from the median plane or outward.

Inversion - Moving the sole of the foot towards the median plane or inward.

Ipsilateral – Same side of the body

Contralateral – Opposite side of the body

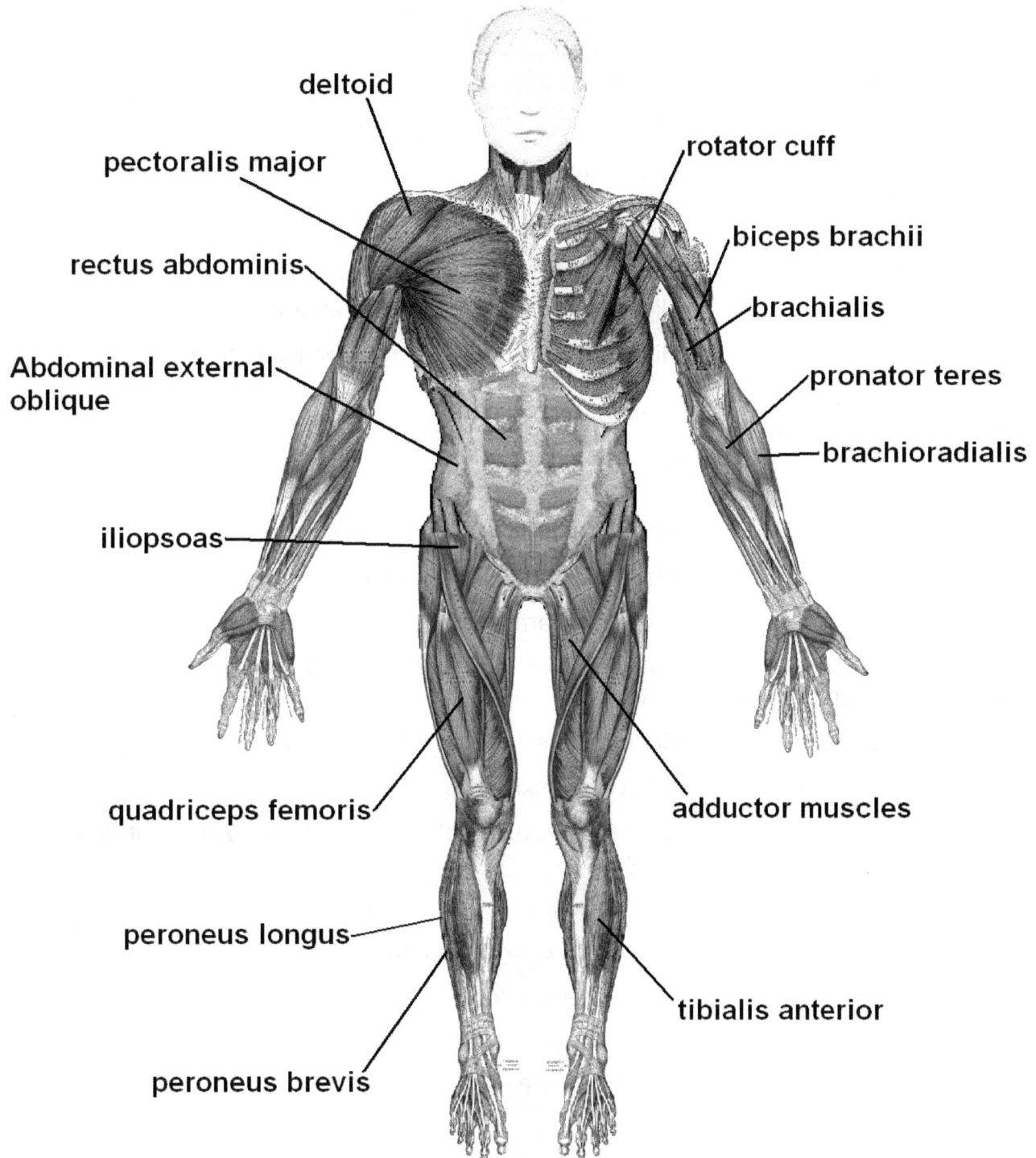

MUSCLES

Grey's Anatomy

ANTERIOR

deltoid

pectoralis major

rectus abdominis

Abdominal external
oblique

iliopsoas

quadriceps femoris

peroneus longus

peroneus brevis

rotator cuff

biceps brachii

brachialis

pronator teres

brachioradialis

adductor muscles

tibialis anterior

Muscle Name (AKA)	Joint Action
Pectoralis major	Shoulder flexion, adduction, internal rotation
Deltoid (anterior)	Shoulder abduction, flexion, internal rotation
Rotator cuff (SITS) Supraspinatus Infraspinatus Teres minor Subscapularis	Shoulder: Supraspinatus: Abduction Infraspinatus: External rotation Teres minor: External rotation Subscapularis: Internal rotation
Biceps brachii	Elbow flexion; Forearm supination
Brachialis	Elbow flexion
Pronator teres	Elbow flexion; Forearm pronation
Brachioradialis	Elbow flexion
Tensor fasciae latae	Hip flexion, medial rotation & abduction
Gracilis*	Hip adduction & internal rotation;Knee flexion & internal rotation
Adductor muscles Adductor magnus, longus & brevis	Hip adduction
Tibialis anterior	Ankle dorsiflexion; foot inversion
Peroneus brevis	Ankle plantarflexion; Foot eversion
Peroneus longus	Ankle plantarflexion; Foot eversion
Rectus femoris (quadriceps femoris)	Hip extension (esp. when knee is extended); Knee flexion
Vastus medialis	Knee extension (esp. when hip is flexed)
Vastus lateralis	Knee extension (esp. when hip is flexed)
Sartorius	Hip flexion & external rotation; Knee flexion & internal rotation
Pectineus	Hip adduction
Iliopsoas, Psosas, Iliacus	Hip flexion & external rotation
Abdominal external oblique	Trunk lateral flexion
Rectus abdominis	Trunk flexion & lateral flexion
Abdominal internal oblique	Trunk lateral flexion

MUSCLES

Grey's Anatomy

POSTERIOR

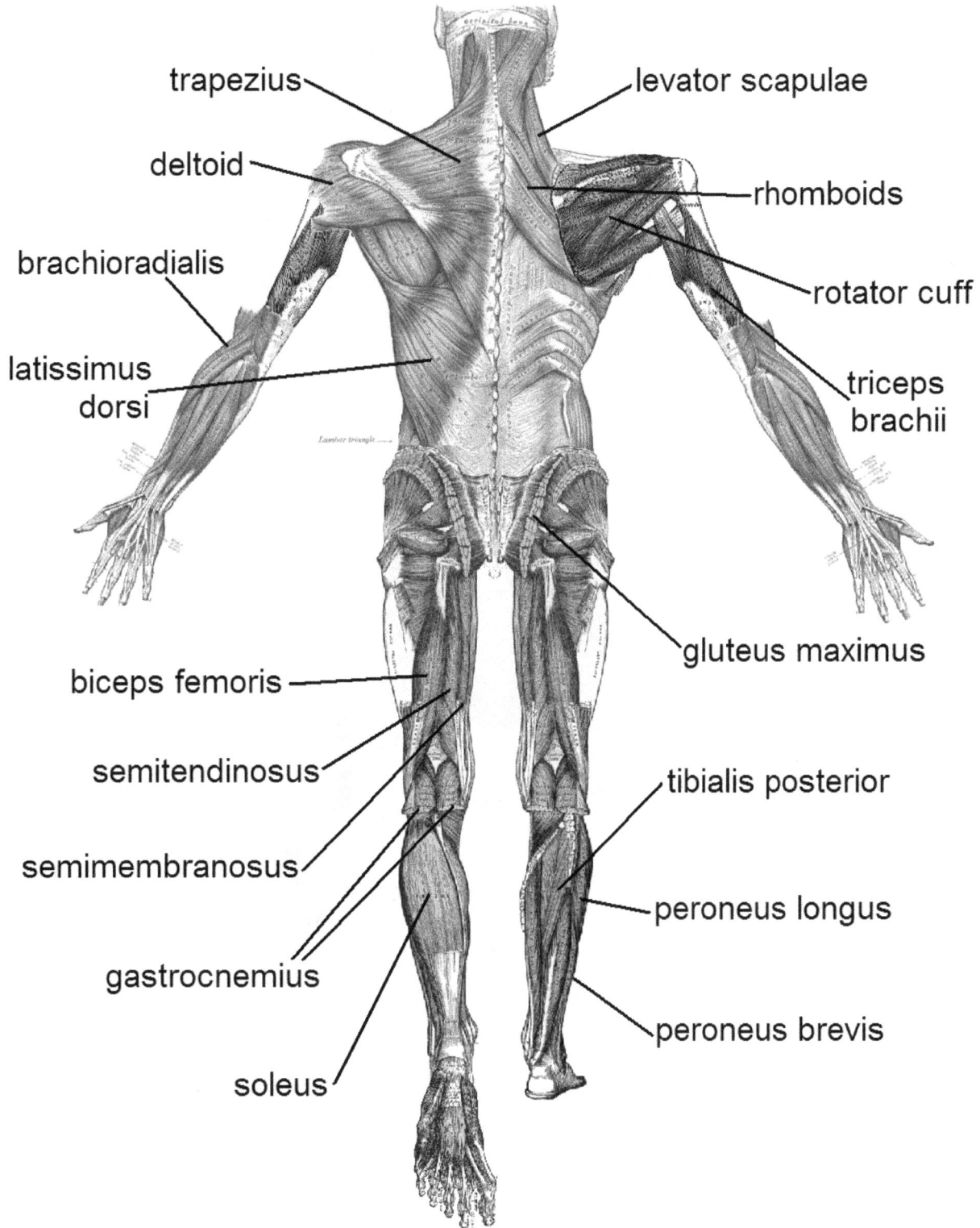

trapezius

levator scapulae

deltoid

rhomboids

brachioradialis

rotator cuff

latissimus
dorsi

triceps
brachii

gluteus maximus

biceps femoris

semitendinosus

tibialis posterior

semimembranosus

peroneus longus

gastrocnemius

peroneus brevis

soleus

Muscle Name (AKA)	Joint Action
Deltoid (posterior)	Shoulder abduction, extension, external rotation
Trapezius	Scapula or Shoulder girdle:, Upper traps: Scapula elevation. Middle traps: Scapula adduction. Lower traps: Scapula depression
Levator scapulae	Scapula elevation
Rhomboids	Scapula adduction & elevation
Triceps brachii	Elbow extension
Gluteus medius	Hip abduction
Gluteus maximus	Hip extension & external rotation
Tibialis, posterior	Inversion, stabilization, assists with plantarflexion
Soleus	Ankle plantarflexion
Gastrocnemius	Knee flexion; Ankle plantarflexion
Semimembranosus	Hip extension & internal rotation; Knee flexion & internal rotation
Semitendinosus	Hip extension & internal rotation; Knee flexion & internal rotation
Biceps femoris (long head)	Hip extension & internal rotation; Knee flexion & external rotation
Latissimus dorsi	Shoulder extension, adduction, internal rotation
Erector spinae, Longissimus, Spinalis, Iliocostalis	Trunk extension, hyperextension & lateral flexion Deep muscle that originate in the posterior iliac crest & sacrum running up the spine and inserts in the transverse process of ribs
Pes anserine, Gracilis, Sartorius, Semimembranosus, Semitendinosus	Internal rotation of tibia when knee is flexed

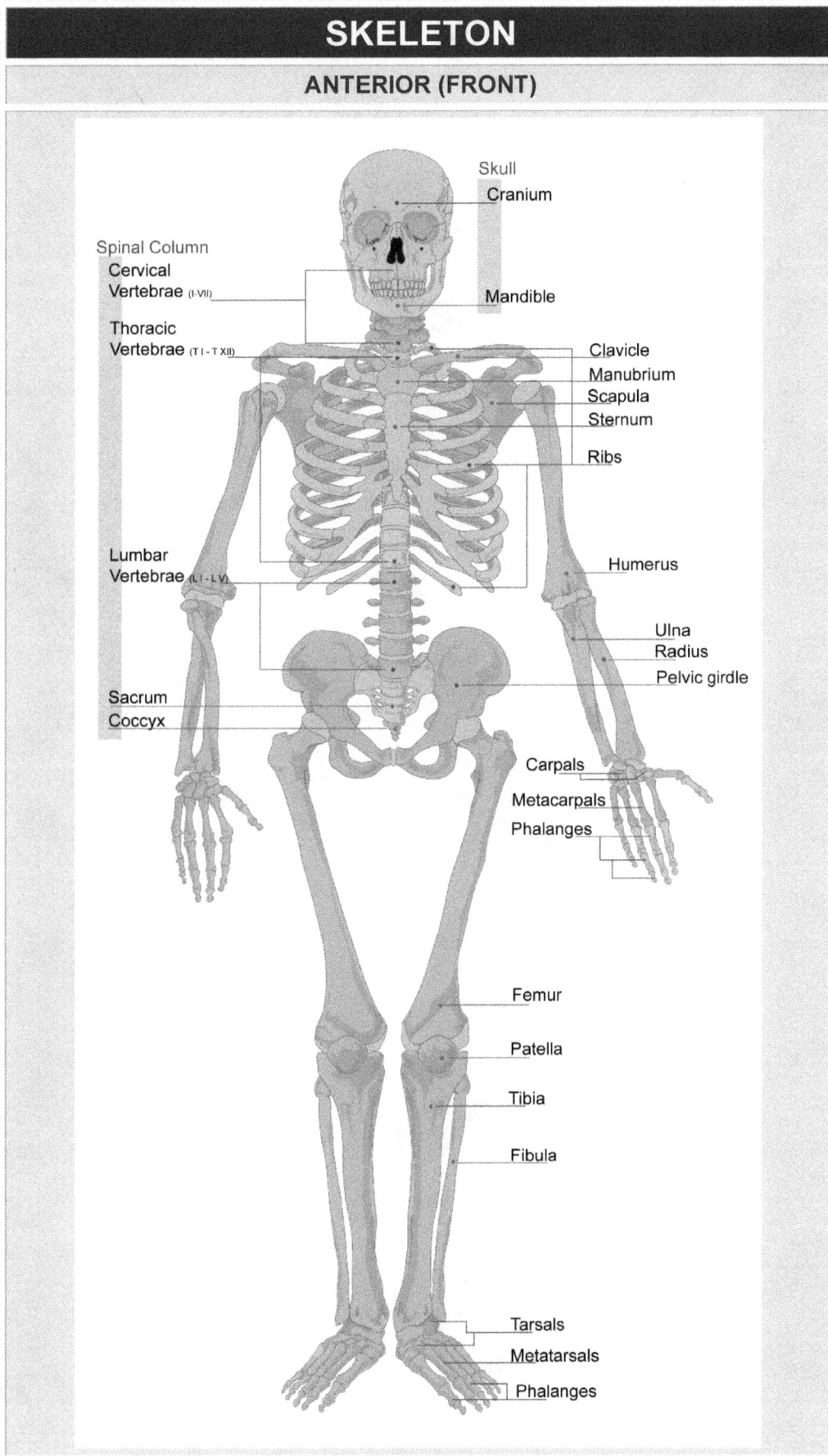

SKELETON

ANTERIOR (FRONT)

Skull
Cranium

Spinal Column
Cervical
Vertebrae (I-VII)

Mandible

Thoracic
Vertebrae (TI - TXII)

Clavicle
Manubrium
Scapula
Sternum

Ribs

Lumbar
Vertebrae (LI - LV)

Humerus

Ulna
Radius
Pelvic girdle

Sacrum
Coccyx

Carpals

Metacarpals

Phalanges

Femur

Patella

Tibia

Fibula

Tarsals

Metatarsals

Phalanges

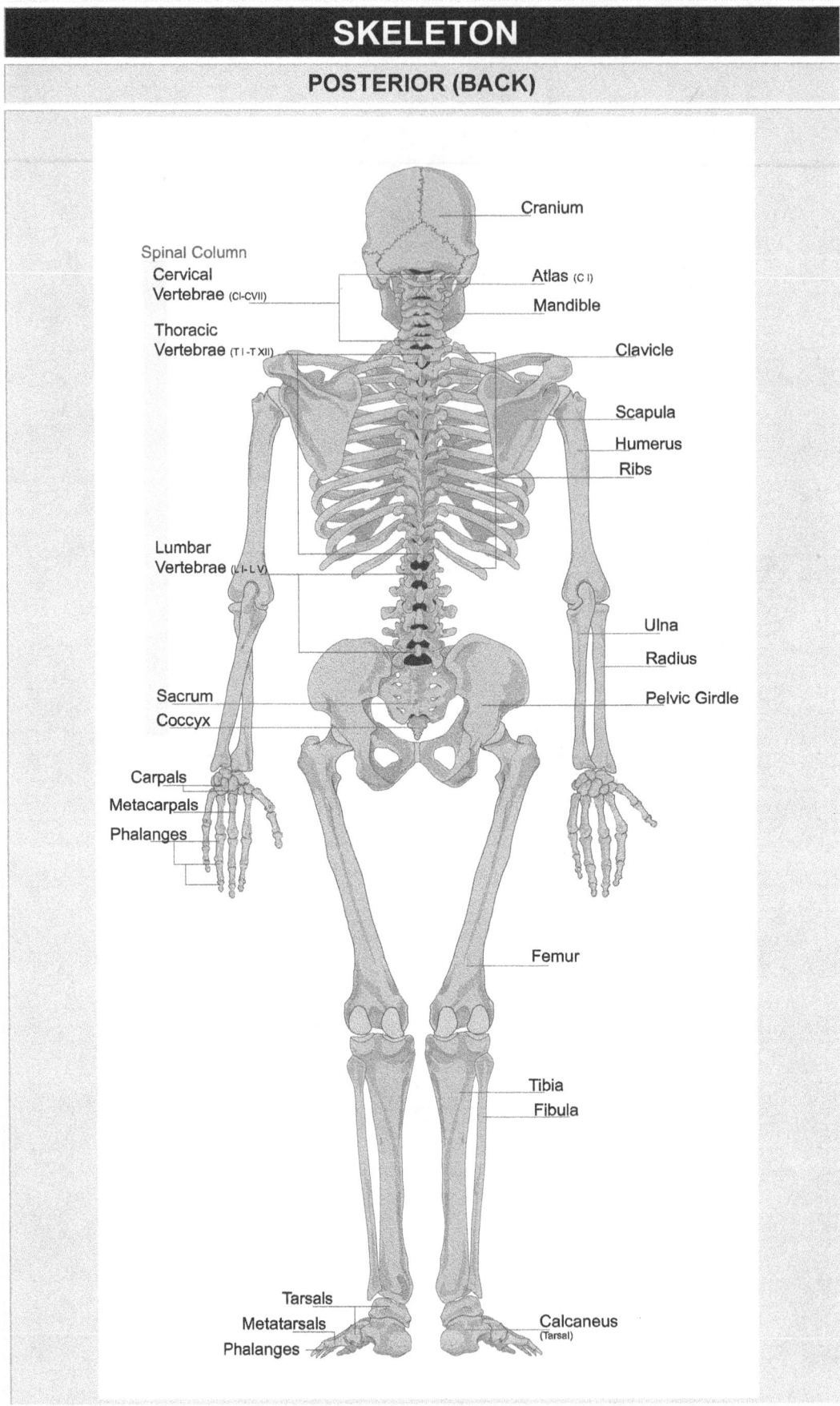

SKELETON

POSTERIOR (BACK)

Cranium

Spinal Column

Cervical
Vertebrae (CI-CVII)

Atlas (C I)

Mandible

Thoracic
Vertebrae (T I -T XII)

Clavicle

Scapula

Humerus

Ribs

Lumbar
Vertebrae (LI-LV)

Ulna

Radius

Sacrum

Coccyx

Pelvic Girdle

Carpals

Metacarpals

Phalanges

Femur

Tibia

Fibula

Tarsals

Metatarsals

Phalanges

Calcaneus
(Tarsal)

Average Joint Range of Motion

Anatomical Positions – Upper Extremity

Joint UPPER EXTREMITY	Movement	Normal Range of Motion (degrees)	Plane
Elbow	Flexion	150	Sagittal
	Extension	0 (neutral)	Sagittal
	Hyperextension	< 10	Sagittal
Shoulder	Flexion	180	Sagittal
	Extension	0 (neutral)	Sagittal
	Hyperextension	60	Sagittal
	Adduction (Add)	0 (neutral)	Frontal
	Abduction (Abd)	180	Frontal
	Horizontal Add/Flexion	130	Transverse
	Horizontal Abd	0 (to neutral)	Transverse
	Horizontal Extension	45	Transverse
	Internal rotation	70	Sagittal
	External rotation	90	Sagittal
Radioulnar	Pronation	90	Transverse
	Supination	90	Transverse

Average Joint Range of Motion

Anatomical Positions – Lower Extremity

Joint LOWER EXTREMITY	Movement	Normal Range of Motion (degrees)	Plane
Knee	Flexion	135	Sagittal
	Extension	0 (neutral)	Sagittal
	Hyperextension	10	Sagittal
Hip	Flexion	120	Sagittal
	Extension	0 (neutral)	Sagittal
	Hyperextension	< 20	Sagittal
	Adduction (Add)	0 (neutral)	Frontal
	Abduction (Abd)	50	Frontal
	Internal rotation	40	Transverse
	External rotation	50	Transverse
Ankle	Dorsiflexion	20	Sagittal
	Plantarflexion	50	Sagittal

EQUIPMENT used in this Book.

Don't buy a lot of equipment before knowing what your goals are.

Stability / Exercise Ball Bosu

These can replace an exercise bench if you do not have the space. It is also used for many of the core strengthening exercises

Should be inflated so that when you sit on it you are at a 90-degree angle.

Dumbbells

Kettle Bell
(optional)

Dowel with/without weight

These will be needed for your strength exercises. See *Strengthening* section on for resistance.

Resistance bands

In different weights/ resistance.

Agility Equipment

Cone hurdles, Speed hurdles, Agility ladder/rings/poles, Bosu, Stair step, Jump rope.

*Balance
Equipment*

Can include
Foam rollers
*(also see
Myofascial below)*

**Balance discs
Balance pad
Cones
Stepper
Bosu**

Exercise Bench (Optional)

The type really depends on what you will use it
for. You can get a plain bench just for support
(as above you can use a stability ball) or you can
get all the bells and whistles. Some have pieces
for leg extensions and curls, as well as arm
pieces for butterflies. If you do not already have
one, I suggest waiting until you start your
exercise program and see what you feel you will
need to advance.

*Examples For
Myofascial*

Massage Ball

*Foam/Textured
Rollers (also
see balance)*

Full Rollers

Half Roller with Flat Bottom

Not Shown

- Exercise mat for floor
  exercises
- **Ankle Weights**
- **Bed, couch or high table/mat**
- **Chair with/without arms -
  High or Low**

- 10-inch play ball
- **Pillow**
- **Towel roll**
- **Strap for stretches**

SELF TESTS

Before starting the exercise program, it is a good idea to see where your baseline is. Taking the following tests will help guide you in the level you will need to start, and help progress by retaking the test periodically. *It is suggested to get a partner to help with both timing and safety, especially with balance tests.* The first 6 tests are modified versions starting at age 60 but are great for adults of any age. Tests 7-10 will help determine how quickly you can advance your balance program.

As with the exercises in this book, these tests should also be performed by those that are otherwise healthy with no chronic or acute ailments OR with supervision of a qualified health coach/personal trainer/physical therapist.

Tests 1-6 should be conducted in the following order if you are doing them at the same time.

A general warm up should be done prior to tests (*see Warm up/Cool down*).
- Stop immediately if any adverse reactions, such as nausea, dizziness, blurred vision, pain of any kind, chest pain, confusion or loss of muscle control.
- Stay hydrated, and do not proceed with testing on days with high temperature/humidity or any other conditions where you would not normally exercise.
- Practice each test several times before attempting to get an accurate score.
- It is advised that you have a second person to time the tests and make sure you are following proper form. Make sure your partner also understands the precautions and goals of these tests.

1. 30 second chair stand - Lower body strength
   - Needed for stair climbing, walking getting up out of tub/chair/car and reduce the risk of falls
2. 30 second arm curl test – Upper body strength
   - Needed to lift and carry everyday items, such as groceries and toolbox
3. 2-minute step test – Aerobic endurance
   - Needed for activities that require endurance, such as walking distance, grocery shopping and climbing stairs
4. Chair sit and reach – Lower body flexibility
   - Needed for normal gait patterns, correct posture, getting in/out of car/tub
5. Back stretch test – Shoulder flexibility
   - Needed to do various activities, such as combing hair and putting on overhead garments
6. 8 foot get up and go – Agility and dynamic balance
   - Needed for pretty much anything you do that requires getting up and walking, such as go to kitchen, bathroom or answering phone.
7. Narrow stance – Balance progression
8. Staggered stance – Balance progression
9. Tandem stance – Balance progression
10. One leg standing – Balance progression

TEST AND PURPOSE	PICTURE	EQUIPMENT NEEDED	EXPLANATION	RESULTS		
30 Second Chair Stand Assess lower body strength *May not want to perform if any chronic pain or back issues. *If you are tall and have had a recent hip replacement skip this or use taller chair.		Straight back or folding chair (~17 inch height) against wall. Stopwatch, wrist watch or clock within view with second hand	*Sit with feet flat on the floor and arms crossed over the chest. *Get up to a full stand and then sit back down. ** Start the time – Immediately repeat as many *full stands* as you can in 30 seconds. *If you cannot stand with hands over chest, try pushing off on your thighs or get a chair with arms and push off arms. If using assist, make sure you note this for progression.*	**Normal Range repetitions**		
				Age	*Men*	*Women*
				60-64	14-19	12-17
				65-69	12-18	11-16
				70-74	12-17	10-15
				75-79	11-17	10-15
				80-84	10-15	9-14
				85-89	8-14	8-13
				90-94	7-12	4-11

TEST AND PURPOSE	PICTURE	EQUIPMENT NEEDED	EXPLANATION	RESULTS		
30 Second Arm Curl Test Upper body strength		Straight back or folding chair without arms. Can be done in standing. Stopwatch or clock within view with second hand Women: 5 lb dumbbell Men: 8 lb dumbbell Can use a wrist weight if arthritis and cannot hold a dumbbell	*Sit with feet flat on the floor towards the edge seat towards dominant side. **Start with the arm extended by your side holding dumbbell in the dominant hand. *Bend elbow with palm facing you keeping the upper arm next to the body (elbow pressed into your side). *Return to starting position. *Keep the wrist straight – do not flex or extend the wrist. **Start the time – Immediately repeat as many arm curls as you can in 30 seconds *with proper form.* *If you cannot hold the suggested weight with proper form, use a lighter weight. Make sure you note this for progression.*	**Normal Range repetitions**		
				Age	*Men*	*Women*
				60-64	16-22	13-19
				65-69	15-21	12-18
				70-74	14-21	12-17
				75-79	13-19	11-17
				80-84	13-19	10-16
				85-89	11-17	10-15
				90-94	10-14	8-13

TEST AND PURPOSE	PICTURE	EQUIPMENT NEEDED	EXPLANATION	RESULTS
2 Minute Step Test Aerobic endurance		Wall for support and to mark step height. Sturdy chair to hold on opposite side if unsteady. Stopwatch or clock within view with second hand	*For accuracy, may need a second person to judge step height and count. *Step with side next to wall. Bring knee up mid-thigh between the knee and the hip. Mark the wall with tape at this height. This will be your minimum step height. *Practice marching in place to this step height. **Start the time – Immediately start marching (not jogging) for 2 minutes. Count the number of *full steps* (both legs) that come up to step height. Every time the right knee reaches proper step height; this is counted as one step. *If shortness of breath, extreme fatigue or unable to continue to step height, stop test and this is your baseline.* *If unable to get to step height, but able to complete 2 minutes. Make sure you note this for progression.* *If unsteady, hold onto chair on opposite side for support.*	**Normal Range steps** See table below

Normal Range steps

Age	Men	Women
60-64	87-115	75-107
65-69	86-116	73-107
70-74	80-110	68-101
75-79	73-109	68-100
80-84	71-103	60-90
85-89	59-91	55-85
90-94	52-86	44-72

TEST AND PURPOSE	PICTURE	EQUIPMENT NEEDED	EXPLANATION	RESULTS
Chair Sit And Reach Lower body flexibility, *primarily hamstrings* *Do not do if recent hip replacement or severe osteoporosis. *Stretch to discomfort, not pain.		Chair (~17 inch height). Make sure chair is secure and does not tip forward. 18 inch ruler or yardstick	*Sit on the edge chair – you should feel the middle of the thigh at the edge of the chair. *Bend one leg with foot flat on floor. *Straighten the target leg in front with heel on the floor and foot flexed up. *Reach forward with one hand over the other and middle fingers even. *Exhale as you bend forward at the hips and reach forward towards or past the toes. Keep the extended knee straight and adjust if it bends. *Practice a few times on both legs to see which one you would prefer for testing. Do two tests and measure as below. **Measure tips of middle fingers to the tip of the shoe (closest to ½ inch). ***The midpoint at the toe of the shoe is considered zero (0), and is scored as such if you reach this point. ***If the reach is short, score this as a minus (-) ***If the reach is past this point, score this as a plus (+)	**Normal Range inches** <table><tr><td>Age</td><td>Men</td><td>Women</td></tr><tr><td>60-64</td><td>-2.5 +4.0</td><td>-0.5 + 5.0</td></tr><tr><td>65-69</td><td>-3.0 +3.0</td><td>-0.5 + 4.5</td></tr><tr><td>70-74</td><td>-3.0 +3.0</td><td>-1.0 + 4.0</td></tr><tr><td>75-79</td><td>-4.0 +2.0</td><td>-1.5 + 3.5</td></tr><tr><td>80-84</td><td>-5.5 +1.5</td><td>2.0 + 3.0</td></tr><tr><td>85-89</td><td>-5.5 +0.5</td><td>-2.5 + 2.5</td></tr><tr><td>90-94</td><td>-6.5 -0.5</td><td>-4.5 + 1.0</td></tr></table>
TEST AND PURPOSE	PICTURE	EQUIPMENT NEEDED	EXPLANATION	RESULTS
Back Stretch Test Shoulder flexibility *Do not do if any upper back, shoulder or neck injuries		18-inch ruler or yardstick	*Will need second person to measure. *Stand and place the target arm over the same shoulder, palm down with fingers extended. Reach down the middle of the back. *Place the opposite arm around the back, palm up reaching up the middle of the back towards other hand. Try to touch middle fingers together or overlap if possible. *Do not overlap fingers and pull.* *Practice a few times on both arms to see which one you would prefer for testing. Do two tests and measure as below. **Measure the distance between tips of middle fingers or overlap. ***If the middle fingers do not touch, score this as a minus (-) ***If the middle fingers just touch, score this as a zero (0) ***If the middle fingers overlap, score this as a plus (+)	**Normal Range inches** <table><tr><td>Age</td><td>Men</td><td>Women</td></tr><tr><td>60-64</td><td>-6.5 +0.0</td><td>-3.0 + 1.5</td></tr><tr><td>65-69</td><td>-7.5 -1.0</td><td>-3.5 + 1.5</td></tr><tr><td>70-74</td><td>-8.0 -1.0</td><td>-4.0 + 1.0</td></tr><tr><td>75-79</td><td>-9.0 -2.0</td><td>-5.0 + 0.5</td></tr><tr><td>80-84</td><td>-9.5 -2.0</td><td>-5.5 + 0.0</td></tr><tr><td>85-89</td><td>-9.5 -3.0</td><td>-7.0 -1.0</td></tr><tr><td>90-94</td><td>-10.5 -4.0</td><td>-8.0 -1.0</td></tr></table>

TEST AND PURPOSE	PICTURE	EQUIPMENT NEEDED	EXPLANATION	RESULTS		
8 Foot Get Up And Go Agility and dynamic balance *If unsteady, have someone by your side in case you lose your balance.		Chair against wall (~17-inch height) Cone or another marker to walk around Stopwatch or clock within view with second hand *Put chair against wall and cone 8 feet in front. Measure from front of chair to back of cone (side facing chair).	*This is done better with a partner watching the clock or a stopwatch. *Sit on chair, back straight, feet flat on floor, one foot slightly in front, torso leaning slightly forward and hands resting on thighs. **Start the time – Immediately get up and walk around the cone (either side) and return to chair. Stopwatch immediately when seated. **Try 2-3x and record the fastest time within 10th /second. *Can use a cane or walker or start from standing position. Make sure you note this for progression.	**Normal Range seconds**		
				Age	*Men*	*Women*
				60-64	5.6-3.8	6.0-4.4
				65-69	5.9-4.3	6.4-4.8
				70-74	6.2-4.4	7.1-4.9
				75-79	7.2-4.6	7.4-5.2
				80-84	7.6-5.2	8.7-5.7
				85-89	8.9-5.5	9.6-6.2
				90-94	10.0-6.2	11.5-7.3

8 feet →

TEST AND PURPOSE	PICTURE	EQUIPMENT NEEDED	EXPLANATION	RESULTS
Narrow Stance Balance progression		Wall, counter or chair within arm's reach for support if needed Stopwatch or clock within view with second hand	Keep your feet together and stand for up to one minute. *Time stops if loss of balance with need to hold on to support.	One minute: Normal *Progress to Staggered Stance Test* *Less than 30 seconds: Continue balance program with wider stance and progress to narrow stance using support. *(See Balance)*
Staggered Stance Balance progression		Wall, counter or chair within arm's reach for support if needed Stopwatch or clock within view with second hand	Stand with one foot in front of the other and slightly off to the side. Stand for up to one minute. Repeat on other side for comparison *Time stops if loss of balance with need to hold on to support.	One minute: Normal *Progress to Tandem Stance Test* *Less than 30 seconds: Continue balance program using support. *(See Balance)*
Tandem Stance Balance progression		Wall, counter or chair within arm's reach for support if needed Stopwatch or clock within view with second hand	Stand with one foot directly in back of the other – toe should be touching the opposite heel. Hold for up to one minute. Repeat on other side for comparison *Time stops if loss of balance with need to hold on to support.	One minute: Normal *Progress to One Leg Standing Balance* *Less than 30 seconds: Continue balance program using support. *(See Balance)*
Single Leg Stance Balance progression		Wall, counter or chair within arm's reach for support if needed Stopwatch or clock within view with second hand	Stand on one leg for up to one minute. Repeat on other side for comparison *Time stops if loss of balance with need to hold on to support or if opposite foot taps the floor	One minute: Normal *Less than 30 seconds: Continue balance program using support. *(See Balance)*

EXERCISE **Myofascial Release**	EXERCISE NUMBER	PAGE	REPS	SETS	X DAY	HOLD
ANTERIOR CHEST - BALL	1					
ANTERIOR CHEST - FOAM ROLL	2					
LATISSIMUS DORSI – BALL	3					
LATISSIMUS DORSI - FOAM ROLL	4					
TRICEP – FOAM ROLL	5					
OCCIPITAL RELEASE - FOAM ROLL	6					
THORACIC MOBILIZATION – SUPINE - FOAM ROLL	7					
THORACIC MOBILIZATION – STANDING - FOAM ROLL	8					
LUMBAR – STANDING – BALL - can do with foam roll	9					
LUMBAR – SUPINE – FOAM ROLLER	10					
HIP FLEXORS - BALL	11					
HIP FLEXORS – FOAM ROLL	12					
QUADRICEPS – BILATERAL - FOAM ROLL	13					
QUADRICEP – SINGLE - FOAM ROLL	14					
GLUTE /PIRIFORMIS - FOAM ROLL	15					
HIP ADDUCTORS – FOAM ROLL	16					
HAMSTRING – BILATERAL - FOAM ROLL	17					
HAMSTRING – SINGLE – FOAM ROLL	18					
CALVES – BILATERAL - FOAM ROLL	19					
CALVES – SINGLE - FOAM ROLL	20					
ILIOTIBIAL BAND (IT Band) - FOAM ROLL	21					
ILIOTIBIAL BAND (IT Band) - BALL	22					
PLANTAR FASCIA ROLLING – BALL	23					
PLANTAR FASCIA ROLLING - COLD SODA CAN	24					

EXERCISE Flexibility (Stretching)	EXERCISE NUMBER	PAGE	REPS	SETS	X DAY	HOLD
INVERSION	1					
EVERSION	2					
ANTERIOR TIBIALIS	3					
PLANTARFLEXION	4					
DORSIFLEXION - STRAP	5					
DORSIFLEXION - FLOOR ASSISTED	6					
STANDING CALF STRETCH - GASTROC	7					
STANDING CALF STRETCH - GASTROC – HAND ON KNEE	8					
GASTROCNEMIUS STAIR STRETCH	9					
STANDING CALF STRETCH - SOLEUS	10					
HAMSTRING STRETCH – TOWEL, BAND, STRAP or BELT	11					
HAMSTRING STRETCH – TOWEL, BAND, STRAP or BELT	12					
HAMSTRING STRETCH - TABLE, BED OR COUCH	13					
HAMSTRING / KNEE EXTENSION STRETCH - SEATED	14					
HAMSTRING STRETCH - STANDING	15					
TOE TOUCH – STANDING - NARROW or WIDE BOS	16					
HEEL SLIDES - SELF ASSISTED	17					
HEEL SLIDES - LONG SIT ASSISTED - TOWEL, BAND, STRAP or BELT	18					
HEEL SLIDES - SUPINE	19					
KNEE BENDS - EXERCISE BALL	20					
KNEE FLEXION – SELF ASSISTED - PRONE	21					
KNEE FLEXION – BELT ASSISTED - PRONE	22					
HEEL SLIDES - SELF ASSISTED	23					
HEEL SLIDES - SEATED	24					
KNEE FLEXION – SCOOT FORWARD - SEATED	25					

EXERCISE Flexibility (Stretching)	EXERCISE NUMBER	PAGE	REPS	SETS	X DAY	HOLD
KNEE FLEXION – STAIR OR STEP	26					
PIRIFORMIS STRETCH	27					
PIRIFORMIS STRETCH - EXERCISE BALL	28					
PIRIFORMIS STRETCH - LONG SIT	29					
PIRIFORMIS STRETCH – STANDING	30					
HIP FLEXOR STRETCH - SIDE OF BALL or CHAIR	31					
HIP FLEXOR STRETCH - STANDING	32					
HIP FLEXOR STRETCH - HALF KNEEL	33					
RUNNER'S STRETCH - MODIFIED	34					
HIP FLEXOR STRETCH – SUPINE	35					
HIP FLEXOR STRETCH – SUPINE - 2	36					
QUAD STRETCH - SIDELYING	37					
QUAD STRETCH - STANDING	38					
KNEE FALL OUT STRETCH or FROG STRETCH	39					
BUTTERFLY STRETCH	40					
HIP ADDUCTOR STRECH – KNEELING	41					
HIP ADDUCTOR STRECH - STANDING	42					
HIP EXTERNAL ROTATION STRETCH - SUPINE	43					
HIP INTERNAL ROTATION STRETCH - SEATED	44					
IT BAND STRETCH - STANDING	45					
IT BAND STRETCH -- SIDELYING	46					
NECK ROTATION and SIDE BENDS	47					
NECK FLEXION AND EXTENSION	48					
TRUNK FLEXION - SEATED	49					
LOW BACK STRETCH - SEATED	50					
LOW BACK STRETCH – STANDING - STRAIGHT & LATERAL	51					
LOW BACK STRETCH – RAIL OR DOORKNOB	52					

EXERCISE Flexibility (Stretching)	EXERCISE NUMBER	PAGE	REPS	SETS	X DAY	HOLD
PRAYER STRETCH and LATERAL	53					
PRAYER STRETCH - EXERCISE BALL	54					
CAT AND CAMEL	55					
KNEE TO CHEST STRETCH - SINGLE and BILATERAL	56					
PRONE ON ELBOWS	57					
PRESS UPS	58					
TRUNK ROTATION STRETCH – SINGLE LEG	59					
LOWER TRUNK ROTATIONS – BILATERAL	60					
TRUNK ROTATION - SEATED	61					
TRUNK ROTATION - STANDING or SEATED – DOWEL	62					
LATERAL TRUNK STRETCH - SINGLE, SEATED or STANDING	63					
LATERAL TRUNK STRETCH - BILATERAL SEATED or STANDING	64					
FLEXION - SUPINE - DOWEL	65					
WALL WALK	66					
FLEXION - TABLE SLIDE	67					
FLEXION - TABLE SLIDE - BALL	68					
EXTERNAL ROTATION - SUPINE – DOWEL *INTERNAL ROTATION ON OPPOSITE ARM*	69					
EXTERNAL ROTATION - 90-90 - DOWEL	70					
EXTERNAL ROTATION – SEATED – DOWEL *INTERNAL ROTATION ON OPPOSITE ARM*	71					
EXTERNAL ROTATION – STANDING – DOWEL *INTERNAL ROTATION ON OPPOSITE ARM*	72					
ABDUCTION - TABLE SLIDE - BALL	75					
ABDUCTION WITH DOWEL	76					
LYING DOWN EXTENSION - TABLE or BED	77					
WAND EXTENSION - STANDING	78					
CHEST STRETCH – SEATED, STANDING, or SUPINE	79					

EXERCISE **Flexibility (Stretching)**	EXERCISE NUMBER	PAGE	REPS	SETS	X DAY	HOLD
TRICEP STRETCH - STRAP or TOWEL	82					
POSTERIOR SHOULDER/DELTOID RELEASE	83					
POSTERIOR CAPSULE STRETCH	84					

EXERCISE Core / Stability	EXERCISE NUMBER	PAGE	REPS	SETS	X DAY	HOLD
ABDOMINAL BRACING TRAINING	1					
ABDOMINAL BRACING - SUPINE	2					
PELVIC TILT - SUPINE	3					
PELVIC TILT - KNEELING	4					
BRIDGING	5					
BRIDGE - BOSU	6					
BRIDGING WITH PILLOW SQUEEZE	7					
BRIDGING WITH PILLOW SQUEEZE - BOSU	8					
BRACE SUPINE MARCHING / BRIDGE LEG UP	9					
BRIDGE LEG UP - BOSU -	10					
SINGLE LEG BRIDGE	11					
BRIDGE SINGLE LEG - BOSU	12					
BRIDGING CROSSED LEG	13					
BRIDGING CROSSED LEG – BOSU	14					
BRIDGING CROSSED LEG - ARMS UP	15					
BRIDGING CROSSED LEG - ARMS UP - BOSU	16					
BRIDGE - ELASTIC BAND	17					
BRIDGING - ABDUCTION - ELASTIC BAND	18					
FLOOR BRIDGE - EXERCISE BALL	19					
FLOOR BRIDGE ALTERNATE LEG LIFT - EXERCISE BALL	20					
BRIDGE UPPER BACK - EXERCISE BALL	21					
BRIDGE UPPER BACK - SINGLE LEG - EXERCISE BALL	22					
QUADRUPED ALTERNATE ARM	23					
QUADRUPED ALTERNATE LEG	24					
QUADRUPED ALTERNATE ARM AND LEG	25					
BIRD DOG ELBOW TOUCHES	26					

EXERCISE	EXERCISE NUMBER	PAGE	REPS	SETS	X DAY	HOLD
Core / Stability						
PRONE BALL	27					
PRONE BALL - ALTERNATE ARM	28					
PRONE BALL - ALTERNATE LEG	29					
PRONE BALL - ALTERNATE ARM AND LEG	30					
MODIFIED PLANK	31					
MODIFIED PLANK - ALTERNATE LEG	32					
FULL PLANK	33					
PLANK - ALTERNATE ARMS	34					
PLANK - ALTERNATE LEGS	35					
PLANK - EXERCISE BALL	36					
PRONE ON ELBOWS	37					
PRESS UPS	38					
SKYDIVER	39					
PRONE SUPERMAN - BOSU	40					
TRUNK EXTENSION - BOSU	41					
TRUNK EXTENSION - HANDS CROSSED IN FRONT - BOSU	43					
SUPERMAN - ARMS BACK- EXERCISE BALL	44					
SUPERMAN – BOTH ARMS IN FRONT - EXERCISE BALL	45					
SUPERMAN – ONE ARM FORWARD / ONE ARM BACK - EXERCISE BALL	46					
LATERAL PLANK MODIFIED	47					
LATERAL PLANK MODIFIED- BOSU	48					
LATERAL PLANK - 1 KNEE 1 FOOT	49					
LATERAL PLANK - 1 KNEE 1 FOOT – BOSU	50					
LATERAL PLANK	51					
LATERAL PLANK - BOSU	52					

EXERCISE Core / Stability	EXERCISE NUMBER	PAGE	REPS	SETS	X DAY	HOLD
LEAN BACK	53					
LEAN BACK - BOSU	54					
LEAN BACK WITH ARMS OUT	55					
LEAN BACK WITH ARMS OUT - BOSU	56					
LEAN BACK WITH TWIST	57					
LEAN BACK WITH TWIST – BOSU	58					
CRUNCHY FROG	59					
SEATED BIKE - FORWARD AND BACKWARDS	60					
CRUNCH – ARMS OUT	61					
CRUNCH – ARMS OUT - BOSU	62					
CRUNCH – ARMS IN BACK OF HEAD	63					
CRUNCH – ARMS IN BACK OF HEAD - BOSU	64					
OBLIQUE CRUNCH	65					
OBLIQUE CRUNCH - BOSU	66					
90 DEGREE CRUNCH	67					
BALL CRUNCH – Can put legs on seat of chair	68					
CURL UPS – ARMS ON LEGS - EXERCISE BALL	69					
CURL UPS- ARMS CROSSED IN FRONT - EXERCISE BALL	70					
CURL UPS – ARMS BEHIND HEAD - EXERCISE BALL	71					
SUPINE CRUNCH TOUCH - EXERCISE BALL	72					
LOWER ABDOMINAL CRUNCH – WITH or WITHOUT BALL	73					
HIGH MARCH CRUNCH	74					
STANDING SIDE CRUNCH	75					
STANDING BIKE CRUNCH	76					

EXERCISE Lower Extremity - Lying & Seated Strengthening and Range of Motion	EXERCISE NUMBER	PAGE	REPS	SETS	X DAY	HOLD
INVERSION – SEATED - ELASTIC BAND	1					
INVERSION – SEATED - ELASTIC BAND - 2	2					
EVERSION – SEATED - ELASTIC BAND	3					
EVERSION – SEATED - ELASTIC BAND - 2	4					
ANKLE PUMPS - SEATED	5					
ANKLE PUMPS – SUPINE or FEET UP ON STOOL	6					
DORSIFLEXION – SEATED - ELASTIC BAND	7					
DORSIFLEXION – SEATED - ELASTIC BAND - 2	8					
PLANTARFLEXION - STRAP	9					
PLANTARFLEXION - SEATED – ELASTIC BAND	10					
HEEL SLIDES - SUPINE	11					
HEEL SLIDES - RESISTED EXTENSION – ELASTIC BAND	12					
QUAD SET –ISOMETRIC	13					
QUAD SET WITH TOWEL UNDER HEEL - ISOMETRIC	14					
SHORT ARC QUAD (SAQ) – SELF ASSISTED	15					
SHORT ARC QUAD - (SAQ)	16					
KNEE EXTENSION - SELF ASSISTED	17					
PARTIAL ARC QUAD - LOW SEAT	18					
LONG ARC QUAD (LAQ) – LOW SEAT (90 deg)	19					
LONG ARC QUAD (LAQ) – LOW SEAT - ANKLE WEIGHTS	20					
LONG ARC QUAD (LAQ) - HIGH SEAT	21					
LONG ARC QUAD (LAQ) - HIGH SEAT - ANKLE WEIGHTS	22					
LONG ARC QUAD - ELASTIC BAND – HAND HELD	23					
LONG ARC QUAD - ELASTIC BAND	24					

EXERCISE Lower Extremity - Lying & Seated Strengthening and Range of Motion	EXERCISE NUMBER	PAGE	REPS	SETS	X DAY	HOLD
HAMSTRING CURLS - PRONE - ASSISTED	25					
HAMSTRING CURLS - PRONE	26					
HAMSTRING CURLS - - PRONE - WEIGHTS	27					
HAMSTRING CURLS – PRONE - ELASTIC BAND	28					
HAMSTRING CURLS – ELASTIC BAND	29					
HAMSTRING CURLS – ELASTIC BAND - 2	30					
HAMSTRING CURLS ON BALL	31					
HAMSTRING CURLS - SINGLE LEG - EXERCISE BALL	32					
HIP FLEXION ISOMETRIC	33					
HIP FLEXION ISOMETRIC BILATERAL	34					
HIP FLEXION – ISOMETRIC	35					
STRAIGHT LEG RAISE (SLR)	36					
STRAIGHT LEG RAISE (SLR) – ANKLE WEIGHTS	37					
STRAIGHT LEG RAISE (SLR) - ELASTIC BAND	38					
SEATED MARCHING	39					
SEATED MARCHING - ELASTIC BAND	40					
HIP EXTENSION - PRONE	41					
HIP EXTENSION – PRONE – ANKLE WEIGHTS	42					
HIP EXTENSION – PRONE – ELASTIC BAND	43					
HIP EXTENSION – QUADRUPED	44					
HIP ABDUCTION - SUPINE	45					
HIP ABDUCTION - SUPINE – ANKLE WEIGHTS	46					
HIP ABDUCTION – SUPINE - ELASTIC BAND	47					
HIP ABDUCTION / CLAMS– SUPINE - ELASTIC BAND	48					
MODIFIED HIP ABDUCTION – SIDELYING	49					

EXERCISE Lower Extremity - Lying & Seated Strengthening and Range of Motion	EXERCISE NUMBER	PAGE	REPS	SETS	X DAY	HOLD
HIP ABDUCTION – SIDELYING	50					
HIP ABDUCTION – SIDELYING - WEIGHTS	51					
HIP ABDUCTION – SIDELYING - ELASTIC BAND	52					
CLAM SHELLS	53					
SIDELYING CLAM - ELASTIC BAND	54					
HIP ABDUCTION - FIRE HYDRANT - QUADRUPED	55					
HIP ABDUCTION - FIRE HYDRANT – QUADRUPED - ELASTIC BAND	56					
HIP ABDUCTION - SEATED - STRAIGHT LEG	57					
HIP ABDUCTION - SEATED - STRAIGHT LEG – ANKLE WEIGHT	58					
HIP ABDUCTION - SINGLE- SEATED	59					
HIP ABDUCTION - SINGLE- SEATED – ELASTIC BAND	60					
HIP ABDUCTION - BILATERAL- SEATED	61					
HIP ABDUCTION - BILATERAL- SEATED - ELASTIC BAND	62					
HIP ADDUCTION SQUEEZE – SUPINE – KNEES BENT	63					
HIP ADDUCTION SQUEEZE – SUPINE – LEGS STRAIGHT	64					
HIP ADDUCTION - SIDELYING	65					
INTERNAL ROTATION - HEEL SQUEEZE - ISOMETRIC	67					
HIP INTERNAL ROTATION - SUPINE	68					
REVERSE CLAMS - SIDELYING	69					
REVERSE CLAMS - SIDELYING - ELASTIC BAND	70					
HIP INTERNAL ROTATION - SEATED	71					
HIP INTERNAL ROTATION - ELASTIC BAND	72					
HIP EXTERNAL ROTATION - SUPINE	73					

EXERCISE **Lower Extremity - Lying & Seated Strengthening and Range of Motion**	EXERCISE NUMBER	PAGE	REPS	SETS	X DAY	HOLD
HIP EXTERNAL ROTATION - ELASTIC BAND	74					
HIP ROTATIONS – BILATERAL - SIDELYING	75					
HIP ROTATION - SEATED - BALL and ELASTIC BAND	76					
PRESS – BILATERAL – ELASTIC BAND	77					
PRESS – SINGLE LEG – ELASTIC BAND	78					
HIP HIKE - STANDING	79					
HIP HIKE – KNEELING	80					
GLUTE SETS - PRONE	81					
GLUTE SET - SUPINE	82					
GLUTE SQUEEZE - SITTING	83					
GLUTE SCULPT (MAX/MEDIUS)	84					

EXERCISE **Upper Extremity Strengthening and Range of Motion**	EXERCISE NUMBER	PAGE	REPS	SETS	X DAY	HOLD
ELBOW FLEXION EXTENSION - SUPINE	1					
ELBOW FLEXION / EXTENSION - GRAVITY ELIMINATED	2					
BICEPS CURLS – ALTERNATING	3					
BICEPS CURL - SELF FIXATION – ELASTIC BAND	4					
SEATED BICEPS CURLS - ALTERNATING	5					
SEATED BICEPS CURLS - BILATERAL	6					
CONCENTRATION CURLS – SITTING	7					
PREACHER CURL ON BALL	8					
BICEPS CURLS	9					
BICEPS CURLS - RADIOBRACHIALIS - HAMMER CURL	10					
BICEPS CURLS - BRACHIALIS	11					
BICEPS CURLS – ROTATE OUTWARD	12					
BICEPS CURLS – ONE ARM - ELASTIC BAND	13					
BICEPS CURLS – BILATERAL - ELASTIC BAND	14					
BICEPS CURLS - RADIOBRACHIALIS - HAMMER CURL – ONE ARM - ELASTIC BAND	15					
BICEPS CURLS - RADIOBRACHIALIS - HAMMER CURL – BILATERAL - ELASTIC BAND	16					
BICEPS CURLS – BRACHIALIS - ONE ARM - ELASTIC BAND	17					
BICEPS CURL – BRACHIALIS – BILATERAL - ELASTIC BAND	18					
TRICEPS - SELF FIXATION - ELASTIC BAND	19					
OVERHEAD TRICEPS - SELF FIXATION –SEATED OR STANDING - ELASTIC BAND	20					
TRICEP EXTENSION – SITTING OR STANDING - WEIGHT	21					
TRICEP EXTENSION – SITTING OR STANDING – BILATERAL - WEIGHT	22					
ELBOW EXTENSION - BALL	23					

EXERCISE **Upper Extremity Strengthening and Range of Motion**	EXERCISE NUMBER	PAGE	REPS	SETS	X DAY	HOLD
ELBOW EXTENSION - SKULL CRUSHER - BALL	24					
TRICEPS - ELASTIC BAND	25					
TRICEPS - BENT OVER	26					
CHAIR DIPS / PUSH UPS	27					
DIPS OFF CHAIR	28					
PENDULUM SHOULDER FORWARD/BACK	29					
PENDULUM SHOULDER – SIDE TO SIDE	30					
PENDULUM SHOULDER CIRCLES	31					
PENDULUMS - SUPINE	32					
ISOMETRIC FLEXION	33					
SHOULDER FLEXION – SIDELYING	34					
FLEXION – SUPINE - SINGLE OR BILATERAL	35					
FLEXION – SUPINE – SINGLE OR BILATERAL - WEIGHT	36					
FLEXION – SUPINE - DOWEL	37					
FLEXION – SUPINE - DOWEL - Weight	38					
FLEXION - SELF FIXATION – ELASTIC BAND	39					
FLEXION – ELASTIC BAND	40					
FLEXION - STANDING - PALMS DOWN / OVERHAND DOWEL	41					
FLEXION - STANDING - PALMS UP / UNDERHAND DOWEL	42					
FLEXION – PALMS FACING INWARD	43					
FLEXION – PALMS DOWN	44					
V RAISE	45					
V RAISE – WEIGHTS	46					
MILITARY PRESS – DOWEL	47					
MILITARY PRESS - FREE WEIGHTS	48					

EXERCISE Upper Extremity Strengthening and Range of Motion	EXERCISE NUMBER	PAGE	REPS	SETS	X DAY	HOLD
ISOMETRIC EXTENSION	49					
PRONE EXTENSION - EXERCISE BALL	50					
SHOULDER EXTENSION - STANDING	51					
SHOULDER EXTENSION - STANDING - WEIGHTS	52					
EXTENSION – STANDING – DOWEL	53					
EXTENSION - SELF FIXATION - ELASTIC BAND	54					
EXTENSION - ELASTIC BAND	55					
EXTENSION - BILATERAL - ELASTIC BAND	56					
INTERNAL ROTATION – ISOMETRIC	57					
INTERNAL ROTATION - ISOMETRIC- ELEVATED	58					
INTERNAL ROTATION - SIDELYING	59					
INTERNAL ROTATION - ELASTIC BAND	60					
INTERNAL / EXTERNAL ROTATION - STANDING – DOWEL	61					
INTERNAL ROTATION – DOWEL	62					
EXTERNAL ROTATION - ISOMETRIC	63					
EXTERNAL ROTATION - ISOMETRIC – ELEVATED	64					
EXTERNAL ROTATION WITH TOWEL - SIDELYING	65					
EXTERNAL ROTATION – 90/90 - WEIGHTS	66					
EXTERNAL ROTATION - BILATERAL - ELASTIC BAND	67					
EXTERNAL ROTATION - ELASTIC BAND	68					
ADDUCTION – ISOMETRIC	69					
ADDUCTION - ELASTIC BAND	70					
ABDUCTION – ISOMETRIC	71					
HORIZONTAL ABDUCTION - DOWEL	72					

EXERCISE Upper Extremity Strengthening and Range of Motion	EXERCISE NUMBER	PAGE	REPS	SETS	X DAY	HOLD
HORIZONTAL ABDUCTION/ADDUCTTION - SUPINE	73					
HORIZONTAL ABDUCTION/ADDUCTTION - SUPINE -WEIGHT	74					
ABDUCTION - SIDELYING	75					
HORIZONTAL ABDUCTION - SIDELYING	76					
ABDUCTION – WEIGHT	77					
ABDUCTION – ELASTIC BAND	78					
HORIZONTAL ABDUCTION – BILATERAL - ELASTIC BAND	79					
90/90 ABDUCTION - WEIGHT	80					
LATERAL RAISES	81					
LATERAL RAISES – LEAN FORWARD	82					
LATERAL RAISES – LEAN FORWARD - ARM ROTATION	83					
FRONTAL RAISE – WEIGHTS	84					
UPRIGHT ROW – WEIGHTS	85					
UPRIGHT ROW – ELASTIC BAND	86					
SHRUGS	87					
SHRUGS - WEIGHTS	88					
SHOULDER ROLLS	89					
SHOULDER ROLLS - WEIGHTS	90					
SCAPULAR RETRACTIONS - BILATERAL	91					
SCAPULAR RETRACTION – SINGLE ARM	92					
ELASTIC BAND SCAPULAR RETRACTIONS WITH MINI SHOULDER EXTENSIONS	93					
PRONE RETRACTION	94					
SCAPULAR PROTRACTION - SUPINE - BILATERAL	95					
SCAPULAR PROTRACTION - SUPINE - WEIGHT	96					

EXERCISE **Upper Extremity Strengthening and Range of Motion**	EXERCISE NUMBER	PAGE	REPS	SETS	X DAY	HOLD
SCAPULAR PROTRACTION - SUPINE - ELASTIC BAND	97					
SCAPULAR PROTRACTION / TABLE PLANK	98					
CHEST PRESS – SEATED or STANDING - ELASTIC BAND	99					
CHEST PRESS – BALL, FLOOR or BENCH- WEIGHTS	100					
DOWEL PRESS – STANDING	101					
CHEST PRESS – STANDING or SEATED	102					
BENT OVER ROWS	103					
ROWS – PRONE	104					
ROWS - ELASTIC BAND	105					
WIDE ROWS - ELASTIC BAND	106					
LOW ROW – ELASTIC BAND	107					
HIGH ROW – ELASTIC BAND	108					
FLY'S – FLOOR - WEIGHT	109					
FLY'S – BALL or BENCH – WEIGHT	110					
WALL PUSH UPS	111					
WALL PUSH UP - BALL	112					
WALL PUSH UP - Triceps uneven	113					
WALL PUSH UP - Hands inverted	114					
WALL PUSH UP - Narrow	115					
WALL PUSH UP – Wide	116					
PUSH UPS - BALL	117					
PUSH UP - MODIFIED	118					
PUSH UP	119					
PUSH UP -DIAMOND	120					
PUSH UP – MODIFIED - BOSU - UNSTABLE	121					

EXERCISE **Upper Extremity Strengthening and Range of Motion**	EXERCISE NUMBER	PAGE	REPS	SETS	X DAY	HOLD
PUSH UP – BOSU - UNSTABLE	122					
PUSH UP – MODIFIED – INVERTED BOSU - UNSTABLE	123					
PUSH UP – INVERTED BOSU - UNSTABLE	124					

EXERCISE Balance / Standing Exercises	EXERCISE NUMBER	PAGE	REPS	SETS	X DAY	HOLD
WIDE BOS DECREASING TO NARROW BOS	1					
NARROW BOS	2					
ARM MOVEMENT	3					
TRUNK ROTATION	4					
EYES SHUTS	5					
HEAD TURNS	6					
READING ALOUD	7					
BALANCE PAD	8					
SPLIT STANCE – SEMI TANDEM	9					
SPLIT STANCE - *Progression*	10					
TANDEM- SHARPENED ROMBERG STANCE	11					
TANDEM STANCE - Progression	12					
SINGLE LEG STANCE (SLS)	13					
SINGLE LEG STANCE (SLS) - *Progression*	14					
SLS – LEG FORWARD	15					
SLS – LEG BACKWARDS	16					
SLS – LEG FORWARD / OPPOSITE ARM UP	17					
SLS – LEG BACKWARDS / OPPOSITE ARM UP	18					
SLS - REACH FORWARD	19					
SLS - REACH TWIST	20					
SINGLE LEG TOE TAP	21					
SINGLE LEG STANCE - CLOCKS	22					
BALL ROLLS - HEEL TOE	23					
BALL ROLLS - LATERAL	24					
SQUAT	25					
SIT TO STAND	26					

EXERCISE Balance / Standing Exercises	EXERCISE NUMBER	PAGE	REPS	SETS	X DAY	HOLD
SQUATS – WALL WITH BALL	27					
SQUATS WITH WEIGHTS	28					
MINI SQUAT - UNSTABLE SUPPORT - FOAM PAD	29					
SQUATS - SINGLE LEG	30					
SIDE TO SIDE WEIGHT SHIFT	31					
FORWARD AND BACKWARDS WEIGHT SHIFTS	32					
SPLIT STANCE WEIGHT SHIFT SIDE TO SIDE	33					
SPLIT STANCE WEIGHT SHIFT FORWARD AND BACKWARDS	34					
WALL FALLS - FORWARD - BALANCE DRILL	35					
WALL FALLS - LATERAL - BALANCE DRILL	36					
WALL FALLS - BACKWARDS - BALANCE DRILL	37					
WALL FALLS - SINGLE LEG - FORWARD - BALANCE DRILL	38					
WALL FALLS - SINGLE LEG - LATERAL - BALANCE DRILL	39					
WALL FALLS - SINGLE LEG - MEDIAL - BALANCE DRILL	40					
WALL FALLS - SINGLE LEG - BACKWARDS - BALANCE DRILL	41					
FALL LATERAL - STEP RECOVERY	42					
FALL FORWARD - STEP RECOVERY	43					
FALL BACKWARD - STEP RECOVERY	44					
TOE TAP ABDUCTION	45					
HIP ABDUCTION - STANDING	46					
HIP EXTENSION – STANDING	47					
HIP FLEXION - STANDING – STRAIGHT LEG RAISE	48					
HIP / KNEE FLEXION - SINGLE LEG	49					
STANDING MARCHING	50					

EXERCISE Balance / Standing Exercises	EXERCISE NUMBER	PAGE	REPS	SETS	X DAY	HOLD
HAMSTRING CURL	51					
TOE RAISES	52					
TOE RAISES IR AND ER	53					
ONE LEGGED TOE RAISE	54					
SINGLE LEG BALANCE FORWARD	55					
SINGLE LEG BALANCE LATERAL	56					
SINGLE LEG BALANCE RETRO	57					
SINGLE LEG STANCE RETROLATERAL	58					
SQUAT	59					
SINGLE LEG SQUAT	60					
LUNGE – STATIC	61					
LUNGE FORWARD/BACKWARD	62					
FOUR CORNER MARCHING IN PLACE	63					
FOUR CORNER MARCHING IN PLACE WITH HEAD TURNS	64					
WALKING ON HEELS FORWARD AND BACKWARDS	65					
WALKING ON TOES FORWARD AND BACKWARDS	66					
TANDEM STANCE AND WALK – FORWARD AND BACKWARDS	67					
RUNNING MAN	68					
HOP STICK - FORWARD	69					
HOP STICK - BACKWARDS	70					
MINI LATERAL LUNGE	71					
SIDE STEPPING	72					
HOP STICK - LATERAL	73					
SINGLE LEG DEAD LIFT	74					

EXERCISE Balance / Standing Exercises	EXERCISE NUMBER	PAGE	REPS	SETS	X DAY	HOLD
CONE TAPS - SINGLE LEG STANCE	75					
CONE TAPS - SINGLE LEG STANCE - UNSTABLE	76					
FIGURE 8 AROUND CONES	77					
FIGURE 8 AROUND CONES – FOOT OR HAND TAP	78					
BALANCE DOUBLE LEG STANCE - WIDE	79					
BALANCE DOUBLE LEG STANCE - NARROW	80					
TANDEM STANCE	81					
TANDEM WALK	82					
SINGLE LEG STANCE - ABDUCTION	83					
SINGLE LEG STANCE - ABDUCTION	84					
SINGLE LEG STANCE – FORWARD KICK	85					
SINGLE LEG STANCE – HAMSTRING CURL	86					
SINGLE LEG SQUAT – LEG FORWARD	87					
SINGLE LEG SQUAT – LEG BACKWARDS	88					
TOE TAP OR HEEL PLACEMENT	89					
PULL UP FOOT TOUCHES ON STEP	90					
ALTERNATING SUSTAINED FOOT TOUCHES ON STEP	91					
STEP UP AND OVER	92					
FORWARD SWING THROUGH STEP	93					
SIDE STEPPING - *REPEAT STEPS 89-93 from a side approach.*	94					

EXERCISE Agility/Reactivity/Speed	EXERCISE NUMBER	PAGE	REPS	SETS	X DAY	HOLD
Four Square Drills	1					
Dots	2					
Ladder Drills	3					
Box Drills	4					
Cones	5					
Hurdles	6					

Myofascial Release

Myofascial release (MFR, self-myofascial release) is an alternative medicine therapy that claims to treat skeletal muscle immobility and pain by relaxing contracted muscles, improving blood and lymphatic circulation, and stimulating the stretch reflex in muscles.

Fascia is a thin, tough, elastic type of connective tissue that wraps most structures within the human body, including muscle. Fascia supports and protects these structures. Osteopathic theory proposes that this soft tissue can become restricted due to psychogenic disease, overuse, trauma, infectious agents, or inactivity, often resulting in pain, muscle tension, and corresponding diminished blood flow. (Wikipedia - *https://en.wikipedia.org/wiki/Myofascial_release*)

Possible Benefits of Myofascial Release

- Muscle relaxation
- Improves muscular and joint range of motion
- Reduces muscle soreness and improves tissue recovery
- Encourages the flow of lymph.
- Improves neuromuscular efficiency.
- Reduces adhesions and scar tissue.
- Releases trigger point (sensitivity and pain) – brings in blood flow and nutrient exchange.
- Maintains normal functional muscular length / Provides optimal length-tension relationship.
- Corrects muscle imbalances

USE

- Roll on foam roller or ball until you find the sore spot or trigger point. When you find this point, stop and rest on it or decrease the range to this particular area and hold for 10-20 seconds.
- Apply pressure to muscle area only. Try not to roll over bones, joints or directly on the spine (you can use a ball over the muscles on the side of the spine).
- Use this as a part of your warmup for particular areas you are exercising that day (for instance the hamstrings, calves and quadricep on leg strengthening day)
- You can use this technique on additional days for trouble areas and can even devote a dedicated session for whole body myofascial release.

Equipment Needed: FOAM ROLLER and/or TEXTURED or SOFT MASSAGE BALL

WARNING POST BREAST SURGERY OR RADIATION THAT INVOLVE LYMPH NODES:
DO NOT perform myofasical release over these regions.
This will compress the areas and potentially worsen lymphedema. Massage can be done by a practitioner that specializes in breast rehab for axillary web syndrome.
Please see entire section on breast cancer

EXERCISE Myofascial Release	EXERCISE NUMBER	NOTES
ANTERIOR CHEST - BALL	1	
ANTERIOR CHEST - FOAM ROLL	2	
LATISSIMUS DORSI – BALL	3	
LATISSIMUS DORSI - FOAM ROLL	4	
TRICEP – FOAM ROLL	5	
OCCIPITAL RELEASE - FOAM ROLL	6	
THORACIC MOBILIZATION – SUPINE - FOAM ROLL	7	
THORACIC MOBILIZATION – STANDING - FOAM ROLL	8	
LUMBAR – STANDING – BALL - can do with foam roll	9	
LUMBAR – SUPINE – FOAM ROLLER	10	
HIP FLEXORS - BALL	11	
HIP FLEXORS – FOAM ROLL	12	
QUADRICEPS – BILATERAL - FOAM ROLL	13	
QUADRICEP – SINGLE - FOAM ROLL	14	
GLUTE /PIRIFORMIS - FOAM ROLL	15	
HIP ADDUCTORS – FOAM ROLL	16	
HAMSTRING – BILATERAL - FOAM ROLL	17	
HAMSTRING – SINGLE – FOAM ROLL	18	
CALVES – BILATERAL - FOAM ROLL	19	
CALVES – SINGLE - FOAM ROLL	20	
ILIOTIBIAL BAND (IT Band) - FOAM ROLL	21	
ILIOTIBIAL BAND (IT Band) - BALL	22	
PLANTAR FASCIA ROLLING – BALL	23	
PLANTAR FASCIA ROLLING - COLD SODA CAN	24	

Myofascial Release

_____ Reps _____ Sets _____X Day _____Hold		_____ Reps _____ Sets _____X Day _____Hold
1	Notes:	**2**	Notes:

ANTERIOR CHEST - BALL

Face towards the wall and place small ball at the outside of chest. Bend knees up and down to find the target point and hold.

ANTERIOR CHEST - FOAM ROLL

Lie face down so that a foam roll is under the upper part of your arm and chest. Using your other arm and legs, roll forward and back across this area.

_____ Reps _____ Sets _____X Day _____Hold		_____ Reps _____ Sets _____X Day _____Hold
3	Notes:	**4**	Notes:

LATISSIMUS DORSI – BALL

Turn with your target side towards the wall and place small ball on the side under the shoulder. Bend knees up and down to find the target point and hold.

LATISSIMUS DORSI - FOAM ROLL

Lie on your side so that a foam roll is under the upper part of your arm and back. Using your other arm and legs, roll forward and back across this area.

_____ Reps _____ Sets _____ X Day _____ Hold	_____ Reps _____ Sets _____ X Day _____ Hold
5 Notes:	**6** Notes:

TRICEP – FOAM ROLL

In a sidelying position, place your tricep on the foam roll. Use the opposite arm and your body to help roll out the arm on the foam roll.

OCCIPITAL RELEASE - FOAM ROLL

Lie on your back and put a foam roll under the back of your head. Turn your head slowly from side to side.

_____ Reps _____ Sets _____ X Day _____ Hold	_____ Reps _____ Sets _____ X Day _____ Hold
7 Notes:	**8** Notes:

THORACIC MOBILIZATION – SUPINE - FOAM ROLL

Lie on a foam roller. While supporting your neck, roll up and down your mid-back.

THORACIC MOBILIZATION – STANDING - FOAM ROLL

Stand with a foam roll behind your upper back. Slowly perform mini-squats and allow the foam roller to roll up and down your back for a self-massage.

	_____ Reps _____ Sets _____ X Day _____ Hold		_____ Reps _____ Sets _____ X Day _____ Hold
9	Notes:	**10**	Notes:

LUMBAR – STANDING – BALL - can do with foam roll

Place small ball in lower back on the side of the spine. DO NOT roll directly over the spine. Slowly perform mini-squats and allow the ball to roll up and down your back for a self-massage.
*Can use foam roll behind lower back and follow above directions.

LUMBAR – SUPINE – FOAM ROLLER

Lie on a foam roll under the lower back. While supporting your upper body, roll up and down your lower back.

	_____ Reps _____ Sets _____ X Day _____ Hold		_____ Reps _____ Sets _____ X Day _____ Hold
11	Notes:	**12**	Notes:

HIP FLEXORS - BALL   **Ball under hip flexor**

Lie on your stomach and place small ball under hip flexor. Roll up and down ball making small movements and hold on the target muscle.

HIP FLEXORS – FOAM ROLL

Lie on your stomach and place foam roll under both hip flexors. Roll up and down avoiding rolling directly over hip bones.

	_____ Reps _____ Sets _____X Day _____Hold
13	Notes:

QUADRICEPS – BILATERAL - FOAM ROLL

Lie face down so that a foam roll is under the top of your thighs. Using your arms propped on your elbows, roll forward and back across this area.

	_____ Reps _____ Sets _____X Day _____Hold
14	Notes:

QUADRICEP – SINGLE - FOAM ROLL

Lie face down so that a foam roll is under the top of your target thigh. Cross your other leg over the top of your target leg. Using your arms propped on your elbows, roll forward and back across this area.

	_____ Reps _____ Sets _____X Day _____Hold
15	Notes:

GLUTE /PIRIFORMIS - FOAM ROLL

Sit on a foam roll and cross your affected leg on top of your other knee. Lean slightly towards your target side. Using your arms and unaffected leg roll forward and back across your buttock area.

	_____ Reps _____ Sets _____X Day _____Hold
16	Notes:

HIP ADDUCTORS – FOAM ROLL

Lie on your stomach supported by arms and lace your inner thigh on the roller. Roll and compress the target thigh muscle.

	_____ Reps _____ Sets _____X Day _____Hold	
17	Notes:	

HAMSTRING – BILATERAL - FOAM ROLL

Sit on a foam roll under both thighs. Using your arms, roll forward and back across this area

	_____ Reps _____ Sets _____X Day _____Hold	
18	Notes:	

HAMSTRING – SINGLE – FOAM ROLL

Sit on a foam roll under thigh. Using your arms, roll forward and back across this area.

	_____ Reps _____ Sets _____X Day _____Hold	
19	Notes:	

CALVES – BILATERAL - FOAM ROLL

Sit with the foam roll under your both your calves. Lift your body up with your arms and roll forward and back across your calf area. Try turning toes in and out to access the inside and outside of calf areas. Do not roll in the crease of your knee.

	_____ Reps _____ Sets _____X Day _____Hold	
20	Notes:	

CALVES – SINGLE - FOAM ROLL

Sit with the foam roll under your target calf and cross your other leg on top. Lift your body up with your arms and roll forward and back across your calf area. Do not roll in the crease of your knee.

_____ Reps _____ Sets _____ X Day _____ Hold

21 | Notes:

ILIOTIBIAL BAND (IT Band) - FOAM ROLL

Lie on your side with a foam roll under your bottom thigh. Use your arms and unaffected leg and then roll up and down the foam roll along the outside of your thigh.

_____ Reps _____ Sets _____ X Day _____ Hold

22 | Notes:

ILIOTIBIAL BAND (IT Band) - BALL

Lie on your side or sit in chair. Hold small ball and move along the outside of the thigh. Hold on the target muscle.

_____ Reps _____ Sets _____ X Day _____ Hold

23 | Notes:

PLANTAR FASCIA ROLLING – BALL

Sit and place ball under foot. Roll plantar fascia over ball back and forth.

_____ Reps _____ Sets _____ X Day _____ Hold

24 | Notes:

PLANTAR FASCIA ROLLING - COLD SODA CAN

Sit and place cold soda can under foot. Roll plantar fascia over can back and forth.

Flexibility (Stretching)

Range of motion within a joint across various planes of motion that can be increased with stretching. This is needed to prevent decreased range of motion in a joint. Joint mobility can be inhibited by body habitués, genetics, connective tissue elasticity, skin that surrounds the joint, or the joint itself.

Some of the benefits of stretching: *(ACE Personal Training Manual)*	• Increased physical efficiency and performance. • Decreased risk of injury by decreasing resistance in various tissues. • Increased blood supply and nutrients to joint structures. • Improved nutrient exchange by increasing the quantity and decreasing the thickness of synovial fluid in the joint. • Increased neuromuscular coordination. • Improved muscular balance and postural awareness. • Reduced muscular tension. *(Bryant & Daniel, Ace Personal Training Manual, 2003, pg 306-307)*
Things to remember when stretching	• It is always better to stretch a warm muscle (*see Warm up and Cool down*) when the tissue temperature is above normal. Think of putting an elastic band in the freezer compared to heating it before stretching. Which do you think will get a better stretch? • Static stretching is best for the type for beginning athletes. Static stretching is a slow, gradual lengthening of the connective tissue (tendon, muscles and ligaments) through a full range of motion to the point of discomfort – not pain. This stretch should be held for at least 30 seconds, but no longer than two minutes. • Dynamic stretching consists of controlled leg and arm swings that take you to the limits of your range of motion. This type of stretching is appropriate to perform part of a warmup and/or cool down. • Ballistic stretching is a rapid, bouncing movement that may be appropriate in some sports. The problem is that there is also a high-risk factor for injury and should only be done with a professional's guidance. • Again, always remember to warm up before stretching. Repeat all stretches 2-3 times and hold for 15-30 seconds up to 60 seconds) unless otherwise indicated. • Some evidence shows that static stretching may be more beneficial at the end of the exercise program when there is more certainty that the muscles have warmed up. • Dynamic stretching may be more beneficial at the beginning of the exercise program as part of your warmup. This can also be done at the end as part of the cool down.

EXERCISE Flexibility (Stretching)	EXERCISE NUMBER	NOTES
INVERSION	1	
EVERSION	2	
ANTERIOR TIBIALIS	3	
PLANTARFLEXION	4	
DORSIFLEXION - STRAP	5	
DORSIFLEXION - FLOOR ASSISTED	6	
STANDING CALF STRETCH - GASTROC	7	
STANDING CALF STRETCH - GASTROC – HAND ON KNEE	8	
GASTROCNEMIUS STAIR STRETCH	9	
STANDING CALF STRETCH - SOLEUS	10	
HAMSTRING STRETCH – TOWEL, BAND, STRAP or BELT	11	
HAMSTRING STRETCH – TOWEL, BAND, STRAP or BELT	12	
HAMSTRING STRETCH - TABLE, BED OR COUCH	13	
HAMSTRING / KNEE EXTENSION STRETCH - SEATED	14	
HAMSTRING STRETCH - STANDING	15	
TOE TOUCH – STANDING - NARROW or WIDE BOS	16	
HEEL SLIDES - SELF ASSISTED	17	
HEEL SLIDES - LONG SIT ASSISTED - TOWEL, BAND, STRAP or BELT	18	
HEEL SLIDES - SUPINE	19	
KNEE BENDS - EXERCISE BALL	20	
KNEE FLEXION – SELF ASSISTED - PRONE	21	
KNEE FLEXION – BELT ASSISTED - PRONE	22	
HEEL SLIDES - SELF ASSISTED	23	
HEEL SLIDES - SEATED	24	
KNEE FLEXION – SCOOT FORWARD - SEATED	25	

EXERCISE Flexibility (Stretching)	EXERCISE NUMBER	NOTES
KNEE FLEXION – STAIR OR STEP	26	
PIRIFORMIS STRETCH	27	
PIRIFORMIS STRETCH - EXERCISE BALL	28	
PIRIFORMIS STRETCH - LONG SIT	29	
PIRIFORMIS STRETCH – STANDING	30	
HIP FLEXOR STRETCH - SIDE OF BALL or CHAIR	31	
HIP FLEXOR STRETCH - STANDING	32	
HIP FLEXOR STRETCH - HALF KNEEL	33	
RUNNER'S STRETCH - MODIFIED	34	
HIP FLEXOR STRETCH – SUPINE	35	
HIP FLEXOR STRETCH – SUPINE - 2	36	
QUAD STRETCH - SIDELYING	37	
QUAD STRETCH - STANDING	38	
KNEE FALL OUT STRETCH or FROG STRETCH	39	
BUTTERFLY STRETCH	40	
HIP ADDUCTOR STRECH – KNEELING	41	
HIP ADDUCTOR STRECH - STANDING	42	
HIP EXTERNAL ROTATION STRETCH - SUPINE	43	
HIP INTERNAL ROTATION STRETCH - SEATED	44	
IT BAND STRETCH - STANDING	45	
IT BAND STRETCH -- SIDELYING	46	
NECK ROTATION and SIDE BENDS	47	
NECK FLEXION AND EXTENSION	48	
TRUNK FLEXION - SEATED	49	
LOW BACK STRETCH - SEATED	50	
LOW BACK STRETCH – STANDING - STRAIGHT & LATERAL	51	
LOW BACK STRETCH – RAIL OR DOORKNOB	52	

EXERCISE **Flexibility (Stretching)**	EXERCISE NUMBER	NOTES
PRAYER STRETCH and LATERAL	53	
PRAYER STRETCH - EXERCISE BALL	54	
CAT AND CAMEL	55	
KNEE TO CHEST STRETCH - SINGLE and BILATERAL	56	
PRONE ON ELBOWS	57	
PRESS UPS	58	
TRUNK ROTATION STRETCH – SINGLE LEG	59	
LOWER TRUNK ROTATIONS – BILATERAL	60	
TRUNK ROTATION - SEATED	61	
TRUNK ROTATION - STANDING or SEATED – DOWEL	62	
LATERAL TRUNK STRETCH - SINGLE, SEATED or STANDING	63	
LATERAL TRUNK STRETCH - BILATERAL SEATED or STANDING	64	
FLEXION - SUPINE - DOWEL	65	
WALL WALK	66	
FLEXION - TABLE SLIDE	67	
FLEXION - TABLE SLIDE - BALL	68	
EXTERNAL ROTATION - SUPINE – DOWEL *INTERNAL ROTATION ON OPPOSITE ARM*	69	
EXTERNAL ROTATION - 90-90 - DOWEL	70	
EXTERNAL ROTATION – SEATED – DOWEL *INTERNAL ROTATION ON OPPOSITE ARM*	71	
EXTERNAL ROTATION – STANDING – DOWEL *INTERNAL ROTATION ON OPPOSITE ARM*	72	
ABDUCTION - TABLE SLIDE - BALL	75	
ABDUCTION WITH DOWEL	76	
LYING DOWN EXTENSION - TABLE or BED	77	
WAND EXTENSION - STANDING	78	
CHEST STRETCH – SEATED, STANDING, or SUPINE	79	

EXERCISE **Flexibility (Stretching)**	EXERCISE NUMBER	NOTES
TRICEP STRETCH - STRAP or TOWEL	82	
POSTERIOR SHOULDER/DELTOID RELEASE	83	
POSTERIOR CAPSULE STRETCH	84	

Stretching / Range of Motion (ROM)

Inversion

	_____ Reps _____ Sets _____X Day _____Hold
1	Notes:

INVERSION

Sit and cross your legs so that the target leg is on top. Hold your foot and pull upwards until a stretch is felt along the side of your ankle.

Eversion

	_____ Reps _____ Sets _____X Day _____Hold
2	Notes:

EVERSION

Sit and cross your legs so that the target leg is on top. Hold your foot and push downward until a stretch is felt along the inner side of your ankle.

Anterior Tibialis (Ant Tib)

	_____ Reps _____ Sets _____X Day _____Hold
3	Notes:

ANTERIOR TIBIALIS

Kneel upright and slowly sit back onto legs forcing heels down towards floor. Sit back until stretch is felt.

Plantarflexion (PF) *DF not shown*

	_____ Reps _____ Sets _____X Day _____Hold
4	Notes:

PLANTARFLEXION

Sit and place your affected foot on a firm surface. Use one hand bend the ankle downward as shown.

DORSIFLEXION – *Not shown*
Sit and place your affected foot on a firm surface. Use one hand under foot to push up towards shin (see #5 for movement)

Dorsiflexion (DF)

_____ Reps _____ Sets _____X Day _____Hold		_____ Reps _____ Sets _____X Day _____Hold
5	**Notes:** *Lymphedema: Do not wrap band around UE or LE	**6**	**Notes:**

DORSIFLEXION - STRAP

Sit with heel on floor and leg straight. Place belt/strap on forefoot and pull back until stretch is felt.

DORSIFLEXION - FLOOR ASSISTED

Sit and slide your foot back towards under the chair until a stretch is felt at the ankle.

Gastroc/Soleus

_____ Reps _____ Sets _____X Day _____Hold		_____ Reps _____ Sets _____X Day _____Hold
7	**Notes:**	**8**	**Notes:**

Target Leg

STANDING CALF STRETCH - GASTROC

Stand in front of a wall, chair, or other sturdy object. Step forward with one foot and maintain your toes on both feet to be pointed straight forward. Keep the leg behind you with a straight knee during the stretch. Lean forward as you allow your front knee to bend until a stretch is felt along the back of your leg. Move closer or further away from the wall to control the stretch of the back leg.

Target Leg

STANDING CALF STRETCH - GASTROC – HAND ON KNEE

Step forward with one foot and place hand on thigh. Maintain your toes on both feet to be pointed straight forward. Keep the leg behind you with a straight knee during the stretch. Lean forward as you allow your front knee to bend until a stretch is felt along the back of your leg. You can adjust the bend of the front knee to control the stretch.

	_____ Reps _____ Sets _____ X Day _____ Hold		_____ Reps _____ Sets _____ X Day _____ Hold
9	Notes:	10	Notes:

GASTROCNEMIUS STAIR STRETCH

Stand with the middle of your foot on the edge of the stairs while holding onto the railing. Slowly drop heels off until you feel a stretch in the back of your legs keeping your knees straight.

STANDING CALF STRETCH - SOLEUS

Stand in front of a wall, chair or other sturdy object. Step forward with one foot and maintain your toes on both feet to be pointed straight forward. Keep the leg behind you with a slightly bent knee during the stretch. Lean forward towards the wall and support yourself with your arms as you allow your front knee to bend until a gentle stretch is felt along the back of your leg. *Move closer or further away from the wall to control the stretch of the back leg. You can also adjust the bend of the front knee to control the stretch.

Hamstring / Knee Extension

	_____ Reps _____ Sets _____ X Day _____ Hold		_____ Reps _____ Sets _____ X Day _____ Hold
11	Notes: *Lymphedema: Do not wrap band around UE or LE	12	Notes: *Lymphedema: Do not wrap band around UE or LE

HAMSTRING STRETCH – TOWEL, BAND, STRAP or BELT

Lie down on your back and hook a towel/strap under your foot and draw up your leg until a stretch is felt under your leg/calf area. Keep your knee in a straightened position during the stretch. To increase stretch move strap to forefoot and flex foot.

HAMSTRING STRETCH – TOWEL, BAND, STRAP or BELT

While pushing down on thigh above knee cap with opposite hand, pull on towel/ strap to lift heel from floor. Keep thigh flat. To increase stretch move strap to forefoot and flex foot and/or lean forward at the hip.

_____ Reps _____ Sets _____ X Day _____ Hold		_____ Reps _____ Sets _____ X Day _____ Hold
13	**Notes:**	**14**	**Notes:**

HAMSTRING STRETCH - TABLE, BED OR COUCH

Sit on a raised flat surface where you can prop your target leg up on it such as a treatment table, couch or bed. While keeping your knee straight, slowly lean forward and reach your hands towards your foot until a gentle stretch is felt along the back of your knee/thigh. Hold and then return to starting position and repeat. Allow gravity to stretch your knee towards a more straightened position.
* Can use strap, towel or belt around forefoot as in #12

HAMSTRING / KNEE EXTENSION STRETCH - SEATED

Sit and tighten your top thigh muscle to press the back of your knee downward towards the ground. You should feel a gentle stretch in the back of your knee.

* To increase stretch put strap to forefoot, flex foot and lean forward at the hip.

_____ Reps _____ Sets _____ X Day _____ Hold		_____ Reps _____ Sets _____ X Day _____ Hold
15	**Notes:**	**16**	**Notes:**

HAMSTRING STRETCH - STANDING

Stand and rest your foot on a stool/box/step with your knee straight. Gently lean forward at the hips until a stretch is felt behind your knee/thigh. Keep your back straight. *To increase stretch, flex your foot at the ankle, and/or put strap to forefoot and flex foot. If on stair, you can put foot on 2nd or 3rd step.

TOE TOUCH – STANDING - NARROW or WIDE BOS

Stand and bend forward at waist keep legs straight and reach for toes. Can perform with either narrow or wide base of support.

Knee Flexion

_____ Reps _____ Sets _____X Day _____Hold		_____ Reps _____ Sets _____X Day _____Hold

17 | Notes: | **18** | Notes:
*Lymphedema: Do not wrap band around UE or LE

HEEL SLIDES - SELF ASSISTED

Lie on your back with knees straight and slide the target heel towards your buttock as you bend your knee. Use the unaffected leg to assist the bending. Hold a gentle stretch in this position and then return to original position.

HEEL SLIDES - LONG SIT ASSISTED - TOWEL, BAND, STRAP or BELT

Sit with legs straight. Can place a small hand towel under your heel to help slide. Loop a band around your foot and pull your knee into a bend position as your foot slides towards your buttock. Hold a gentle stretch and then return back to original position.

_____ Reps _____ Sets _____X Day _____Hold		_____ Reps _____ Sets _____X Day _____Hold

19 | Notes: | **20** | Notes:

HEEL SLIDES - SUPINE

Lie on your back with knees straight and slide the target heel towards your buttock as you bend your knee. Hold a gentle stretch in this position and then return to original position.

KNEE BENDS - EXERCISE BALL

Lie on your back and place your heels on an exercise ball. Roll it closer to your buttocks as your knees and hips bend as shown. Hold and then return to original position. *If you have limited range in one knee, use the other leg to help increase range of motion.

	_____ Reps _____ Sets _____X Day _____Hold

21	Notes:

KNEE FLEXION – SELF ASSISTED - PRONE

Lie face down and bend your target knee with the assistance of your unaffected leg.

	_____ Reps _____ Sets _____X Day _____Hold

22	Notes: *Lymphedema: Do not wrap band around UE or LE

KNEE FLEXION – BELT ASSISTED - PRONE

Lie face down with a strap looped around your target side ankle or foot. Use the belt to pull the knee into a bent position allowing for a stretch.

	_____ Reps _____ Sets _____X Day _____Hold

23	Notes:

HEEL SLIDES - SELF ASSISTED

It and slide your heel towards your buttock with the assist of the unaffected leg. Hold a gentle stretch and then return foot forward to original position.

	_____ Reps _____ Sets _____X Day _____Hold

24	Notes:

HEEL SLIDES - SEATED – can use towel or paper under foot to help slide

Sit and place your feet on the floor (can put target foot on a towel or paper to help slide if needed). Slowly slide your foot closer towards you. Hold a gentle stretch and then return foot forward to original position.

	_____ Reps _____ Sets _____X Day _____Hold		_____ Reps _____ Sets _____X Day _____Hold
25	Notes:	**26**	Notes:

Plant foot.
Scoot hips
forward.

KNEE FLEXION – SCOOT FORWARD - SEATED

Sit and slide your foot back to a bent knee position. Keep your foot planted on the ground and scoot forward until a stretch is felt at the knee. Hold the stretch and then scoot back to original position.

KNEE FLEXION – STAIR OR STEP

Place target foot on stool or step with bent knee. Gently bend forward keeping heel on step. Hold the stretch and then return to original position.

Piriformis

	_____ Reps _____ Sets _____X Day _____Hold		_____ Reps _____ Sets _____X Day _____Hold
27	Notes:	**28**	Notes:

PIRIFORMIS STRETCH

Lie on your back with both knees bent. Cross your target leg on the other knee. Hold your unaffected thigh and pull it up towards your chest until a stretch is felt in the buttock.

PIRIFORMIS STRETCH - EXERCISE BALL

Lie on your back with one foot placed on the ball. Cross your other leg over the knee of the leg on the ball and gently roll the ball back towards your chest until a stretch is felt in the buttock.

_____ Reps _____ Sets _____X Day _____Hold		_____ Reps _____ Sets _____X Day _____Hold
29	Notes:	**30**	Notes:

PIRIFORMIS STRETCH - LONG SIT

Sit with one knee straight and the other bent and placed over the opposite knee. Gentle turn your body towards the bend knee side.

PIRIFORMIS STRETCH – STANDING

Stand with unaffected leg crossed in front of target side. Lean forward reaching for foot on target side until stretch is felt in the buttock.

Hip Flexors

_____ Reps _____ Sets _____X Day _____Hold		_____ Reps _____ Sets _____X Day _____Hold
31	Notes:	**32**	Notes:

HIP FLEXOR STRETCH - SIDE OF BALL or CHAIR

Sit on edge of chair or ball. Bend your front knee (unaffected side) and lean forward until a stretch is felt along the front of the target hip.

HIP FLEXOR STRETCH - STANDING

Stand and bend one knee forward (unaffected side) and the other in back. Stand up straight leaning slightly backward until a stretch is felt along the front of the target hip.

_____ Reps _____ Sets _____X Day _____Hold		_____ Reps _____ Sets _____X Day _____Hold
33	Notes:	**34**	Notes:

HIP FLEXOR STRETCH - HALF KNEEL – with or without pad under knee

Begin in a half-kneeling position (you may want to use a pad or pillow for cushion). Bend your front knee (unaffected side) and lean forward until a stretch is felt along the front of the target hip.

RUNNER'S STRETCH - MODIFIED

Stretch target leg in back and bend other knee in front. Bend your front knee (unaffected side) and lean forward until a stretch is felt along the front of the target hip.

_____ Reps _____ Sets _____X Day _____Hold		_____ Reps _____ Sets _____X Day _____Hold
35	Notes:	**36**	Notes:

HIP FLEXOR STRETCH – SUPINE

Lie on a table, high bed or matt and let the affected leg lower towards the floor until a stretch is felt along the front of your thigh.

HIP FLEXOR STRETCH – SUPINE

Lie on a table, high bed or matt and let the affected leg lower towards the floor until a stretch is felt along the front of your thigh. At the same time, grasp your opposite knee and pull it towards your chest.

Quadriceps (Quad)

_____ Reps _____ Sets _____X Day _____Hold	_____ Reps _____ Sets _____X Day _____Hold
37 Notes:	**38** Notes:

QUAD STRETCH - SIDELYING

Lie on your side and reach back holding the top of your foot with bent knee until a stretch is felt.

QUAD STRETCH - STANDING

Stand straight up and bend your knee in back holding your ankle/foot. Gently pull your knee/thigh back in alignment with the standing leg.

Adductor

_____ Reps _____ Sets _____X Day _____Hold	_____ Reps _____ Sets _____X Day _____Hold
39 Notes:	**40** Notes:

One Leg

Both Legs

KNEE FALL OUT STRETCH or FROG STRETCH

Lie on your back with one knee bent. Slowly lower your knee to the side as you stretch the inner thigh/hip area. Frog Stretch: Let both knees fall to the side at the same time.

BUTTERFLY STRETCH

Sit on the floor or mat and bend your knees placing the bottom of your feet together. Slowly let your knees lower towards the floor until a stretch is felt at your inner thighs.

	_____ Reps _____ Sets _____ X Day _____ Hold		_____ Reps _____ Sets _____ X Day _____ Hold
41	Notes:	**42**	Notes:

HIP ADDUCTOR STRECH – KNEELING

Kneel down on your target side knee. Place the opposite leg directly out to the side. Lean towards the side as you bend the knee for a stretch to the inner thigh of the target leg.

HIP ADDUCTOR STRECH - STANDING

Stand with feet spread wide apart. Slowly bend your knee to allow for a gentle stretch of the opposite leg. Maintain a straight knee on the target leg the entire time. You should feel a stretch on the inner thigh.

External Rotation / Internal Rotation

	_____ Reps _____ Sets _____ X Day _____ Hold		_____ Reps _____ Sets _____ X Day _____ Hold
43	Notes:	**44**	Notes:

HIP EXTERNAL ROTATION STRETCH - SUPINE

Lie on your back with your leg crossed over your knee. Use your hand and push the crossed knee away from you.

HIP INTERNAL ROTATION STRETCH - SEATED

Sit on a chair with your legs spread apart and feet planted on the ground. Use your hand to draw your knee inward as shown.

Iliotibial Band (IT Band)

_____ Reps _____ Sets _____ X Day _____ Hold	_____ Reps _____ Sets _____ X Day _____ Hold
45 Notes:	**46** Notes:

IT BAND STRETCH - STANDING

Stand and cross the target leg behind your unaffected leg. Lean forward and towards the unaffected side while using your arm for balance support.

IT BAND STRETCH -- SIDELYING

Lie on bed or couch on unaffected side with target side towards ceiling. Bend lower leg for support. Allow upper leg to drop over side of bed. Keep knee straight and point toe towards floor. May need to roll upper hip backwards in order to feel stretch on side of hip/thigh/knee.

NECK

_____ Reps _____ Sets _____ X Day _____ Hold	_____ Reps _____ Sets _____ X Day _____ Hold
47 Notes:	**48** Notes:

NECK ROTATION and SIDE BENDS

SIDE BENDS: (_Top_) Tilt your head as if you are trying to touch your ear to your shoulder. For extra stretch gently use your hand to increase range and hold.
ROTATION: (_Bottom_) Turn your head to the side as if looking over your shoulder. For an extra stretch gently use your hand on your chin to increase range and hold.

NECK FLEXION AND EXTENSION

EXTENSION: Look up as if you are looking at the sky moving your neck only.
FLEXION: Look down as if you are looking at the floor. For an extra stretch gently put both hands behind your head to move chin towards the chest and hold.

BACK	

	_____ Reps _____ Sets _____X Day _____Hold		_____ Reps _____ Sets _____X Day _____Hold
49	**Notes:**	**50**	**Notes:**

TRUNK FLEXION - SEATED

Sit and cross your arms over your chest. Slowly curl your back forward in order to round your upper back.

LOW BACK STRETCH - SEATED

Sit and slowly bend forward reaching your hands for the floor. Bend your trunk and head forward and down.

	_____ Reps _____ Sets _____X Day _____Hold		_____ Reps _____ Sets _____X Day _____Hold
51	**Notes:**	**52**	**Notes:**

LOW BACK STRETCH – STANDING - STRAIGHT & LATERAL

Stand in front of a table / chair or other surface and bend forward at the waist. Support yourself with your hands on a surface.

Reach to the side for a lateral bend (see #53)

LOW BACK STRETCH – RAIL OR DOORKNOB

Hold onto doorknob, rail or other unmovable surface and pull while moving hips back and hold.

	_____ Reps _____ Sets _____X Day _____Hold
53	**Notes:**

Lateral

Straight

PRAYER STRETCH and LATERAL

STRAIGHT: Start on your hands and knees. Slowly lower your buttocks towards your feet until a stretch is felt along your back and or buttocks.

LATERAL: Start on your hands and knees. Slowly lower your buttocks towards your feet. Lower your chest towards the floor as you reach out towards the side.

	_____ Reps _____ Sets _____X Day _____Hold
54	**Notes:**

PRAYER STRETCH - EXERCISE BALL

Kneel with an exercise ball in front of you. Slowly lean forward and roll the ball forward until a stretch is felt.

*Can do lateral movement as in #53

	_____ Reps _____ Sets _____X Day _____Hold
55	**Notes:**

CAT AND CAMEL

Start on your hands and knees. Raise up your back and arch it towards the ceiling (cat). Return to a lowered position and arch your back the opposite direction (camel).

	_____ Reps _____ Sets _____X Day _____Hold
56	**Notes:**

Both Legs

One Leg

KNEE TO CHEST STRETCH - SINGLE and BILATERAL

BILATERAL: Lie on your back and hold your knees while pulling up towards your chest and hold.
SINGLE: Lie on your back and hold your knee while pulling up towards your chest and hold. Opposite leg can be straight or bent.

Trunk Extension

_____ Reps _____ Sets _____X Day _____Hold	_____ Reps _____ Sets _____X Day _____Hold
57 Notes:	**58** Notes:

PRONE ON ELBOWS

Lie on your stomach. Slowly press up and prop yourself up on your elbows. Keep hips on floor/mat.

PRESS UPS

Lie on your stomach. Slowly press up and arch your back using your arms. Keep hips on floor/mat.

Trunk Rotation

_____ Reps _____ Sets _____X Day _____Hold	_____ Reps _____ Sets _____X Day _____Hold
59 Notes:	**60** Notes:

TRUNK ROTATION STRETCH – SINGLE LEG

Lie on your back with arms to the sides. Bend one knee and then raise it up and across your body. Allow your trunk to rotate for a gentle stretch to the spine. Hold and then repeat.

LOWER TRUNK ROTATIONS – BILATERAL

Lie on your back with your knees bent and gently move your knees side-to-side.

	_____ Reps _____ Sets _____ X Day _____ Hold	_____ Reps _____ Sets _____ X Day _____ Hold
61	Notes:	**62** Notes:

TRUNK ROTATION - SEATED

Sit up as tall with erect posture. Rotate in one direction, using your hand to press against the opposite thigh to aide in further rotation. Exhale to increase the rotation and stretch. Return to the starting position, maintain an upright posture -repeat in the opposite direction.

TRUNK ROTATION - STANDING or SEATED – DOWEL

Stand or sit holding dowel in hands. Slowly rotate trunk in one direction and then in the opposite direction.

Lateral

	_____ Reps _____ Sets _____ X Day _____ Hold	_____ Reps _____ Sets _____ X Day _____ Hold
63	Notes:	**64** Notes:

LATERAL TRUNK STRETCH - SINGLE SEATED or STANDING

Raise your arm and bend to the opposite side for a stretch. Hold and repeat with opposite arm.

LATERAL TRUNK STRETCH - BILATERAL SEATED or STANDING

Clasp hands together and raise arms over head. Bend to one side. Hold and repeat in opposite direction.

Shoulder Flexion

	_____ Reps _____ Sets _____X Day _____Hold
65	**Notes:**

FLEXION - SUPINE - DOWEL

Lie on your back and hold a dowel/cane. Slowly raise the dowel overhead.

*If you have a weak or injured arm, you can use your unaffected arm to assist with the movement.

	_____ Reps _____ Sets _____X Day _____Hold
66	**Notes:**

WALL WALK

Place your target hand on the wall with the palm facing the wall. Walk your fingers up the wall towards overhead. Slide or walk your hand back down the wall to the starting position.

	_____ Reps _____ Sets _____X Day _____Hold
67	**Notes:**

FLEXION - TABLE SLIDE

Sit or stand and rest your target arm on a table and gently slide it forward and then back.

	_____ Reps _____ Sets _____X Day _____Hold
68	**Notes:**

FLEXION - TABLE SLIDE - BALL

Stand and rest your target arm on top of a ball on a table. Gently roll the ball forward and then back.

Shoulder External Rotation (ER)

_____ Reps _____ Sets _____X Day _____Hold		_____ Reps _____ Sets _____X Day _____Hold

69 | Notes:

70 | Notes:

Starting
Position

EXTERNAL ROTATION - SUPINE – DOWEL
INTERNAL ROTATION ON OPPOSITE ARM

Lie on your back holding a dowel/cane with both hands. On the target side, maintain approx. 90-degree bend at the elbow with your arm approximately 30-45 degrees away from your side. Use your other arm to push the dowel/cane to rotate the affected arm back into a stretch. Hold and then return to starting position. Repeat

EXTERNAL ROTATION - 90-90 - DOWEL

Lie on your back and hold a dowel with your elbows out to the side and rested down. Roll your arms back towards overhead until a stretch is felt. Keep elbows bent at a 90-degree angle.

_____ Reps _____ Sets _____X Day _____Hold		_____ Reps _____ Sets _____X Day _____Hold

71 | Notes:

72 | Notes:

EXTERNAL ROTATION – SEATED – DOWEL
INTERNAL ROTATION ON OPPOSITE ARM

Using the unaffected arm, push the dowel into the hand of the target arm. Keep the arm at a 90-degree angle and push until a stretch is felt. Hold and repeat.

EXTERNAL ROTATION – STANDING – DOWEL
INTERNAL ROTATION ON OPPOSITE ARM

Using the unaffected arm, push the dowel into the hand of the target arm. Keep the arm at a 90-degree angle and push until a stretch is felt. Hold and repeat.

Shoulder Internal Rotation (IR) - *also see #69, 71, 72*

	_____ Reps _____ Sets _____X Day _____Hold		_____ Reps _____ Sets _____X Day _____Hold
73	Notes:	**74**	Notes:

INTERNAL ROTATION – TOWEL OR STRAP

Hold one end of the towel in front and with the target arm behind your back. Gently pull up your target arm behind your back with the assist of a towel.

INTERNAL ROTATION – DOWEL

Hold a dowel/cane behind your back. Slowly pull the target arm towards the center of your back.

Shoulder Abduction

	_____ Reps _____ Sets _____X Day _____Hold		_____ Reps _____ Sets _____X Day _____Hold
75	Notes:	**76**	Notes:

ABDUCTION - TABLE SLIDE - BALL

Stand and rest your target arm on top of a ball on a table and gently roll it to the side and back.

ABDUCTION WITH DOWEL

Hold a dowel/cane in front. Slowly push the dowel of the unaffected arm towards the target arm upward and to the side.

Shoulder Extension

_____ Reps _____ Sets _____ X Day _____ Hold		_____ Reps _____ Sets _____ X Day _____ Hold
77	Notes:	**78**

LYING DOWN EXTENSION - TABLE or BED

Lie on your back and gently let target arm drop off table or bed.

WAND EXTENSION - STANDING

Stand and hold a dowel/cane. Use the unaffected arm to help push the target arm back. The elbow should remain straight the entire time.

Chest/Pec Stretch

_____ Reps _____ Sets _____ X Day _____ Hold		_____ Reps _____ Sets _____ X Day _____ Hold
79	Notes:	**80**

CHEST STRETCH – SEATED, STANDING, or SUPINE

TOP: Bend arms at a 90-degree angle. Move elbows back until feeling a stretch in front of shoulders/chest.

BOTTOM: Clasp hands in back of head. Move elbows back until feeling a stretch in front of shoulders/chest.

CHEST STRETCH - STEP THROUGH

Stand with arms in doorway at a 90-degree angle. Step through until you feel a stretch through the chest and hold. Keep shoulders down and back. Take another step to increase stretch.

Triceps

_____ Reps _____ Sets _____X Day _____Hold	_____ Reps _____ Sets _____X Day _____Hold
81 Notes:	**82** Notes: *Lymphedema: Do not wrap band around UE or LE

TRICEP STRETCH

With your target elbow bent and shoulder raised, use your other hand and gently push your target elbow back towards overhead until a stretch is felt.

TRICEP STRETCH - STRAP or TOWEL

Hold strap of target arm with your hand above your head. Use the other hand to pull downward on the strap, allowing the elbow to bend until a stretch is in the back of the arm.

Posterior Capsule

_____ Reps _____ Sets _____X Day _____Hold	_____ Reps _____ Sets _____X Day _____Hold
83 Notes:	**84** Notes:

POSTERIOR SHOULDER/DELTOID RELEASE

Bring your target arm across your body. Use the opposite hand to grasp the back of your shoulder and further pull the arm. Hold.

POSTERIOR CAPSULE STRETCH

Lie on your side and grasp the elbow of the arm closest to the floor. Gently pull it upward and across the front of your body.

Core/Stability Training

Core strengthening is the foundation of all the other exercises that follow, especially balance. Core training is not only an important step in conditioning, but also helps other issues, including neurological, orthopedic, weight, or overall weakness

The core includes muscles of the thoraco-lumbar spine (trunk), cervical spine., erector spinae, abdomen, pelvis, shoulder/scapulae, and your lower lats.

Static core functionality is the ability of one's core to align the skeleton to resist a force that does not change. The core is used to stabilize the thorax and the pelvis during dynamic movement. The nature of dynamic movement must consider our skeletal structure (as a lever) in addition to the force of external resistance and consequently incorporates a vastly different complex of muscles and joints versus a static position.

The core is traditionally assumed to originate most full-body functional movement, including most sports. In addition, the core determines to a large part a person's posture. In all, human anatomy is built to take force upon the bones and direct autonomic force, through various joints, in the desired direction. The core muscles align the spine, ribs, and pelvis of a person to resist a specific force, whether static or dynamic.
(Wikipedia: *https://en.wikipedia.org/wiki/Core_(anatomy)*)

These muscles work as stabilizers for the entire body. Core training is simply doing specific exercises to develop and strengthen these stabilizer muscles. If any of these core muscles are weakened, it could result in lower back pain or a protruding waistline. Keeping these core muscles strong can do wonders for your posture and help give you more strength in other exercises like running and walking.
(Bodybuilding.com - *https://www.bodybuilding.com/fun/mielke12.htm*)

There is a saying 'form follows function'. This is especially true with core stability and how it affects your balance. Gravity influences all movement, so effective core training must be done against gravity. The rectus abdominus muscle that you are isolating with those crunches flexes the spine/abs only when you are lying on your back or returning the torso to an upright position from hyperextension in standing. "In the upright position, flexion is controlled by eccentric contraction of the back extensors as the lower the weight of the torso in the same direction as gravity". (*Bryant & Green, 2003, p. 84*)

Being able to engage the core with not only your balance exercises but also arm and leg exercises will help prevent injury.

Step 1: First learn to brace the abdomen *(see pictures 1 and 2 on next page)* Think of this as trying to either brace for a punch to the stomach or trying to put on a tight pair of pants (not just sucking in your stomach)

Step 2: After getting a good feel for bracing, try doing a pelvic tilt *(see pictures 3 and 4 on next page)* and then progress to bridging *(see picture 5)*

Step 3: These two basic movements should be done while you progress your abdominal and core training, continuing through the balance section, and to some extent with arm and leg strengthening.

*** **When doing floor work, such as crunches, make sure you are on a soft surface, such as a mat, Bosu, stability ball, etc. Pushing your back into a hard surface, such as a wood floor, can do more damage than good to the spine.**

*** **Breathe – Never hold your breath.**

EXERCISE	EXERCISE NUMBER	NOTES
Core / Stability		
ABDOMINAL BRACING TRAINING	1	
ABDOMINAL BRACING - SUPINE	2	
PELVIC TILT - SUPINE	3	
PELVIC TILT - KNEELING	4	
BRIDGING	5	
BRIDGE - BOSU	6	
BRIDGING WITH PILLOW SQUEEZE	7	
BRIDGING WITH PILLOW SQUEEZE - BOSU	8	
BRACE SUPINE MARCHING / BRIDGE LEG UP	9	
BRIDGE LEG UP - BOSU -	10	
SINGLE LEG BRIDGE	11	
BRIDGE SINGLE LEG - BOSU	12	
BRIDGING CROSSED LEG	13	
BRIDGING CROSSED LEG – BOSU	14	
BRIDGING CROSSED LEG - ARMS UP	15	
BRIDGING CROSSED LEG - ARMS UP - BOSU	16	
BRIDGE - ELASTIC BAND	17	
BRIDGING - ABDUCTION - ELASTIC BAND	18	
FLOOR BRIDGE - EXERCISE BALL	19	
FLOOR BRIDGE ALTERNATE LEG LIFT - EXERCISE BALL	20	
BRIDGE UPPER BACK - EXERCISE BALL	21	
BRIDGE UPPER BACK - SINGLE LEG - EXERCISE BALL	22	
QUADRUPED ALTERNATE ARM	23	
QUADRUPED ALTERNATE LEG	24	
QUADRUPED ALTERNATE ARM AND LEG	25	
BIRD DOG ELBOW TOUCHES	26	

EXERCISE Core / Stability	EXERCISE NUMBER	NOTES
PRONE BALL	27	
PRONE BALL - ALTERNATE ARM	28	
PRONE BALL - ALTERNATE LEG	29	
PRONE BALL - ALTERNATE ARM AND LEG	30	
MODIFIED PLANK	31	
MODIFIED PLANK - ALTERNATE LEG	32	
FULL PLANK	33	
PLANK - ALTERNATE ARMS	34	
PLANK - ALTERNATE LEGS	35	
PLANK - EXERCISE BALL	36	
PRONE ON ELBOWS	37	
PRESS UPS	38	
SKYDIVER	39	
PRONE SUPERMAN - BOSU	40	
TRUNK EXTENSION - BOSU	41	
TRUNK EXTENSION - HANDS CROSSED IN FRONT - BOSU	43	
SUPERMAN - ARMS BACK- EXERCISE BALL	44	
SUPERMAN – BOTH ARMS IN FRONT - EXERCISE BALL	45	
SUPERMAN – ONE ARM FORWARD / ONE ARM BACK - EXERCISE BALL	46	
LATERAL PLANK MODIFIED	47	
LATERAL PLANK MODIFIED- BOSU	48	
LATERAL PLANK - 1 KNEE 1 FOOT	49	
LATERAL PLANK - 1 KNEE 1 FOOT – BOSU	50	
LATERAL PLANK	51	
LATERAL PLANK - BOSU	52	

EXERCISE	EXERCISE NUMBER	NOTES
Core / Stability		
LEAN BACK	53	
LEAN BACK - BOSU	54	
LEAN BACK WITH ARMS OUT	55	
LEAN BACK WITH ARMS OUT - BOSU	56	
LEAN BACK WITH TWIST	57	
LEAN BACK WITH TWIST – BOSU	58	
CRUNCHY FROG	59	
SEATED BIKE - FORWARD AND BACKWARDS	60	
CRUNCH – ARMS OUT	61	
CRUNCH – ARMS OUT - BOSU	62	
CRUNCH – ARMS IN BACK OF HEAD	63	
CRUNCH – ARMS IN BACK OF HEAD - BOSU	64	
OBLIQUE CRUNCH	65	
OBLIQUE CRUNCH - BOSU	66	
90 DEGREE CRUNCH	67	
BALL CRUNCH – Can put legs on seat of chair	68	
CURL UPS – ARMS ON LEGS - EXERCISE BALL	69	
CURL UPS- ARMS CROSSED IN FRONT - EXERCISE BALL	70	
CURL UPS – ARMS BEHIND HEAD - EXERCISE BALL	71	
SUPINE CRUNCH TOUCH - EXERCISE BALL	72	
LOWER ABDOMINAL CRUNCH – WITH or WITHOUT BALL	73	
HIGH MARCH CRUNCH	74	
STANDING SIDE CRUNCH	75	
STANDING BIKE CRUNCH	76	

Core/Abdominal

Abdominal Bracing – Pelvic Tilt

_____ Reps _____ Sets _____ X Day _____ Hold		_____ Reps _____ Sets _____ X Day _____ Hold	
1	Notes:	**2**	Notes:

ABDOMINAL BRACING TRAINING

Press your fingertips into your relaxed abdomen lateral of your navel. Tighten and brace your abdomen so that the muscles push your fingertips away from the center of your body. Hold, relax and repeat.
Think of this as trying to either brace for a punch to the stomach or trying to put on a tight pair of pants (not just sucking in your stomach)

Starting Position

ABDOMINAL BRACING - SUPINE

Lie on your back. Tighten your stomach muscles as you draw your navel down towards the floor.

Think of this as trying to either brace for a punch to the stomach or trying to put on a tight pair of pants (not just sucking in your stomach)

_____ Reps _____ Sets _____ X Day _____ Hold		_____ Reps _____ Sets _____ X Day _____ Hold	
3	Notes:	**4**	Notes:

Starting Position

PELVIC TILT - SUPINE

Lie on your back with your knees bent. Next, arch your low back and then flatten it repeatedly (bracing as above). Your pelvis should tilt forward and back during the movement. Move through a comfortable range of motion.

Starting Position

PELVIC TILT - KNEELING

Kneel on the floor (you can kneel on a pillow or pad if needed). Arch your lower back and then flatten it repeatedly (bracing as above). Your pelvis should tilt forward and back during the movement. Move through a comfortable range of motion.

Bridging

	_____ Reps _____ Sets _____ X Day _____ Hold		_____ Reps _____ Sets _____ X Day _____ Hold
5	**Notes:**	**6**	**Notes:**

Starting

Position

BRIDGING

Lie on your back. Tighten your lower abdominals (as with abdominal bracing), squeeze your buttocks and then raise your buttocks off the floor/bed. Hold and then lower yourself slowly and repeat. Brace the stomach muscles to keep your spine from moving, trying to keep the pelvis level the entire time.

Starting

Position

BRIDGE - BOSU – Can use foam pad, stair step or box

Lie on your back with your feet planted on top of the Bosu and knees bent. Lift up your buttocks as shown. Hold and then lower yourself slowly and repeat.
Brace the stomach muscles to keep your spine from moving, trying to keep the pelvis level the entire time.

	_____ Reps _____ Sets _____ X Day _____ Hold		_____ Reps _____ Sets _____ X Day _____ Hold
7	**Notes:**	**8**	**Notes:**

Starting

Position

BRIDGING WITH PILLOW SQUEEZE - Use pillow, ball or rolled towel between knees

Lie on your back and place a pillow, towel roll or ball between your knees and squeeze. Hold this and then tighten your lower abdominals, squeeze your buttocks and raise your buttocks off the floor/bed. Brace the stomach muscles to keep your spine from moving, trying to keep the pelvis level.

Starting

Position

BRIDGING WITH PILLOW SQUEEZE - BOSU - Can use foam pad, stair step or box

Lie on your back with your feet planted on top of the Bosu and knees bent. Place a pillow, towel roll or ball between your knees and squeeze. Lift up your buttocks as shown. Hold and then lower yourself slowly and repeat. Brace the stomach muscles to keep your spine from moving, trying to keep the pelvis level.

	_____ Reps _____ Sets _____ X Day _____ Hold
9	**Notes:**

Starting Position

BRACE SUPINE MARCHING / BRIDGE LEG UP

Lie on your back with your knees bent, slowly lift up one foot a few inches and then set it back down. Perform on your other leg. Brace the stomach muscles to keep your spine from moving, trying to keep the pelvis level the entire time.

*To increase challenge, go into bridge position as with #5, then continue march – can bring leg higher to advance

	_____ Reps _____ Sets _____ X Day _____ Hold
10	**Notes:**

Starting Position

BRIDGE LEG UP - BOSU - Can use foam pad, stair step or box

Lie on your back with your feet planted on top of the Bosu and knees bent. Slowly lift up one foot a few inches and then set it back down. Next, perform on your other leg. Brace the stomach muscles to keep your spine from moving, trying to keep the pelvis level the entire time. *To increase challenge, go into bridge position as with #6, then continue march – can bring leg higher to advance

	_____ Reps _____ Sets _____ X Day _____ Hold
11	**Notes:**

Starting Position

SINGLE LEG BRIDGE

Lie on your back, raise your buttocks off the floor/bed into a bridge position. Straighten a leg so that only one leg is supporting your body. Then, return that leg back to the ground and change to the other side. Brace the stomach muscles to keep your spine from moving, trying to keep the pelvis level the entire time.

	_____ Reps _____ Sets _____ X Day _____ Hold
12	**Notes:**

Starting Position

BRIDGE SINGLE LEG - BOSU - can use foam pad, stair step or box

Lie on your back with your feet planted on top of the Bosu and knees bent, lift up your buttocks and then straighten one knee in the air. Return that leg back to the ground and change to the other side. Brace the stomach muscles to keep your spine from moving, trying to keep the pelvis level the entire time.

	_____ Reps _____ Sets _____ X Day _____ Hold
13	**Notes:**

Starting
Position

BRIDGING CROSSED LEG

Lie on your back, cross your leg. Tighten your lower abdomen, squeeze your buttocks and raise your buttocks off the floor/bed. Brace the stomach muscles to keep your spine from moving, trying to keep the pelvis level the entire time.

	_____ Reps _____ Sets _____ X Day _____ Hold
14	**Notes:**

Starting Position

BRIDGING CROSSED LEG – BOSU - can use foam pad, stair step or box

Lie on your back with your feet planted on top of the Bosu cross your leg. Tighten your lower abdomen, squeeze your buttocks and raise your buttocks. Brace the stomach muscles to keep your spine from moving, trying to keep the pelvis level the entire time.

	_____ Reps _____ Sets _____ X Day _____ Hold
15	**Notes:**

Starting
Position

BRIDGING CROSSED LEG - ARMS UP

Lie on your back, cross your leg and put your hands together as shown. Next, tighten your lower abdomen, squeeze your buttocks and raise your buttocks off the floor/bed. Brace the stomach muscles to keep your spine from moving, trying to keep the pelvis level the entire time.

	_____ Reps _____ Sets _____ X Day _____ Hold
16	**Notes:**

BRIDGING CROSSED LEG - ARMS UP - BOSU - can use foam pad, stair step or box

Lie on your back with your feet planted on top of the Bosu and hands together and leg crossed. Tighten your lower abdomen, squeeze your buttocks and raise your buttocks. Brace the stomach muscles to keep your spine from moving, trying to keep the pelvis level.

_____ Reps _____ Sets _____ X Day _____ Hold		_____ Reps _____ Sets _____ X Day _____ Hold
17	Notes:	**18** Notes:

Starting

Position

BRIDGE - ELASTIC BAND

Lie on your back, hold an elastic band down around your waist for resistance. Tighten your lower abdomen, squeeze your buttocks and then raise your buttocks off the floor/bed. Brace the stomach muscles to keep your spine from moving, trying to keep the pelvis level the entire time.

Starting

Position

BRIDGING - ABDUCTION - ELASTIC BAND – can be done with feet on BOSU, foam, stair step or box

Lie on your back, place an elastic band around your knees and pull your knees apart. Hold this and then tighten your lower abdomen, squeeze your buttocks and raise your buttocks off the floor/bed. Brace the stomach muscles to keep your spine from moving, trying to keep the pelvis level the entire time.

_____ Reps _____ Sets _____ X Day _____ Hold		_____ Reps _____ Sets _____ X Day _____ Hold
19	Notes:	**20** Notes:

Starting

Position

FLOOR BRIDGE - EXERCISE BALL

Lie on the floor, place an exercise ball under your lower legs and then raise up your buttocks. Hold and repeat. Brace the stomach muscles to keep your spine from moving, trying to keep the pelvis level the entire time.

Starting

Position

FLOOR BRIDGE ALTERNATE LEG LIFT - EXERCISE BALL

Lie on the floor, place an exercise ball under your lower legs and then raise up your buttocks. While holding this position raise up a leg off the ball towards the ceiling then lower back to the ball and alternate to lift the other leg. Brace the stomach muscles to keep your spine from moving, trying to keep the pelvis level.

_____ Reps _____ Sets _____ X Day _____ Hold	_____ Reps _____ Sets _____ X Day _____ Hold
21 Notes:	**22** Notes:

BRIDGE UPPER BACK - EXERCISE BALL

Start in a seated position on the ball and slowly walk your feet forward so that the ball is on your upper back. Keep your buttocks and pelvis up off the ball and straight with your thighs. Brace the stomach muscles to keep your spine from moving, trying to keep the pelvis level the entire time.
*To increase the challenge, you can do a supine march or perform some arm exercises, such as Fly's or Chest Presses (*See Upper Extremity exercises*)

Starting Position

BRIDGE UPPER BACK - SINGLE LEG - EXERCISE BALL

Start in a seated position on the ball and slowly walk your feet forward so that the ball is on your upper back. Keep your buttocks and pelvis up off the ball and straight with your thighs. Raise up one leg so that you straighten your knee in the air. Return it back to the floor and then switch to raise up the other side. Brace the stomach muscles to keep your spine from moving, trying to keep the pelvis level the entire time.

Quadruped

_____ Reps _____ Sets _____ X Day _____ Hold	_____ Reps _____ Sets _____ X Day _____ Hold
23 Notes:	**24** Notes:

QUADRUPED ALTERNATE ARM

While in a crawling position, slowly raise up an arm out in front of you.

QUADRUPED ALTERNATE LEG

While in a crawling position, slowly draw your leg back behind you as you straighten your knee. Either repeat on same side or alternate.

_____ Reps _____ Sets _____ X Day _____ Hold	_____ Reps _____ Sets _____ X Day _____ Hold
25 Notes:	**26** Notes:

QUADRUPED ALTERNATE ARM AND LEG

While in a crawling position, brace at your abdominals and then slowly lift a leg and opposite arm upwards. Maintain a level and stable pelvis and spine the entire time. Either repeat on same side or alternate.

Touch your elbow to your opposite knee

Starting Position

BIRD DOG ELBOW TOUCHES

While in a crawling position, slowly lift your leg and opposite arm upwards. When returning your arm and leg down, do not touch the floor but instead touch your elbow to your opposite knee and lift and straighten them again. Then set them down on the floor. Either repeat on same side or alternate.

_____ Reps _____ Sets _____ X Day _____ Hold	_____ Reps _____ Sets _____ X Day _____ Hold
27 Notes:	**28** Notes:

PRONE BALL

Lie face down over a ball, support your self with your feet and hands.

PRONE BALL - ALTERNATE ARM

Lie face down over a ball, support your self with your feet and hands. Next, slowly raise up one arm. Return arm back to floor and then raise up the other arm. Keep alternating arms.

_____ Reps _____ Sets _____ X Day _____ Hold		_____ Reps _____ Sets _____ X Day _____ Hold	
29	Notes:	**30**	Notes:

PRONE BALL - ALTERNATE LEG

Lie face down over a ball, support yourself with your arms and legs. Next slowly raise up a leg. Return leg back to floor and then raise up the other leg.

PRONE BALL - ALTERNATE ARM AND LEG

Lie face down over a ball, support yourself with your feet and hands. Next, slowly raise up one arm and opposite leg. Return arm and leg back to floor and then raise up the opposite arm/leg.

Plank

_____ Reps _____ Sets _____ X Day _____ Hold		_____ Reps _____ Sets _____ X Day _____ Hold	
31	Notes:	**32**	Notes:

MODIFIED PLANK

Lie face down, lift your body up on your elbows and toes. Try and maintain a straight spine the entire time. Do not allow your low back sag downward.

Starting

Position

MODIFIED PLANK - ALTERNATE LEG

Lie face down, lift your body up on your elbows and toes. Next, lift one leg off the ground and then set it back down. Then repeat on the other leg. Try and maintain a straight spine the entire time.

_____ Reps _____ Sets _____ X Day _____ Hold

33 | Notes:

FULL PLANK

Lie face down, lift your body up on your elbows and toes. Straighten your arms in full elbow extension and hold in full plank position. Do not let your back arch down. Try and maintain a straight spine the entire time.

_____ Reps _____ Sets _____ X Day _____ Hold

34 | Notes:

PLANK - ALTERNATE ARMS

Hold a plank position as previous (#33). Raise one arm out in front of you as shown. Return to the starting position and then raise your other arm out in front of you and repeat.
Try and maintain a straight spine the entire time.

_____ Reps _____ Sets _____ X Day _____ Hold

35 | Notes:

PLANK - ALTERNATE LEGS

Hold a plank position as previous (#33). Raise one leg off the floor as shown. Return to the starting position and then raise your other leg and repeat. Try and maintain a straight spine the entire time.

_____ Reps _____ Sets _____ X Day _____ Hold

36 | Notes:

PLANK - EXERCISE BALL

While kneeling on the floor with an exercise ball in front of you, place your elbows and hands on the ball and lift your body up. Try and maintain a straight spine. Do not allow your hips or pelvis on either side to drop.

Back Extension

_____ Reps _____ Sets _____ X Day _____ Hold

37 | **Notes:**

PRONE ON ELBOWS

Lie face down, slowly press up and prop yourself up on your elbows.

_____ Reps _____ Sets _____ X Day _____ Hold

38 | **Notes:**

PRESS UPS

Lie face down, slowly press up and arch your back using your arms.

_____ Reps _____ Sets _____ X Day _____ Hold

39 | **Notes:**

SKYDIVER

Lie face down with arms by your side. Next, lift your upper body, lower legs, thighs, and arms off the ground at the same time as shown. You can place a pillow under your stomach/hips for comfort.

_____ Reps _____ Sets _____ X Day _____ Hold

40 | **Notes:**

PRONE SUPERMAN - BOSU

Lie face down over the Bosu. Slowly raise your arms and legs upward off the ground. Then lower slowly back to the ground.

_____ Reps _____ Sets _____ X Day _____ Hold

41 | Notes:

TRUNK EXTENSION - BOSU

Lie face down with your upper body on a Bosu and slowly raise your head and chest upwards as shown.
Your arms can be behind your back or alongside your body.

Starting Position

_____ Reps _____ Sets _____ X Day _____ Hold

42 | Notes:

Starting Position

TRUNK EXTENSION - HANDS BEHIND HEAD - BOSU

Lie face down with your upper body on a Bosu.
Touch the back of your head with both hands and slowly raise your head and chest upwards.

_____ Reps _____ Sets _____ X Day _____ Hold

43 | Notes:

Starting Position

TRUNK EXTENSION - HANDS CROSSED IN FRONT - BOSU

While lying face down with your upper body on a Bosu, slowly raise your head and chest upwards.
Keep your arms crossed on your chest as you perform.

_____ Reps _____ Sets _____ X Day _____ Hold

44 | Notes:

SUPERMAN - ARMS BACK- EXERCISE BALL

Start in a kneeling position with an exercise ball in front of you. Roll forward so that you are face down on the ball with your feet on the ground and your stomach on the ball. Hold up your head and chest so that a straight line exists between your feet and head. Also bring your arms back along side of your body and hold this position.

_____ Reps _____ Sets _____ X Day _____ Hold		_____ Reps _____ Sets _____ X Day _____ Hold
45	Notes:	**46**	Notes:

SUPERMAN – BOTH ARMS IN FRONT - EXERCISE BALL

Start in a kneeling position with an exercise ball in front of you. Next, roll forward so that you are face down on the ball with your feet on the ground and your stomach on the ball. Hold up your head and chest so that a straight line exists between your feet and head. Also bring your arms up and forward out in front of you and hold this position.

SUPERMAN – ONE ARM FORWARD / ONE ARM BACK - EXERCISE BALL

Start in a kneeling position with an exercise ball in front of you. Next, roll forward so that you are face down on the ball with your feet on the ground and your stomach on the ball. Hold up your head and chest so that a straight line exists between your feet and head. Raise one arm up and out in front of you as you bring the other arm back and along side your body as in a swimming motion.

Lateral Plank

_____ Reps _____ Sets _____ X Day _____ Hold		_____ Reps _____ Sets _____ X Day _____ Hold
47	Notes:	**48**	Notes:

Starting

Position

LATERAL PLANK MODIFIED

Lie on your side with your knees bent, lift your body up on your elbow and knees. Try and maintain a straight spine.

LATERAL PLANK MODIFIED- BOSU- can be anything unstable

Lie on your side with your knees bent and your elbow on the Bosu, lift your body up on your elbow and knees. Try and maintain a straight spine.

	_____ Reps _____ Sets _____X Day _____Hold
49	**Notes:**

LATERAL PLANK - 1 KNEE 1 FOOT

Lie on your side with bottom knee bent and top knee straight. Lift your body up on your elbow and knee on one side and foot on the other side. Try and maintain a straight spine.

	_____ Reps _____ Sets _____X Day _____Hold
50	**Notes:**

LATERAL PLANK - 1 KNEE 1 FOOT – BOSU- Can be anything unstable

Lie on your side with elbow on Bosu with bottom knee bent and the top knee straight. Lift your body up on your elbow and knee on one side and foot on the other side. Try and maintain a straight spine.

	_____ Reps _____ Sets _____X Day _____Hold
51	**Notes:**

Starting

Position

LATERAL PLANK

Lie on your side with both legs straight and lift your body up on your elbow and feet. Try and maintain a straight spine.

	_____ Reps _____ Sets _____X Day _____Hold
52	**Notes:**

LATERAL PLANK - BOSU - Can be anything unstable

Lie on your side with your elbow on the Bosu and both legs straight. Lift your body up on your elbow and feet. Try and maintain a straight spine.

Backward Lean

	_____ Reps _____ Sets _____X Day _____Hold		_____ Reps _____ Sets _____X Day _____Hold
53	Notes:	**54**	Notes:

LEAN BACK

Start in an upright seated position with knees bent. Hold onto thighs and lean back keeping spine as straight as possible.

LEAN BACK - BOSU

Start in an upright seated position on Bosu with knees bent. Hold onto thighs or Bosu and lean back keeping spine as straight as possible.

	_____ Reps _____ Sets _____X Day _____Hold		_____ Reps _____ Sets _____X Day _____Hold
55	Notes:	**56**	Notes:

LEAN BACK WITH ARMS OUT

Start in an upright seated position with knees bent. Hold arms straight out or overhead, brace core and lean back keeping spine as straight as possible

LEAN BACK WITH ARMS OUT - BOSU

Start in an upright seated position on Bosu with knees bent. Hold arms straight out or overhead, brace core and lean back keeping spine as straight as possible.

_____ Reps _____ Sets _____ X Day _____ Hold	_____ Reps _____ Sets _____ X Day _____ Hold

57   Notes:

58   Notes:

Starting

Position

Starting

Position

LEAN BACK WITH TWIST

Start in an upright seated position with knees bent. Hold arms straight out, brace core and lean back keeping spine as straight as possible. Rotate trunk/arms to one side and then repeat to the other side.

LEAN BACK WITH TWIST – BOSU

Start in an upright seated position on Bosu with knees bent. Hold arms straight out, brace core and lean back keeping spine as straight as possible. Rotate trunk/arms to one side - repeat to the other side

_____ Reps _____ Sets _____ X Day _____ Hold	_____ Reps _____ Sets _____ X Day _____ Hold

59   Notes:

60   Notes:

CRUNCHY FROG

Sit on floor or edge of couch/bench. Lean back and with arms wide apart and legs straight. Next, bring knees towards chest and arms forward and return to starting position.

SEATED BIKE - FORWARD AND BACKWARDS

Sit on floor and lean back. With arms on floor or off ground, peddle feet forward for 15-30 repetitions, rest and then reverse. *Progress by moving hands forward near hips or remove arm support*

Abdominal Crunch Variations

	_____ Reps _____ Sets _____ X Day _____ Hold
61	Notes:

CRUNCH – ARMS OUT

Lie on your back with your arms outstretched forward, brace core and curl up lifting your shoulder blades off the ground. Exhale as you come up and squeeze/tighten your abdominal muscles.

	_____ Reps _____ Sets _____ X Day _____ Hold
62	Notes:

CRUNCH – ARMS OUT - BOSU

Lie on your back on Bosu with your arms outstretched forward, brace core and curl up lifting your shoulder blades off the ground. Exhale as you come up and squeeze/tighten your abdominal muscles.

	_____ Reps _____ Sets _____ X Day _____ Hold
63	Notes:

CRUNCH – ARMS IN BACK OF HEAD

Lie on your back with your arms behind your head, brace core and curl up lifting your shoulder blades off the ground. Exhale as you come up and squeeze/tighten your abdominal muscles. Do not pull on your neck/head.

	_____ Reps _____ Sets _____ X Day _____ Hold
64	Notes:

CRUNCH – ARMS IN BACK OF HEAD - BOSU

Lie on your back on Bosu with your arms behind your head, brace core and curl up lifting your shoulder blades off the ground. Exhale as you come up and squeeze/tighten your abdominal muscles. Do not pull on your neck/head.

_____ Reps _____ Sets _____ X Day _____ Hold

65   Notes:

OBLIQUE CRUNCH

Lie on your back with one or both hands in back of head. Brace core and curl up targeting elbow to opposite knee as shown. Keep shoulders off floor. Exhale as you come up and squeeze/tighten your abdominal muscles. Do not pull on your neck/head.

_____ Reps _____ Sets _____ X Day _____ Hold

66   Notes:

OBLIQUE CRUNCH - BOSU

Lie back on Bosu with one or both hands in back of head. Brace core and curl up targeting elbow to opposite knee as shown. Keep shoulders off Bosu. Exhale as you come up and squeeze/tighten your abdominal muscles. Do not pull on your neck/head.

_____ Reps _____ Sets _____ X Day _____ Hold

67   Notes:

90 DEGREE CRUNCH

Lie on your back with legs straight in air. Reach your hands towards toes, crunching shoulders off ground. Exhale as you come up and squeeze/tighten your abdominal muscles.

_____ Reps _____ Sets _____ X Day _____ Hold

68   Notes:

BALL CRUNCH – Can put legs on seat of chair

Lie on back with legs up on ball so knees and hips are at ~ 90 degrees. Cross hands over chest or behind head. Brace core and curl up lifting your shoulder blades off the ground. Exhale as you come up and squeeze/tighten your abdominal muscles. Do not pull on your neck/head.

	_____ Reps _____ Sets _____X Day _____Hold

69   Notes:

Starting Position

CURL UPS – ARMS ON LEGS - EXERCISE BALL

While sitting on an exercise ball, roll forward so that your back lies against the ball. Put hands on thighs/legs. Brace core and curl up lifting your shoulder blades off the ball. Exhale as you come up and squeeze/tighten your abdominal muscles.

	_____ Reps _____ Sets _____X Day _____Hold

70   Notes:

CURL UPS- ARMS CROSSED IN FRONT - EXERCISE BALL

While sitting on an exercise ball, roll forward so that your back lies against the ball. Cross hands over your chest. Brace core and curl up lifting your shoulder blades off the ball. Exhale as you come up and squeeze/tighten your abdominal muscles.

	_____ Reps _____ Sets _____X Day _____Hold

71   Notes:

CURL UPS – ARMS BEHIND HEAD - EXERCISE BALL

While sitting on an exercise ball, roll forward so that your back lies against the ball. Place your hands behind your head. Brace core and curl up lifting your shoulder blades off the ball. Exhale as you come up and squeeze/tighten your abdominal muscles. Do not pull on your neck/head.

	_____ Reps _____ Sets _____X Day _____Hold

72   Notes:

Starting Position

SUPINE CRUNCH TOUCH - EXERCISE BALL

Lie on the floor with your knees bend and holding a ball over your head. Bring both your knees and ball towards each other above your chest and touch your knees to the ball. Slowly return both to original positions and repeat.

_____ Reps _____ Sets _____ X Day _____ Hold

73   Notes:

LOWER ABDOMINAL CRUNCH – WITH or WITHOUT BALL

Sit on a solid surface with or without a ball/pillow between your knees. Maintaining a straight spine, contract your lower abdominals. Lift both knees up. Hold and control movement back to starting position. Repeat. Can be done holding onto surface for added stability with or without ball (3rd picture)

_____ Reps _____ Sets _____ X Day _____ Hold

74   Notes:

HIGH MARCH CRUNCH

Lift knee towards chest keeping hips forward in a high march position. Continue to alternate sides while standing in place. Exhale as you come up and squeeze/tighten your abdominal muscles.

_____ Reps _____ Sets _____ X Day _____ Hold

75   Notes:

Starting Position

STANDING SIDE CRUNCH

Standing with hip rotated out bring knee up towards same side elbow squeezing your obliques. Continue alternating sides while standing in place. Exhale as you come up and squeeze/tighten muscles.

_____ Reps _____ Sets _____ X Day _____ Hold

76   Notes:

Starting Position

STANDING BIKE CRUNCH

Lift knee to chest and rotate pulling opposite elbow towards knee. Continue to alternate sides while standing in place. Exhale as you come up and squeeze/tighten muscles.

Strengthening

Anaerobic - without oxygen: Single repetition with maximum resistance
Lifting lighter weights with a high number of repetitions will result in 'toning', whereas lifting heavier weights with a lower number of repetitions will result in 'bulking up'.

Benefits of strengthening	<ul><li>Increases muscle fiber size and contractile strength</li><li>Increases tendon and ligament strength</li><li>Increases bone strength / bone mineral density</li><li>Improves hormonal balances-decreased cortisol</li><li>Increases Peripheral (PNS) and Central (CNS) Nervous System communication/proprioception</li><li>Improves function for ADL's (Activities of Daily Living)</li></ul>
Range of Motion (ROM)	Refers to the distance and direction a joint can move between the flexed position and the extended position (stretching from flexion to extension for physiological gain). It is important to be able to complete full ROM before adding resistance. ***Before strengthening (adding resistance), make sure you can go through full ROM*** unless being followed by an MD or physical/occupational therapist or other professional.
Forms of strengthening exercise	<ul><li>**Isometric** – Muscles contract with no motion at the joint or change in length of the muscle. The exercises usually consist of maximal effort against an object that does not move, like a wall.</li><li>**Isotonic** – Muscles contract with motion at the joint; muscles either lengthen or shorten (*see **concentric/eccentric** below*). Tension is not constant through the range of motion. (During a bicep curl, holding a 5 lb weight, the contraction is not constant during the entire movement). Most common form of isotonic exercises use free weights with either dumbbells or a barbell.</li><li>**Concentric** – Muscle shortens, positive phase of lift. Bending the elbow in a bicep curl</li><li>**Eccentric** – Muscle lengthens, negative phase of lift or lowering. Straightening the elbow in a bicep curl.</li><li>**Isokinetic** – Muscles contract with motion at the joint; muscles either lengthen or shorten. Machines or equipment control the speed of the movement, so tension is constant providing the maximum amount of resistance throughout the entire movement.</li></ul>
Repetition (Reps)	Single cycle of lifting and lowering a weight in a controlled manner, moving through the form of the exercise. Example: 12 Bicep curls per set.
Set	Several repetitions performed one after another with no break between. There can be a number of reps per set and sets per exercise depending on the goal of the individual. Example: 12 reps x3 sets
Rep Maximum (RM)	The number of repetitions one can perform at a certain weight is called the Rep Maximum (RM). For example, if one could perform 10 repetitions with a 75 lbs dumbbell, then their RM for that weight would be 10RM. 1RM is the maximum weight that someone can lift in a given exercise - i.e. a weight that they can only lift once. (*Wikipedia*) (*See Bulk Up or Tone Up Below*)
Bulk up or Tone up	Do you want to 'bulk up' or 'tone up'? Although much of this depends on genetics and your ratio of slow and fast twitch fibers, discussed in the *Endurance* section, it is good to know what your goals are before starting. The average person should be able to perform at about 75% of their maximum resistance for 10 repetitions. If you can do ONE bicep curl with a 20-pound dumbbell/weight, then you should be able to do 10 with a 15 lbs. weight. (See *Set*) 20 lbs. x 75% = 15 lbs. Once you get into a routine, it will be easy for you to know when to increase the weight.

General rule of thumb	<ul><li>Work from the Ground up</li><li>Order: Isometric > ROM > Eccentric > Concentric</li><li>Use assistance before resistance – Start without weight to complete range of motion and then add weight with proper form. *(See ROM above)*</li><li>Add weight: 8-12 reps x 2-3 sets of each exercise at 75% of one repetition maximum (one-rep max).</li><li>Once you reach 12 easily, you can then recheck your one-rep max. If it has increased, then increase your weight as above.</li><li>If you are looking to 'bulk up', perform low repetitions at a higher weight – up to 85-90% of the one-rep maximum. 5-8 reps x 2-3 sets. With increased weight, there is a higher risk of injury.</li><li>If you are looking to 'tone up', perform high repetitions with 65-75% of the one-rep max. 12-20 reps x 2-3 sets.</li><li>Do NOT exercise the same muscle group every day. The muscles need about 48-72 hours to repair. This includes the abdomen. **Muscle strengthening, if you are lifting weights, alternate upper and lower body with isolated abdomen exercises every other day as well. For those working out several days a week, find a schedule that works for you, but give each muscle group 48-72 hours to recover.</li><li>Cardiac/aerobic conditioning can be done daily.</li><li>Breathe!! Always exhale on the exertion. For example, when you are doing a crunch, exhale as you flexing the abs or 'curling'. Do not hold your breath.</li><li>Engage your core. Don't forget what you learned under core and balance.</li></ul>

Duration, Frequency, Intensity and Movement Patterns

Intensity: How *much* mental and physical *effort* it takes to sustain an activity.	This can be done using the target heart rate range THR (optimum exercise intensity levels through beats per minute, talk test or rate of perceived exertion.
Duration: How *long* the training lasts.	The higher the intensity, the shorter the duration. The American College of Sports Medicine guidelines recommend all healthy adults aged 18–65 yr should participate in moderate intensity aerobic physical activity for a minimum of 30 min on five days per week, or vigorous intensity aerobic activity for a minimum of 20 min on three days per week.
Frequency: How *often* the training occurs.	Strength training should be performed every other day or 2-3 days a week. It is important to give each muscle group 48-72 hours to recover. Alternate upper and lower body with isolated abdomen/core exercises every other day. For those working out several days a week, find a schedule that works for you as long as you give each muscle group 48 hours of recovery time.
Movement Patterns and Examples Basic movements that help to increase overall body strengthening	<ul><li>Bend and Lift: Squats, Dead Lifts and Leg presses<ul><li>Picking up item off floor</li></ul></li><li>Single Leg: Step ups, Single leg stance, Lunges<ul><li>Walking up steps</li></ul></li><li>Push: Shoulder press, Bench press, Push up<ul><li>Pushing Shopping cart or Lawn mower</li></ul></li><li>Pull: Lat pull downs, Seated rows<ul><li>Vacuuming, Raking</li></ul></li><li>Rotational<ul><li>Shoveling snow</li></ul></li></ul>

EXERCISE Lower Extremity - Lying & Seated Strengthening and Range of Motion	EXERCISE NUMBER	NOTES
INVERSION – SEATED - ELASTIC BAND	1	
INVERSION – SEATED - ELASTIC BAND - 2	2	
EVERSION – SEATED - ELASTIC BAND	3	
EVERSION – SEATED - ELASTIC BAND - 2	4	
ANKLE PUMPS - SEATED	5	
ANKLE PUMPS – SUPINE or FEET UP ON STOOL	6	
DORSIFLEXION – SEATED - ELASTIC BAND	7	
DORSIFLEXION – SEATED - ELASTIC BAND - 2	8	
PLANTARFLEXION - STRAP	9	
PLANTARFLEXION - SEATED – ELASTIC BAND	10	
HEEL SLIDES - SUPINE	11	
HEEL SLIDES - RESISTED EXTENSION – ELASTIC BAND	12	
QUAD SET –ISOMETRIC	13	
QUAD SET WITH TOWEL UNDER HEEL - ISOMETRIC	14	
SHORT ARC QUAD (SAQ) – SELF ASSISTED	15	
SHORT ARC QUAD - (SAQ)	16	
KNEE EXTENSION - SELF ASSISTED	17	
PARTIAL ARC QUAD - LOW SEAT	18	
LONG ARC QUAD (LAQ) – LOW SEAT (90 deg)	19	
LONG ARC QUAD (LAQ) – LOW SEAT - ANKLE WEIGHTS	20	
LONG ARC QUAD (LAQ) - HIGH SEAT	21	
LONG ARC QUAD (LAQ) - HIGH SEAT - ANKLE WEIGHTS	22	
LONG ARC QUAD - ELASTIC BAND – HAND HELD	23	
LONG ARC QUAD - ELASTIC BAND	24	

EXERCISE Lower Extremity - Lying & Seated Strengthening and Range of Motion	EXERCISE NUMBER	NOTES
HAMSTRING CURLS - PRONE - ASSISTED	25	
HAMSTRING CURLS - PRONE	26	
HAMSTRING CURLS - - PRONE - WEIGHTS	27	
HAMSTRING CURLS – PRONE - ELASTIC BAND	28	
HAMSTRING CURLS – ELASTIC BAND	29	
HAMSTRING CURLS – ELASTIC BAND - 2	30	
HAMSTRING CURLS ON BALL	31	
HAMSTRING CURLS - SINGLE LEG - EXERCISE BALL	32	
HIP FLEXION ISOMETRIC	33	
HIP FLEXION ISOMETRIC BILATERAL	34	
HIP FLEXION – ISOMETRIC	35	
STRAIGHT LEG RAISE (SLR)	36	
STRAIGHT LEG RAISE (SLR) – ANKLE WEIGHTS	37	
STRAIGHT LEG RAISE (SLR) - ELASTIC BAND	38	
SEATED MARCHING	39	
SEATED MARCHING - ELASTIC BAND	40	
HIP EXTENSION - PRONE	41	
HIP EXTENSION – PRONE – ANKLE WEIGHTS	42	
HIP EXTENSION – PRONE – ELASTIC BAND	43	
HIP EXTENSION – QUADRUPED	44	
HIP ABDUCTION - SUPINE	45	
HIP ABDUCTION - SUPINE – ANKLE WEIGHTS	46	
HIP ABDUCTION – SUPINE - ELASTIC BAND	47	
HIP ABDUCTION / CLAMS– SUPINE - ELASTIC BAND	48	
MODIFIED HIP ABDUCTION – SIDELYING	49	

EXERCISE Lower Extremity - Lying & Seated Strengthening and Range of Motion	EXERCISE NUMBER	NOTES
HIP ABDUCTION – SIDELYING	50	
HIP ABDUCTION – SIDELYING - WEIGHTS	51	
HIP ABDUCTION – SIDELYING - ELASTIC BAND	52	
CLAM SHELLS	53	
SIDELYING CLAM - ELASTIC BAND	54	
HIP ABDUCTION - FIRE HYDRANT - QUADRUPED	55	
HIP ABDUCTION - FIRE HYDRANT – QUADRUPED - ELASTIC BAND	56	
HIP ABDUCTION - SEATED - STRAIGHT LEG	57	
HIP ABDUCTION - SEATED - STRAIGHT LEG – ANKLE WEIGHT	58	
HIP ABDUCTION - SINGLE- SEATED	59	
HIP ABDUCTION - SINGLE- SEATED – ELASTIC BAND	60	
HIP ABDUCTION - BILATERAL- SEATED	61	
HIP ABDUCTION - BILATERAL- SEATED - ELASTIC BAND	62	
HIP ADDUCTION SQUEEZE – SUPINE – KNEES BENT	63	
HIP ADDUCTION SQUEEZE – SUPINE – LEGS STRAIGHT	64	
HIP ADDUCTION - SIDELYING	65	
INTERNAL ROTATION - HEEL SQUEEZE - ISOMETRIC	67	
HIP INTERNAL ROTATION - SUPINE	68	
REVERSE CLAMS - SIDELYING	69	
REVERSE CLAMS - SIDELYING - ELASTIC BAND	70	
HIP INTERNAL ROTATION - SEATED	71	
HIP INTERNAL ROTATION - ELASTIC BAND	72	
HIP EXTERNAL ROTATION - SUPINE	73	

EXERCISE Lower Extremity - Lying & Seated Strengthening and Range of Motion	EXERCISE NUMBER	NOTES
HIP EXTERNAL ROTATION - ELASTIC BAND	74	
HIP ROTATIONS – BILATERAL - SIDELYING	75	
HIP ROTATION - SEATED - BALL and ELASTIC BAND	76	
PRESS – BILATERAL – ELASTIC BAND	77	
PRESS – SINGLE LEG – ELASTIC BAND	78	
HIP HIKE - STANDING	79	
HIP HIKE – KNEELING	80	
GLUTE SETS - PRONE	81	
GLUTE SET - SUPINE	82	
GLUTE SQUEEZE - SITTING	83	
PT (MAX/MEDIUS)	84	

LOWER EXTREMITY - Range Of Motion > Isometric > Strength
Lying and Seated

Inversion (IV) / Eversion (EV)

_____ Reps _____ Sets _____ X Day _____ Hold	_____ Reps _____ Sets _____ X Day _____ Hold

1 | **Notes:**
*Lymphedema: Do not wrap band around UE or LE

2 | **Notes:**
*Lymphedema: Do not wrap band around UE or LE

INVERSION – SEATED - ELASTIC BAND

In a seated position, cross your legs and using an elastic band attached to your foot, hook it under your opposite foot and up to your hand. Draw the resisted foot inward. Keep your heel in contact with the floor the entire time.

INVERSION – SEATED - ELASTIC BAND - 2

In a seated position, use an elastic band secured to a steady object and the other end attached to your foot. Draw the resisted foot inward. Keep your heel in contact with the floor the entire time.

_____ Reps _____ Sets _____ X Day _____ Hold	_____ Reps _____ Sets _____ X Day _____ Hold

3 | **Notes:**
*Lymphedema: Do not wrap band around UE or LE

4 | **Notes:**
*Lymphedema: Do not wrap band around UE or LE

EVERSION – SEATED - ELASTIC BAND

In a seated position, use an elastic band attached to your foot, hook it under your opposite foot and up to your hand. Draw the resisted foot outward. Keep your heel in contact with the floor the entire time.

EVERSION – SEATED - ELASTIC BAND - 2

In a seated position, use an elastic band secured to a steady object and the other end attached to your foot. Draw the resisted foot outward. Keep your heel in contact with the floor the entire time.

Dorsiflexion (DF) / Plantarflexion (PF)

	_____ Reps _____ Sets _____X Day _____Hold
5	**Notes:**

ANKLE PUMPS - SEATED

In a seated position keeping feet on the floor, first go up on toes (toes pointed towards the ground – PF). Then point toes up keeping heels on the ground (DF). Alternate back and forth in a pumping motion.

	_____ Reps _____ Sets _____X Day _____Hold
6	**Notes:**

ANKLE PUMPS – SUPINE or FEET UP ON STOOL

Lying or with feet up on stool first point the toes forward (PF) and then back up with toes facing the ceiling. Alternate back and forth in a pumping motion.

	_____ Reps _____ Sets _____X Day _____Hold
7	**Notes:** *Lymphedema: Do not wrap band around UE or LE

DORSIFLEXION – SEATED - ELASTIC BAND

In a seated position, use an elastic band attached to your target foot, hook it under your opposite foot and up to your hand. Draw the band upwards with the resisted foot as shown. Keep your heel in contact with the floor the entire time.

	_____ Reps _____ Sets _____X Day _____Hold
8	**Notes:** *Lymphedema: Do not wrap band around UE or LE

DORSIFLEXION – SEATED - ELASTIC BAND - 2

In a seated position, use an elastic band secured to a steady object and the other end attached to your foot. Draw the resisted foot upward. Keep your heel in contact with the floor the entire time.

	_____ Reps _____ Sets _____X Day _____Hold
9	**Notes:** *Lymphedema: Do not wrap band around UE or LE

PLANTARFLEXION - STRAP

In a seated position, attach one loop of the strap to your foot and hold the other end. Move your foot forward and back at the ankle as shown. Keep your heel in contact with the floor the entire time.

	_____ Reps _____ Sets _____X Day _____Hold
10	**Notes:** *Lymphedema: Do not wrap band around UE or LE

PLANTARFLEXION - SEATED – ELASTIC BAND

In a seated position, hold an elastic band and attach the other end to your foot. Press your foot downward towards the floor. Keep your heel in contact with the floor the entire time.

Heel Slides

	_____ Reps _____ Sets _____X Day _____Hold
11	**Notes:**

HEEL SLIDES - SUPINE

Lie on your back with knees straight and slide the target heel towards your buttock as you bend your knee. Hold a gentle stretch in this position and then return to original position.

	_____ Reps _____ Sets _____X Day _____Hold
12	**Notes:** *Lymphedema: Do not wrap band around UE or LE

HEEL SLIDES - RESISTED EXTENSION – ELASTIC BAND

Long sit with band around bottom of target foot. Slide the target heel towards your buttock as you bend your knee. Push your foot to straighten knee against resistance to the original position.

Quadriceps (QUAD) / Knee Extension

	_____ Reps _____ Sets _____ X Day _____ Hold
13	Notes:

QUAD SET –ISOMETRIC

Tighten your top thigh muscle as you attempt to press the back of your knee downward towards the table. Hold 5-10 seconds. Repeat.

	_____ Reps _____ Sets _____ X Day _____ Hold
14	Notes:

Starting Position

QUAD SET WITH TOWEL UNDER HEEL - ISOMETRIC

Lying or sitting with a small towel roll under your ankle, tighten your top thigh muscle to press the back of your knee downward towards the ground. Hold 5-10 seconds. Repeat.

	_____ Reps _____ Sets _____ X Day _____ Hold
15	Notes:

Starting Position

SHORT ARC QUAD (SAQ) – SELF ASSISTED

Place a rolled-up towel or other rounded object under your knee. Hook one foot under the other to assist the affected leg. Slowly straighten your knee as your raise up your foot tightening the top thigh muscle.

	_____ Reps _____ Sets _____ X Day _____ Hold
16	Notes:

SHORT ARC QUAD - (SAQ) - Can add ankle weight

Place a rolled-up towel or object under your knee and slowly straighten your knee as your raise up your foot tightening the top thigh muscle. Flex your foot to increase the stretch.

_____ Reps _____ Sets _____ X Day _____ Hold		_____ Reps _____ Sets _____ X Day _____ Hold
17	Notes:	**18** Notes:

KNEE EXTENSION - SELF ASSISTED

In a seated position, place the unaffected leg under the target leg. Use the unaffected leg to assist the target leg up to a straightened knee position.

PARTIAL ARC QUAD - LOW SEAT - Can add ankle weight

Sit with your knee in a semi bent position and your heel touching the ground and then slowly straighten your knee as you raise your foot upwards as shown. Lower your foot back down slowly controling the muscle until your heel touches the ground and then repeat.

_____ Reps _____ Sets _____ X Day _____ Hold		_____ Reps _____ Sets _____ X Day _____ Hold
19	Notes:	**20** Notes:

LONG ARC QUAD (LAQ) – LOW SEAT (90 deg)

Sit with your knee in a bent position and then tighten the quadricep. Slowly straighten your knee as you raise your foot upwards as shown. Lower your foot back down to original bent knee position slowly controlling the muscle and then repeat.

LONG ARC QUAD (LAQ) – LOW SEAT - ANKLE WEIGHTS

Attach and ankle weight. Sit with your knee in a bent position and then tighten the quadricep. Slowly straighten your knee as you raise your foot upwards as shown. Lower your foot back down to original bent knee position slowly controlling the muscle - repeat.

	_____ Reps _____ Sets _____ X Day _____ Hold		_____ Reps _____ Sets _____ X Day _____ Hold
21	Notes:	**22**	Notes:

LONG ARC QUAD (LAQ) - HIGH SEAT

Sit with your knee in a bent position and then tighten the quadricep. Slowly straighten your knee as you raise your foot upwards as shown. Lower your foot back down to original bent knee position slowly controlling the muscle and then repeat.

LONG ARC QUAD (LAQ) - HIGH SEAT - ANKLE WEIGHTS

Attach and ankle weight. Sit with your knee in a bent position and then tighten the quadricep. Slowly straighten your knee as you raise your foot upwards as shown. Lower your foot back down to original bent knee position slowly controlling the muscle and then repeat.

	_____ Reps _____ Sets _____ X Day _____ Hold		_____ Reps _____ Sets _____ X Day _____ Hold
23	Notes: *Lymphedema: Do not wrap band around UE or LE	**24**	Notes: *Lymphedema: Do not wrap band around UE or LE

LONG ARC QUAD - ELASTIC BAND – HANDHELD

Attach a looped elastic band to your ankle and to the opposite foot or hold with your hand. Sit with your knee in a bent position and then tighten the quadricep. Draw your lower leg upwards to a straighten knee position while your other foot or hand secures the band. Lower your foot back down to original bent knee position slowly controlling the muscle and then repeat.

LONG ARC QUAD - ELASTIC BAND

Attach a looped elastic band to your ankle and to a steady object behind you. Sit with your knee in a bent position and then tighten the quadricep. Draw your lower leg upwards to a straightened knee position. Lower your foot back down to original bent knee position slowly controlling the muscle and then repeat.

Hamstrings

_____ Reps _____ Sets _____ X Day _____ Hold		_____ Reps _____ Sets _____ X Day _____ Hold
25	Notes:	**26**	Notes:

HAMSTRING CURLS - PRONE - ASSISTED

Lie face down and hook one foot under the other to assist the affected leg. Bend the target leg with the assistance of your unaffected leg.

HAMSTRING CURLS - PRONE

Lie face down and slowly bend your knee as you bring your foot towards your buttock.

_____ Reps _____ Sets _____ X Day _____ Hold		_____ Reps _____ Sets _____ X Day _____ Hold
27	Notes:	**28**	Notes: *Lymphedema: Do not wrap band around UE or LE

HAMSTRING CURLS - - PRONE - WEIGHTS

Attach and ankle weight. Lie face down and slowly bend your knee as you bring your foot towards your buttock.

HAMSTRING CURLS – PRONE - ELASTIC BAND

Attach an elastic band around your foot and opposite ankle as shown. While lying face down, slowly bend your target knee as you bring your foot towards your buttock. Keep your other foot on the floor to fixate the band.

_____ Reps _____ Sets _____X Day _____Hold		_____ Reps _____ Sets _____X Day _____Hold
29	**Notes:** *Lymphedema: Do not wrap band around UE or LE	**30**	**Notes:** *Lymphedema: Do not wrap band around UE or LE

HAMSTRING CURLS – ELASTIC BAND

Sit and use an elastic band secured to a steady object and the other end attached to your ankle. Bend your knee and draw back your foot.

HAMSTRING CURLS – ELASTIC BAND - 2

Attach a looped elastic band to your ankle and to the opposite foot while one leg is propped on stool or another raised object. Draw your lower leg downwards to a bent knee position while your other ankle anchors the band on the chair.

_____ Reps _____ Sets _____X Day _____Hold		_____ Reps _____ Sets _____X Day _____Hold
31	**Notes:**	**32**	**Notes: **Advanced**

HAMSTRING CURLS ON BALL – can add ankle weight.

Lie prone on an exercise ball as shown. Slowly bend your knee as you bring your foot towards your buttock.

Starting

Position

HAMSTRING CURLS - SINGLE LEG - EXERCISE BALL

Lie on the floor and place your heel on an exercise ball.
Lift your buttocks and then bend your knees to draw the ball towards your buttocks. Keep your buttocks elevated off the floor the entire time.

Hip Flexion

	_____Reps _____Sets _____X Day _____Hold		_____Reps _____Sets _____X Day _____Hold
33	Notes:	**34**	Notes:

HIP FLEXION ISOMETRIC

Lie on your back, lift up your knee and press it into your hand. Hold. Return to the original position and repeat.

HIP FLEXION ISOMETRIC - ALTERNATING
Lie on your back, lift up your knee and press it into your hand. Hold. Return to the original position and repeat on the other side.

HIP FLEXION ISOMETRIC BILATERAL

Lie on your back, lift up your knees and press them into your hands. Hold. Return to the original position and repeat.

	_____Reps _____Sets _____X Day _____Hold		_____Reps _____Sets _____X Day _____Hold
35	Notes:	**36**	Notes:

HIP FLEXION – ISOMETRIC - Can use towel roll for comfort

While standing in front of a wall, draw your knee forward and press it into the wall. Place a folded towel between your knee and the wall for comfort if needed.

STRAIGHT LEG RAISE (SLR)

Lie on your back, tighten the quad of the target leg and lift up with a straight knee. Keep the opposite knee bent with the foot planted on the ground. (see #37 for starting position)

_____ Reps _____ Sets _____ X Day _____ Hold

37	Notes:

Starting
Position

STRAIGHT LEG RAISE (SLR) – ANKLE WEIGHTS

Attach ankle weights. Lie on your back and lift up your leg with a straight knee. Keep the opposite knee bent with the foot planted on the ground

_____ Reps _____ Sets _____ X Day _____ Hold

38	Notes:
	*Lymphedema: Do not wrap band around UE or LE

STRAIGHT LEG RAISE (SLR) - ELASTIC BAND

Lie on your back with an elastic band looped around your ankles, lift the target leg upwards.

_____ Reps _____ Sets _____ X Day _____ Hold

39	Notes:

SEATED MARCHING - can add ankle weights for resistance

Sit in a chair and move a knee upward, set it back down and then alternate to the other side

_____ Reps _____ Sets _____ X Day _____ Hold

40	Notes:
	*Lymphedema: Do not wrap band around UE or LE

SEATED MARCHING - ELASTIC BAND

Sit in a chair with an elastic band wrapped around your thighs. Move a knee upward, set it back down and then alternate to the other side.

Hip Extension

_____ Reps _____ Sets _____X Day _____Hold	_____ Reps _____ Sets _____X Day _____Hold
41 **Notes:**	**42** **Notes:**

HIP EXTENSION - PRONE

Lie face down with your knee straight and slowly lift up leg off the ground. Maintain a straight knee the entire time.

HIP EXTENSION – PRONE – ANKLE WEIGHTS

Attach ankle weights. Lie face down with your knee straight and slowly lift up leg off the ground. Maintain a straight knee the entire time.

_____ Reps _____ Sets _____X Day _____Hold	_____ Reps _____ Sets _____X Day _____Hold
43 **Notes:** ***Lymphedema: Do not wrap band around UE or LE**	**44** **Notes:**

HIP EXTENSION – PRONE – ELASTIC BAND

Lie on your stomach with an elastic band looped around your ankles and lift the targeted leg upwards. Maintain a straight knee the entire time.

HIP EXTENSION – QUADRUPED with or without ankle weights

Start in a crawl position and then raise your leg up behind you as shown. Keep your knee bent at 90 degrees the entire time.

Hip Abduction (ABD)

_____ Reps _____ Sets _____ X Day _____ Hold	_____ Reps _____ Sets _____ X Day _____ Hold
45 Notes:	**46** Notes:

HIP ABDUCTION - SUPINE

Lie on your back and slowly bring your leg out to the side. Return to original position and repeat. Keep your knee straight the entire time.

HIP ABDUCTION - SUPINE – ANKLE WEIGHTS

Attach and weights. Lie on your back and slowly bring your leg up slightly and then out to the side. Return to original position and repeat. Keep your knee straight the entire time.

_____ Reps _____ Sets _____ X Day _____ Hold	_____ Reps _____ Sets _____ X Day _____ Hold
47 Notes: *Lymphedema: Do not wrap band around UE or LE	**48** Notes: *Lymphedema: Do not wrap band around UE or LE

HIP ABDUCTION – SUPINE - ELASTIC BAND

Lie on your back and slowly bring your leg out to the side. Return to original position and repeat. Keep your knee straight the entire time.

HIP ABDUCTION / CLAMS– SUPINE - ELASTIC BAND

Lie down on your back with your knees bent. Place an elastic band around your knees and then draw your knees apart. Return to original position and repeat.

_____ Reps _____ Sets _____ X Day _____ Hold		_____ Reps _____ Sets _____ X Day _____ Hold
49	Notes:	**50**	Notes:

MODIFIED HIP ABDUCTION – SIDELYING can add weights

Lie on your side and slowly lift up your top leg to the side. The bottom leg can be bent to stabilize your body. Keep your knee straight and maintain your toes pointed forward the entire time. Keep your leg in-line with your body. Return to original position and repeat.

HIP ABDUCTION – SIDELYING

Lie on your side and slowly lift up your top leg to the side. Keep your knee straight and maintain your toes pointed forward the entire time. Keep your leg in-line with your body. Return to original position and repeat.

_____ Reps _____ Sets _____ X Day _____ Hold		_____ Reps _____ Sets _____ X Day _____ Hold
51	Notes:	**52**	Notes: *Lymphedema: Do not wrap band around UE or LE

HIP ABDUCTION – SIDELYING - WEIGHTS

Attach ankle weights. Lie on your side and slowly lift up your top leg to the side. Keep your knee straight and maintain your toes pointed forward the entire time. Keep your leg in-line with your body. Return to original position and repeat.

HIP ABDUCTION – SIDELYING - ELASTIC BAND

Lie on your side with an elastic band looped around your ankles. Lift the top leg upwards keeping your knee straight and maintaining your toes pointed forward the entire time. Keep your leg in-line with your body. Return to original position and repeat.

| _____ Reps _____ Sets _____ X Day _____ Hold | | _____ Reps _____ Sets _____ X Day _____ Hold | |

53   **Notes:**

54   **Notes:**
*Lymphedema: Do not wrap band around UE or LE

Starting

Position

CLAM SHELLS

Lie on your side with your knees bent, draw up the top knee while keeping contact of your feet together.
Do not let your pelvis roll back during the lifting movement.

Starting

Position

SIDELYING CLAM - ELASTIC BAND

Lie on your side with your knees bent and an elastic band wrapped around your knees, draw up the top knee while keeping contact of your feet together as shown. Do not let your pelvis roll back during the lifting movement.

| _____ Reps _____ Sets _____ X Day _____ Hold | | _____ Reps _____ Sets _____ X Day _____ Hold | |

55   **Notes:**

56   **Notes:**
*Lymphedema: Do not wrap band around UE or LE

Starting

Position

HIP ABDUCTION - FIRE HYDRANT - QUADRUPED

Start in a crawl position and raise your leg out to the side as shown. Maintain a straight upper and mid back.

Starting

Position

HIP ABDUCTION - FIRE HYDRANT – QUADRUPED - ELASTIC BAND

Start in a crawl position with an elastic band around your thighs. Raise your leg out to the side as shown. Maintain a straight upper and mid back.

_____ Reps _____ Sets _____X Day _____Hold		
57	**Notes:**	

HIP ABDUCTION - SEATED - STRAIGHT LEG

Sit close to the edge of a chair with your target leg straight at the knee. Move your target leg to the side lifting slightly off the ground and then return to straight ahead.. You can slide your heel across the floor as you move and then return to straight ahead if unable to lift. Maintain your toes pointed up the entire time.

_____ Reps _____ Sets _____X Day _____Hold		
58	**Notes:**	

HIP ABDUCTION - SEATED - STRAIGHT LEG – ANKLE WEIGHT

Attach an ankle weight. Sit close to the edge of a chair with your target leg straight at the knee. Move your target leg to the side lifting slightly off the ground and then return to straight ahead. Maintain your toes pointed up the entire time.

_____ Reps _____ Sets _____X Day _____Hold		
59	**Notes:**	

HIP ABDUCTION - SINGLE- SEATED

Sit close to the edge of a chair with knees bent and both feet on the floor. Move your target knee out to the side as shown and then return to straight ahead. Maintain contact of your feet on the floor the entire time.

_____ Reps _____ Sets _____X Day _____Hold		
60	**Notes:** *Lymphedema: Do not wrap band around UE or LE	

HIP ABDUCTION - SINGLE- SEATED – ELASTIC BAND

With band tied around the thighs, sit close to the edge of a chair with knees bent and both feet on the floor. Move your target knee out to the side as shown and then return to straight ahead. Maintain contact of your feet on the floor the entire time.tact of your feet on the floor the entire time.

_____ Reps _____ Sets _____X Day _____Hold		_____ Reps _____ Sets _____X Day _____Hold

61 | Notes: | **62** | Notes:
| | | *Lymphedema: Do not wrap band around UE or LE

HIP ABDUCTION - BILATERAL- SEATED

Sit close to the edge of a chair with knees bent and both feet on the floor. Move your knees out to the side as shown and then return to straight ahead. Maintain contact of your feet on the floor the entire time.

HIP ABDUCTION - BILATERAL- SEATED - ELASTIC BAND

Sit close to the edge of a chair with an elastic band wrapped around your knees. Move both knees to the sides to separate your legs. Keep contact of your feet on the floor the entire time.

Hip Adduction (ADD)

_____ Reps _____ Sets _____X Day _____Hold		_____ Reps _____ Sets _____X Day _____Hold

63 | Notes: | **64** | Notes:

HIP ADDUCTION SQUEEZE – SUPINE – KNEES BENT

Lie on your back with legs bent and place a rolled up towel, ball or pillow between your knees. Press your knees together so that you squeeze the object firmly. Hold, release and repeat.

HIP ADDUCTION SQUEEZE – SUPINE – LEGS STRAIGHT

Lie on your back and place a rolled up towel, ball or pillow between your knees. Squeeze the object with your knees. Hold, release and repeat.

_____ Reps _____ Sets _____ X Day _____ Hold	_____ Reps _____ Sets _____ X Day _____ Hold
65 Notes:	**66** Notes:

HIP ADDUCTION - SIDELYING

Lie on your side, slowly lift up your bottom leg towards the ceiling. Keep your knee straight the entire time. Your top leg should be bent at the knee and your foot planted on the ground supporting your body.

BALL SQUEEZE - SEATED

Sit and place a rolled-up towel, ball or pillow between your knees and squeeze the object firmly. Hold, release and repeat.

Hip Internal Rotation (IR)

_____ Reps _____ Sets _____ X Day _____ Hold	_____ Reps _____ Sets _____ X Day _____ Hold
67 Notes:	**68** Notes:

INTERNAL ROTATION - HEEL SQUEEZE - ISOMETRIC

Lie face down, spead your knees apart and press your heels together. Hold, release and repeat.

HIP INTERNAL ROTATION - SUPINE

Lie on your back with your knees straight, roll your hip in so that your toes point inward. Be sure that your knee cap faces inward as well.

_____ Reps _____ Sets _____ X Day _____ Hold

69 | **Notes:**

Starting
Position

REVERSE CLAMS - SIDELYING

Lie on your side with your knees bent and raise your top foot towards the ceiling while keeping contact of your knees together. Lower back down to original position. Do not let your pelvis roll forward during the lifting movement.

_____ Reps _____ Sets _____ X Day _____ Hold

70 | **Notes:**
*Lymphedema: Do not wrap band around UE or LE

Starting Position

REVERSE CLAMS - SIDELYING - ELASTIC BAND

Lie on your side with your knees bent and an elastic band around your ankles. Raise your top foot towards the ceiling while keeping contact of your knees together. Lower back down to original position. Do not let your pelvis roll forward during the lifting movement.

_____ Reps _____ Sets _____ X Day _____ Hold

71 | **Notes:**

HIP INTERNAL ROTATION - SEATED

Sit on a chair with your legs spread apart and feet planted on the ground. Use your hand on the inside of your knee to resist the movement inward.

_____ Reps _____ Sets _____ X Day _____ Hold

72 | **Notes:**
*Lymphedema: Do not wrap band around UE or LE

HIP INTERNAL ROTATION - ELASTIC BAND - High chair

Attach one end of an elastic band at your ankle and the other to a sturdy object. Pull away from your other leg while keeping your thigh from moving.

Hip External Rotation (ER)

_____ Reps _____ Sets _____X Day _____Hold		_____ Reps _____ Sets _____X Day _____Hold

73	**Notes:**	**74**	**Notes:** *Lymphedema: Do not wrap band around UE or LE

HIP EXTERNAL ROTATION - SUPINE

Lie on your back with your knees straight and roll your hip out so that your toes point outward. Be sure that your knee cap faces outward as well.

HIP EXTERNAL ROTATION - ELASTIC BAND

Sit and use an elastic band secured to a steady object and the other end attached to your ankle from the side.
Pull towards your other leg while keeping your thigh from moving across the table.

Bilateral Hip Rotation

_____ Reps _____ Sets _____X Day _____Hold		_____ Reps _____ Sets _____X Day _____Hold

75	**Notes:**	**76**	**Notes:** *Lymphedema: Do not wrap band around UE or LE

HIP ROTATIONS – BILATERAL - SIDELYING

Lie on your side in fetal position with knees and hips bent.
Slowly raise up both lower legs and feet as shown.
Your feet and knees should be touching the entire time.

HIP ROTATION - SEATED - BALL and ELASTIC BAND – High chair

Sit and place a rolled-up towel, ball or pillow between your knees and an elastic band around your ankles. Squeeze the ball, sustain and hold. Next, pull the band as you move your feet apart from each other.

Leg Press		

	_____ Reps _____ Sets _____ X Day _____ Hold		_____ Reps _____ Sets _____ X Day _____ Hold
77	Notes: *Lymphedema: Do not wrap band around UE or LE	78	Notes: *Lymphedema: Do not wrap band around UE or LE

Starting Position

PRESS – BILATERAL – ELASTIC BAND

Lie on back put elastic band on bottom of both feet. Start with knees bent and push with feet to straighten both legs.

PRESS – SINGLE LEG – ELASTIC BAND

Lie on back put elastic band on bottom of one foot. Start with knees bent and push with foot to straighten leg.

Hip Hikes (Gluteus Medius)		

	_____ Reps _____ Sets _____ X Day _____ Hold		_____ Reps _____ Sets _____ X Day _____ Hold
79	Notes:	80	Notes:

HIP HIKE - STANDING on Step or Pad

Stand with one foot on a step or pad and the other hanging off as shown. Raise and lower the side of your pelvis that is hanging off the edge.

HIP HIKE – KNEELING on towel or pad

Kneel on both knees with one knee on a folded towel or pad. Raise and lower the side of your pelvis that is not on the towel/pad.

Glutes (Glute Max)		

	_____ Reps _____ Sets _____X Day _____Hold	
81	Notes:	

GLUTE SETS - PRONE

Lie face down, squeeze your buttocks and hold. Repeat.

	_____ Reps _____ Sets _____X Day _____Hold	
82	Notes:	

GLUTE SET - SUPINE

Lie on your back, squeeze your buttocks and hold. Repeat.

	_____ Reps _____ Sets _____X Day _____Hold	
83	Notes:	

GLUTE SQUEEZE - SITTING

While sitting, squeeze your buttocks and hold. Repeat.

	_____ Reps _____ Sets _____X Day _____Hold	
84	Notes:	

GLUTE SCULPT (MAX/MEDIUS)

Lie on your side leaning towards your stomach. Bend leg on target side, raise up and hold.

EXERCISE Upper Extremity Strengthening and Range of Motion	EXERCISE NUMBER	NOTES
ELBOW FLEXION EXTENSION - SUPINE	1	
ELBOW FLEXION / EXTENSION - GRAVITY ELIMINATED	2	
BICEPS CURLS – ALTERNATING	3	
BICEPS CURL - SELF FIXATION – ELASTIC BAND	4	
SEATED BICEPS CURLS - ALTERNATING	5	
SEATED BICEPS CURLS - BILATERAL	6	
CONCENTRATION CURLS – SITTING	7	
PREACHER CURL ON BALL	8	
BICEPS CURLS	9	
BICEPS CURLS - RADIOBRACHIALIS - HAMMER CURL	10	
BICEPS CURLS - BRACHIALIS	11	
BICEPS CURLS – ROTATE OUTWARD	12	
BICEPS CURLS – ONE ARM - ELASTIC BAND	13	
BICEPS CURLS – BILATERAL - ELASTIC BAND	14	
BICEPS CURLS - RADIOBRACHIALIS - HAMMER CURL – ONE ARM - ELASTIC BAND	15	
BICEPS CURLS - RADIOBRACHIALIS - HAMMER CURL – BILATERAL - ELASTIC BAND	16	
BICEPS CURLS – BRACHIALIS - ONE ARM - ELASTIC BAND	17	
BICEPS CURL – BRACHIALIS – BILATERAL - ELASTIC BAND	18	
TRICEPS - SELF FIXATION - ELASTIC BAND	19	
OVERHEAD TRICEPS - SELF FIXATION –SEATED OR STANDING - ELASTIC BAND	20	
TRICEP EXTENSION – SITTING OR STANDING - WEIGHT	21	
TRICEP EXTENSION – SITTING OR STANDING – BILATERAL - WEIGHT	22	
ELBOW EXTENSION - BALL	23	

EXERCISE Upper Extremity Strengthening and Range of Motion	EXERCISE NUMBER	NOTES
ELBOW EXTENSION - SKULL CRUSHER - BALL	24	
TRICEPS - ELASTIC BAND	25	
TRICEPS - BENT OVER	26	
CHAIR DIPS / PUSH UPS	27	
DIPS OFF CHAIR	28	
PENDULUM SHOULDER FORWARD/BACK	29	
PENDULUM SHOULDER – SIDE TO SIDE	30	
PENDULUM SHOULDER CIRCLES	31	
PENDULUMS - SUPINE	32	
ISOMETRIC FLEXION	33	
SHOULDER FLEXION – SIDELYING	34	
FLEXION – SUPINE - SINGLE OR BILATERAL	35	
FLEXION – SUPINE – SINGLE OR BILATERAL - WEIGHT	36	
FLEXION – SUPINE - DOWEL	37	
FLEXION – SUPINE - DOWEL - Weight	38	
FLEXION - SELF FIXATION – ELASTIC BAND	39	
FLEXION – ELASTIC BAND	40	
FLEXION - STANDING - PALMS DOWN / OVERHAND DOWEL	41	
FLEXION - STANDING - PALMS UP / UNDERHAND DOWEL	42	
FLEXION – PALMS FACING INWARD	43	
FLEXION – PALMS DOWN	44	
V RAISE	45	
V RAISE – WEIGHTS	46	
MILITARY PRESS – DOWEL	47	
MILITARY PRESS - FREE WEIGHTS	48	

EXERCISE Upper Extremity Strengthening and Range of Motion	EXERCISE NUMBER	NOTES
ISOMETRIC EXTENSION	49	
PRONE EXTENSION - EXERCISE BALL	50	
SHOULDER EXTENSION - STANDING	51	
SHOULDER EXTENSION - STANDING - WEIGHTS	52	
EXTENSION – STANDING – DOWEL	53	
EXTENSION - SELF FIXATION - ELASTIC BAND	54	
EXTENSION - ELASTIC BAND	55	
EXTENSION - BILATERAL - ELASTIC BAND	56	
INTERNAL ROTATION – ISOMETRIC	57	
INTERNAL ROTATION - ISOMETRIC- ELEVATED	58	
INTERNAL ROTATION - SIDELYING	59	
INTERNAL ROTATION - ELASTIC BAND	60	
INTERNAL / EXTERNAL ROTATION - STANDING – DOWEL	61	
INTERNAL ROTATION – DOWEL	62	
EXTERNAL ROTATION - ISOMETRIC	63	
EXTERNAL ROTATION - ISOMETRIC – ELEVATED	64	
EXTERNAL ROTATION WITH TOWEL - SIDELYING	65	
EXTERNAL ROTATION – 90/90 - WEIGHTS	66	
EXTERNAL ROTATION - BILATERAL - ELASTIC BAND	67	
EXTERNAL ROTATION - ELASTIC BAND	68	
ADDUCTION – ISOMETRIC	69	
ADDUCTION - ELASTIC BAND	70	
ABDUCTION – ISOMETRIC	71	
HORIZONTAL ABDUCTION - DOWEL	72	

EXERCISE Upper Extremity Strengthening and Range of Motion	EXERCISE NUMBER	NOTES
HORIZONTAL ABDUCTION/ADDUCTTION - SUPINE	73	
HORIZONTAL ABDUCTION/ADDUCTTION - SUPINE -WEIGHT	74	
ABDUCTION - SIDELYING	75	
HORIZONTAL ABDUCTION - SIDELYING	76	
ABDUCTION – WEIGHT	77	
ABDUCTION – ELASTIC BAND	78	
HORIZONTAL ABDUCTION – BILATERAL - ELASTIC BAND	79	
90/90 ABDUCTION - WEIGHT	80	
LATERAL RAISES	81	
LATERAL RAISES – LEAN FORWARD	82	
LATERAL RAISES – LEAN FORWARD - ARM ROTATION	83	
FRONTAL RAISE – WEIGHTS	84	
UPRIGHT ROW – WEIGHTS	85	
UPRIGHT ROW – ELASTIC BAND	86	
SHRUGS	87	
SHRUGS - WEIGHTS	88	
SHOULDER ROLLS	89	
SHOULDER ROLLS - WEIGHTS	90	
SCAPULAR RETRACTIONS - BILATERAL	91	
SCAPULAR RETRACTION – SINGLE ARM	92	
ELASTIC BAND SCAPULAR RETRACTIONS WITH MINI SHOULDER EXTENSIONS	93	
PRONE RETRACTION	94	
SCAPULAR PROTRACTION - SUPINE - BILATERAL	95	
SCAPULAR PROTRACTION - SUPINE - WEIGHT	96	

EXERCISE Upper Extremity Strengthening and Range of Motion	EXERCISE NUMBER	NOTES
SCAPULAR PROTRACTION - SUPINE - ELASTIC BAND	97	
SCAPULAR PROTRACTION / TABLE PLANK	98	
CHEST PRESS – SEATED or STANDING - ELASTIC BAND	99	
CHEST PRESS – BALL, FLOOR or BENCH- WEIGHTS	100	
DOWEL PRESS – STANDING	101	
CHEST PRESS – STANDING or SEATED	102	
BENT OVER ROWS	103	
ROWS – PRONE	104	
ROWS - ELASTIC BAND	105	
WIDE ROWS - ELASTIC BAND	106	
LOW ROW – ELASTIC BAND	107	
HIGH ROW – ELASTIC BAND	108	
FLY'S – FLOOR - WEIGHT	109	
FLY'S – BALL or BENCH – WEIGHT	110	
WALL PUSH UPS	111	
WALL PUSH UP - BALL	112	
WALL PUSH UP - Triceps uneven	113	
WALL PUSH UP - Hands inverted	114	
WALL PUSH UP - Narrow	115	
WALL PUSH UP – Wide	116	
PUSH UPS - BALL	117	
PUSH UP - MODIFIED	118	
PUSH UP	119	
PUSH UP -DIAMOND	120	
PUSH UP – MODIFIED - BOSU - UNSTABLE	121	

EXERCISE **Upper Extremity Strengthening and Range of Motion**	EXERCISE NUMBER	NOTES
PUSH UP – BOSU - UNSTABLE	122	
PUSH UP – MODIFIED – INVERTED BOSU - UNSTABLE	123	
PUSH UP – INVERTED BOSU - UNSTABLE	124	

UPPER EXTREMITY - Range Of Motion > Isometric > Strength

Elbow Flexion/Extension

	_____ Reps _____ Sets _____X Day _____Hold		_____ Reps _____ Sets _____X Day _____Hold
1	**Notes:**	**2**	**Notes:**

Flexion   Extension

Extension

Flexion

ELBOW FLEXION EXTENSION - SUPINE

Lie on your back and rest your elbow on a small rolled up towel. Bend at your elbow and then lower back down.

ELBOW FLEXION / EXTENSION - GRAVITY ELIMINATED

Sit and hold your arm up with the help of your other arm. Bend and straighten your elbow.

Elbow Flexion (Biceps)

	_____ Reps _____ Sets _____X Day _____Hold		_____ Reps _____ Sets _____X Day _____Hold
3	**Notes:**	**4**	**Notes:** *Lymphedema: Do not wrap band around UE or LE

BICEPS CURLS – ALTERNATING

Bend your elbow and move your forearm upwards. As you lower back down, begin bending the opposite elbow upwards.

BICEPS CURL - SELF FIXATION – ELASTIC BAND

Sit and hold an elastic band with one hand. Hold the other end of elastic band with the opposite hand and fixate hand on your knee. Slowly draw up your hand by bending at the elbow. Return to starting position and repeat.

*Can increase resistance by doubling band as shown.

	_____ Reps _____ Sets _____X Day _____Hold			

5	**Notes:** *Neuropathy/Hands – Precaution holding weights

SEATED BICEPS CURLS - ALTERNATING

Sit in a chair and hold free weights on each thigh. Lift one side while bending at the elbow and squeezing bicep muscle. Perform on one side and then alternate to the other side.

	_____ Reps _____ Sets _____X Day _____Hold			

6	**Notes:** *Neuropathy/Hands – Precaution holding weights

SEATED BICEPS CURLS - BILATERAL

Sit in a chair and hold free weights on each thigh. Lift both sides while bending at the elbows and squeezing bicep muscles. Lower back down and repeat.

	_____ Reps _____ Sets _____X Day _____Hold			

7	**Notes:** *Neuropathy/Hands – Precaution holding weights

CONCENTRATION CURLS – SITTING

Sit in a chair, lean slightly forward and hold a free weight with arm straight with elbow on inside of thigh. Bend elbow squeezing bicep muscle. Lower back down - repeat.

	_____ Reps _____ Sets _____X Day _____Hold			

8	**Notes:** *Neuropathy/Hands – Precaution holding weights

Starting Position

PREACHER CURL ON BALL

Lie on stomach over ball in crawling position. Hold weights in both hands with back of arms against ball. Lift both sides while bending at the elbows and squeezing bicep muscles. Lower back down - repeat.

	_____ Reps _____ Sets _____X Day _____Hold
9	**Notes:** *Neuropathy/Hands – Precaution holding weights

BICEPS CURLS

Holding weights and keeping your arm at your side, draw up your hand by bending at the elbow squeezing bicep muscle. Keep your palm face up the entire time. Can perform set on one side and then other or alternate arms.

	_____ Reps _____ Sets _____X Day _____Hold
10	**Notes:** *Neuropathy/Hands – Precaution holding weights

BICEPS CURLS - RADIOBRACHIALIS - HAMMER CURL

Holding weights and keeping your arm at your side, draw up your hand by bending at the elbow squeezing bicep muscle. Keep your wrist in a neutral position as shown above the entire time. Can perform set on one side and then other or alternate arms.

	_____ Reps _____ Sets _____X Day _____Hold
11	**Notes:** *Neuropathy/Hands – Precaution holding weights

BICEPS CURLS - BRACHIALIS

Holding weights and keeping your arm at your side, draw up your hand by bending at the elbow squeezing bicep muscle. Keep your palm face down the entire time. Can perform set on one side and then other or alternate arms.

	_____ Reps _____ Sets _____X Day _____Hold
12	**Notes:** *Neuropathy/Hands – Precaution holding weights

BICEPS CURLS – ROTATE OUTWARD

Holding weights and keeping your arm at your side, draw up your hand by bending at the elbow squeezing bicep muscle. Keep your palm face up the entire time. You can do this one arm at a time or bilateral.

	_____ Reps _____ Sets _____X Day _____Hold		_____ Reps _____ Sets _____X Day _____Hold
13	**Notes:** *Lymphedema: Do not wrap band around UE or LE	**14**	**Notes:** *Lymphedema: Do not wrap band around UE or LE

BICEPS CURLS – ONE ARM - ELASTIC BAND

In a standing position, step on the band with one leg. Keep your arm at your side holding an elastic band and draw up your hand by bending at the elbow squeezing bicep muscle. Keep your palm face up the entire time.

BICEPS CURLS – BILATERAL - ELASTIC BAND

In a standing position, step on the band with both feet, shoulder width apart. Keep your arms at your side holding an elastic band and draw up your hands by bending at the elbows squeezing bicep muscles. Keep your palms facing upward the entire time.

	_____ Reps _____ Sets _____X Day _____Hold		_____ Reps _____ Sets _____X Day _____Hold
15	**Notes:** *Lymphedema: Do not wrap band around UE or LE	**16**	**Notes:** *Lymphedema: Do not wrap band around UE or LE

BICEPS CURLS - RADIOBRACHIALIS - HAMMER CURL – ONE ARM - ELASTIC BAND

In a standing position, step on the band with one leg. Keep your arm at your side holding an elastic band and draw up your hand by bending at the elbow squeezing bicep muscle. Keep your palm facing inward the entire time.

BICEPS CURLS - RADIOBRACHIALIS - HAMMER CURL – BILATERAL - ELASTIC BAND

In a standing position, step on the band with both feet, shoulder width apart. Keep your arms at your side holding an elastic band and draw up your hands by bending at the elbows squeezing bicep muscles. Keep your palms facing inward the entire time.

_____ Reps _____ Sets _____ X Day _____ Hold		_____ Reps _____ Sets _____ X Day _____ Hold
17	**Notes:** *Lymphedema: Do not wrap band around UE or LE	**18**	**Notes:** *Lymphedema: Do not wrap band around UE or LE

BICEPS CURLS – BRACHIALIS - ONE ARM - ELASTIC BAND

In a standing position, step on the band with one leg. Keep your arm at your side holding an elastic band and draw up your hand by bending at the elbow squeezing bicep muscle. Keep your palm face down the entire time.

BICEPS CURL – BRACHIALIS – BILATERAL - ELASTIC BAND

In a standing position, step on the band with both feet, shoulder width apart. Keep your arms at your side holding an elastic band and draw up your hands by bending at the elbows squeezing bicep muscles. Keep your palms facing downward the entire time.

Elbow Extension (Triceps)

_____ Reps _____ Sets _____ X Day _____ Hold		_____ Reps _____ Sets _____ X Day _____ Hold
19	**Notes:** *Lymphedema: Do not wrap band around UE or LE	**20**	**Notes:** *Lymphedema: Do not wrap band around UE or LE

TRICEPS - SELF FIXATION - ELASTIC BAND

Hold an elastic band across your chest with the unaffected arm. Pull the band downward with the other arm so that the elbow goes from a bent position to a straightened position as shown.

OVERHEAD TRICEPS - SELF FIXATION –SEATED OR STANDING - ELASTIC BAND

Hold an elastic band with one arm fixated behind back as shown and other hand behind head. Extend elbow with arm overhead and return to starting position.

_____ Reps _____ Sets _____ X Day _____ Hold

21	Notes: *Neuropathy/Hands – Precaution holding weights

Starting
Position

TRICEP EXTENSION – SITTING OR STANDING - WEIGHT

Start with hand behind head holding free weight. Extend your elbow as shown. Maintain your upper arm in an upward direction and only bend and straighten at your elbow.
*Can hold the triceps area with opposite arm to stabilize.

_____ Reps _____ Sets _____ X Day _____ Hold

22	Notes: *Neuropathy/Hands – Precaution holding weights

Starting
Position

TRICEP EXTENSION – SITTING OR STANDING – BILATERAL - WEIGHT

Start with hands behind head holding free weight Extend your elbows while holding a free weight in both hands. Maintain your upper arms in an upward direction and only bend and straighten at your elbows.

_____ Reps _____ Sets _____ X Day _____ Hold

23	Notes: *Neuropathy/Hands – Precaution holding weights

Starting
Position

ELBOW EXTENSION - BALL

Lie on your back on ball. Extend your elbow as shown while holding a free weight in each hand. Maintain your upper arms in an upward direction and only bend and straighten at your elbows.

_____ Reps _____ Sets _____ X Day _____ Hold

24	Notes: *Neuropathy/Hands – Precaution holding weights

ELBOW EXTENSION - SKULL CRUSHER - BALL

Lie on your back on ball with a free weight in each hand. Bend your elbows to lower the weight towards the side of your head and then extend arms straight up towards the ceiling.

	_____ Reps _____ Sets _____ X Day _____ Hold		_____ Reps _____ Sets _____ X Day _____ Hold
25	**Notes:** *Lymphedema: Do not wrap band around UE or LE	**26**	**Notes:** *Neuropathy/Hands – Precaution holding weights

TRICEPS - ELASTIC BAND

Fixate the band at top of door. Start with your elbow bent and holding an elastic band as shown. Pull the elastic band downward as you extend your elbow. Keep your elbow by your side the entire time.

TRICEPS - BENT OVER

Stand and bend over with either support or placing your unaffected arm on thigh for support. With your targeted arm and elbow at your side, extend your elbow as you straighten your arm as shown. Keep your elbow at your side and back flat the entire time.

	_____ Reps _____ Sets _____ X Day _____ Hold		_____ Reps _____ Sets _____ X Day _____ Hold
27	**Notes:**	**28**	**Notes:**

CHAIR DIPS / PUSH UPS

While sitting in a chair with arm rests, push yourself upawards so that you lift your buttocks of the chair and then lower down controlled back to normal seated position.   *If you are unable to lift yourself up, you can perform "pressure releases" so that you simply push to take some weight off your buttocks.

DIPS OFF CHAIR

Push yourself up to a straight elbow position as shown. Then lower your buttocks down towards the floor by bending your elbows.

Shoulder PENDULUMS

_____ Reps _____ Sets _____ X Day _____ Hold	_____ Reps _____ Sets _____ X Day _____ Hold
29 **Notes:**	**30** **Notes:**

PENDULUM SHOULDER FORWARD/BACK

Shift your body weight forward then back to allow your injured arm to swing forward and back freely. Your affected arm should be fully relaxed.

PENDULUM SHOULDER – SIDE TO SIDE

Shift your body weight side to side to allow your injured arm to swing side to side freely. Your affected arm should be fully relaxed.

_____ Reps _____ Sets _____ X Day _____ Hold	_____ Reps _____ Sets _____ X Day _____ Hold
31 **Notes:**	**32** **Notes:** *Neuropathy/Hands – Precaution holding weights

PENDULUM SHOULDER CIRCLES
Shift your body weight in circles to allow your injured arm to swing in circles freely. Your injured arm should be fully relaxed.
REVERSE PENDULUM SHOULDER CIRCLES
Shift your body weight into reverse circles to allow your injured arm to swing in circles freely. Your injured arm should be fully relaxed.

PENDULUMS - SUPINE

Lie on your back and straighten your arm towards the ceiling. Move your arm in small circles in a clockwise motion. After a few seconds, reverse the direction to a counterclockwise motion. Change directions every few seconds.

Shoulder Flexion

_____Reps _____Sets _____X Day _____Hold		_____Reps _____Sets _____X Day _____Hold
33	Notes:	**34**

ISOMETRIC FLEXION - Can use towel roll for comfort

Gently push your fist forward into a wall with your elbow bent. Hold for 5-10 seconds. Repeat.

34 Notes:	

Starting Position

SHOULDER FLEXION – SIDELYING - Can add weight

Lie on your side with arm at your side. Slowly raise the arm forward towards overhead and in front of your body.

_____Reps _____Sets _____X Day _____Hold		_____Reps _____Sets _____X Day _____Hold
35	Notes:	**36**

Starting Position

FLEXION – SUPINE - SINGLE OR BILATERAL

Lie on your back with your arm at your side. Slowly raise arm up and forward towards overhead.

36 Notes:
*Neuropathy/Hands – Precaution holding weights

Starting Position

FLEXION – SUPINE – SINGLE OR BILATERAL - WEIGHT

Lie on your back with your arm at your side. Holding a weight, slowly raise arm up and forward towards overhead.

_____ Reps _____ Sets _____ X Day _____ Hold		_____ Reps _____ Sets _____ X Day _____ Hold
37	Notes:	**38**	Notes:

Starting Position

FLEXION – SUPINE - DOWEL

Lie on your back holding dowel with both hands. Slowly raise up and forward towards overhead. Return to starting position. Repeat.
*If you have an injury/weakness, allow your unaffected arm to perform most of the effort. Your affected arm should be partially relaxed.

Starting Position

FLEXION – SUPINE - DOWEL – Add weight only if equal strength

Attach ankle weight to dowel. Lie on your back holding dowel with both hands. Slowly raise up and forward towards overhead. Return to starting position. Repeat.

_____ Reps _____ Sets _____ X Day _____ Hold		_____ Reps _____ Sets _____ X Day _____ Hold
39	Notes: *Lymphedema: Do not wrap band around UE or LE	**40**	Notes: *Lymphedema: Do not wrap band around UE or LE

FLEXION - SELF FIXATION – ELASTIC BAND

Hold an elastic band in front and fixate unaffected arm straight by your side or on your leg. Pull the band upward towards the ceiling with your target arm.

Starting Position

FLEXION – ELASTIC BAND

In a standing position, step on the band with one leg. Keep your arm at your side holding an elastic band and draw up your arm up in front of you keeping your elbow straight.

| _____ Reps _____ Sets _____ X Day _____ Hold | | _____ Reps _____ Sets _____ X Day _____ Hold | |

41

Notes:

42

Notes:

FLEXION - STANDING - PALMS DOWN / OVERHAND DOWEL - Add weight only if equal strength

Hold a dowel/cane with both arms, palm down on both sides. Raise the dowel forward and up. (see #39/40) *Do not use weight if you have an injury/weakness. Allow your unaffected arm to perform most of the work. Your affected arm should be partially relaxed.

FLEXION - STANDING - PALMS UP /UNDERHAND DOWEL - Add weight only if equal strength

Hold a dowel/cane with both arms and palms up on both sides. Raise the dowel forward and up. *Do not use weight if you have an injury/weakness. Allow your unaffected arm to perform most of the work. Your affected arm should be partially relaxed.

| _____ Reps _____ Sets _____ X Day _____ Hold | | _____ Reps _____ Sets _____ X Day _____ Hold | |

43

Notes:
*Neuropathy/Hands – Precaution holding weights

44

Notes:
*Neuropathy/Hands – Precaution holding weights

FLEXION – PALMS FACING INWARD - Can remove weight BILATERAL or ALTERNATE ARMS.

Sit or stand with your arm at your side. Hold a free weight with your palm facing your side and your elbows straight. Raise up your arm forward as shown then return to starting position. Do not let your shoulder shrug upwards unless instructed to go over shoulder level height.

FLEXION – PALMS DOWN - Can remove weight BILATERAL or ALTERNATE ARMS.

Sit or stand with your arm at your side. Hold a weight with your palm facing down and your elbows straight. Raise up your arm forward as shown then return to starting position. Do not let your shoulder shrug upwards unless instructed to go over shoulder height.

V Raises

	_____ Reps _____ Sets _____ X Day _____ Hold
45	Notes:

	_____ Reps _____ Sets _____ X Day _____ Hold
46	Notes: *Neuropathy/Hands – Precaution holding weights

V RAISE

Start with your arms down by your side, palms facing inward, thumbs up and your elbows straight. Raise up your arms in the form of a V to shoulder height as shown keeping elbows straight then return to starting position.

Starting Position

V RAISE – WEIGHTS

Holding free weights, start with your arms down by your side, palms facing inward and your elbows straight. Raise up your arms in the form of a V to shoulder height keeping elbows straight – return.

Shoulder Press

	_____ Reps _____ Sets _____ X Day _____ Hold
47	Notes:

	_____ Reps _____ Sets _____ X Day _____ Hold
48	Notes: *Neuropathy/Hands – Precaution holding weights

Starting Position

MILITARY PRESS – DOWEL- Add weight only if equal strength

Hold a dowel or cane at chest height. Slowly push the wand upwards towards the ceiling until your elbows become fully straightened. Return to the original position.

Starting Position

MILITARY PRESS - FREE WEIGHTS

Hold free weights at 90-degree angle as shown above.
Slowly push your arms upwards towards the ceiling until your elbows become fully straightened. Return to the original position.

Shoulder Extension								

	_____ Reps _____ Sets _____X Day _____Hold		_____ Reps _____ Sets _____X Day _____Hold
49	Notes:	**50**	Notes:

ISOMETRIC EXTENSION - Can use towel roll for comfort

Gently push your bent elbow back into a wall. Hold for 5-10 seconds. Relax and repeat.

PRONE EXTENSION - EXERCISE BALL – Can add weights.

Lie face down over an exercise ball with your elbows straight and along the side of your body. Slowly raise your arms upward along your side and then return to original position.

	_____ Reps _____ Sets _____X Day _____Hold		_____ Reps _____ Sets _____X Day _____Hold
51	Notes:	**52**	Notes: *Neuropathy/Hands – Precaution holding weights

SHOULDER EXTENSION - STANDING

Start with arms by your side. Draw your arm back behind your waist. Keep your elbows straight.

SHOULDER EXTENSION - STANDING - WEIGHTS

Hold a weight by your side and draw your arm back. Keep your elbows straight.

	_____ Reps _____ Sets _____ X Day _____ Hold
53	**Notes:**

	_____ Reps _____ Sets _____ X Day _____ Hold
54	**Notes:** *Lymphedema: Do not wrap band around UE or LE

Starting Position

EXTENSION – STANDING – DOWEL - Add weight only if equal strength

Hold a dowel or cane behind your back with both arms. Draw your arms back.

EXTENSION - SELF FIXATION - ELASTIC BAND

Hold an elastic band out in front of you with your fixated arm. Pull the band downward towards the ground and backwards with your target arm.

	_____ Reps _____ Sets _____ X Day _____ Hold
55	**Notes:** *Lymphedema: Do not wrap band around UE or LE

	_____ Reps _____ Sets _____ X Day _____ Hold
56	**Notes:** *Lymphedema: Do not wrap band around UE or LE

EXTENSION - ELASTIC BAND

Fixate the end of an elastic band at top of door. Hold the elastic band in front of you with your elbows straight. Slowly pull the band down and back towards your side.

EXTENSION - BILATERAL - ELASTIC BAND

Fixate the middle of an elastic band at top of door. Hold the elastic band with both arms in front of you with your elbows straight. Slowly pull the band downwards and back towards your side.

Shoulder Internal Rotation (IR)

_____ Reps _____ Sets _____X Day _____Hold	_____ Reps _____ Sets _____X Day _____Hold
57 Notes:	**58** Notes:

INTERNAL ROTATION – ISOMETRIC - Can use towel roll for comfort

Press your hand into a wall using the palm side of your hand and hold. Maintain a bent elbow the entire time.

INTERNAL ROTATION - ISOMETRIC- ELEVATED - Can use towel roll for comfort

Push the front of your hand into a wall with your elbow bent and arm elevated and hold.

_____ Reps _____ Sets _____X Day _____Hold	_____ Reps _____ Sets _____X Day _____Hold
59 Notes:	**60** Notes: *Lymphedema: Do not wrap band around UE or LE

INTERNAL ROTATION - SIDELYING

Lie on your side with your shoulder flexed to 90 degrees and elbow bent and rested on the table/bed/matt. Your forearm should be pointing up towards the ceiling. Allow your forearm to lower toward the table as shown. Place a rolled-up towel under your elbow if needed.

INTERNAL ROTATION - ELASTIC BAND

Hold an elastic band at your side with your elbow bent. Start with your hand away from your stomach and then pull the band towards your stomach. Keep your elbow near your side the entire time.

	_____ Reps _____ Sets _____X Day _____Hold
61	Notes:

INTERNAL / EXTERNAL ROTATION - STANDING – DOWEL
Add weight only if equal strength

Stand and hold a dowel/cane with both hands keeping
your elbows bent. Move your arms and dowel/cane side-
to-side. _If you have an injury/weakness, the affected arm
should be partially relaxed while your unaffected arm
performs most of the effort._

	_____ Reps _____ Sets _____X Day _____Hold
62	Notes:

Starting
Position

INTERNAL ROTATION – DOWEL - Add weight only if
equal strength

While holding a dowel/cane behind your back,
slowly pull the wand up.

Shoulder External Rotation (ER)

	_____ Reps _____ Sets _____X Day _____Hold
63	Notes:

EXTERNAL ROTATION - ISOMETRIC – Can use towel roll for
comfort

Gently press your hand into a wall using the back side of
your hand. Maintain a bent elbow the entire time.

	_____ Reps _____ Sets _____X Day _____Hold
64	Notes:

EXTERNAL ROTATION - ISOMETRIC – ELEVATED -
Can use towel roll for comfort

Gently push the back of your hand/arm into a wall
with your arm elevated.

_____ Reps _____ Sets _____ X Day _____ Hold

65	Notes:

Starting
Position

EXTERNAL ROTATION WITH TOWEL - SIDELYING

Lie on your side with your elbow bent to 90 degrees. Place a rolled-up towel between your arm and the side your body as shown. Squeeze your shoulder blade back and rotate arm up and hold this position. Slowly rotate back to original position and repeat.

_____ Reps _____ Sets _____ X Day _____ Hold

66	Notes: *Neuropathy/Hands – Precaution holding weights

Starting
Position

EXTERNAL ROTATION – 90/90 - WEIGHTS

Hold weights with elbows bent to 90 degrees and away from your side. Rotate your shoulders back so that the palms of your hands face forward and then return as shown.

_____ Reps _____ Sets _____ X Day _____ Hold

67	Notes: *Lymphedema: Do not wrap band around UE or LE

EXTERNAL ROTATION - BILATERAL - ELASTIC BAND
Can put a towel between side and elbow (see #68)

Hold an elastic band with your elbows bent, pull your hands away from your stomach area. Keep your elbows near the side of your body.

_____ Reps _____ Sets _____ X Day _____ Hold

68	Notes: *Lymphedema: Do not wrap band around UE or LE

EXTERNAL ROTATION - ELASTIC BAND – Can add roll between side and arm

Fixate an elastic band to the door at elbow height. Hold the other end of the band at your side with your elbow bent. Start with your hand near your stomach and then pull the band away. Keep your elbow at your side the entire time.

Shoulder Adduction (ADD)

	_____ Reps _____ Sets _____ X Day _____ Hold		_____ Reps _____ Sets _____ X Day _____ Hold
69	**Notes:**	**70**	**Notes:** ***Lymphedema: Do not wrap band around UE or LE**

ADDUCTION – ISOMETRIC - Can use towel roll for comfort

Place a towel roll between your bent elbow and body. Gently push your elbow into the side of your body.

ADDUCTION - ELASTIC BAND

Fixate an elastic band to the door and hold the other end of the band away from your side. Pull the band towards your side keeping your elbow straight.

Shoulder Abduction (ABD)

	_____ Reps _____ Sets _____ X Day _____ Hold		_____ Reps _____ Sets _____ X Day _____ Hold
71	**Notes:**	**72**	**Notes:**

ABDUCTION – ISOMETRIC - Can use towel roll for comfort

Gently push your elbow out to the side into a wall with your elbow bent.

HORIZONTAL ABDUCTION - DOWEL

Lie on your back holding a dowel/cane straight up towards the ceiling with your elbows straight. Bring your arms and wand to the side and then towards the other.

_____ Reps _____ Sets _____X Day _____Hold		_____ Reps _____ Sets _____X Day _____Hold
73	Notes:	**74**

Notes: (73)

Notes: (74)
*Neuropathy/Hands – Precaution holding weights

HORIZONTAL ABDUCTION/ADDUCTTION - SUPINE
Lie on your back with arm straight up in front of your body. Slowly lower your arm out towards the side. Return to original position.

HORIZONTAL ABDUCTION/ADDUCTTION - SUPINE - WEIGHT

Hold a weight. Lie on your back with arm straight up in front of your body. Slowly lower your arm out towards the side. Return to original position

_____ Reps _____ Sets _____X Day _____Hold		_____ Reps _____ Sets _____X Day _____Hold
75	Notes:	**76**

Notes: (76)

ABDUCTION - SIDELYING - Can add weight

Lie on your side with arm at your side. Slowly raise the target arm up towards head and away from your side.

HORIZONTAL ABDUCTION - SIDELYING - Can add weight

Lie on your side with arm out in front of your body. Slowly raise up the arm overhead towards the ceiling.

_____ Reps _____ Sets _____X Day _____Hold		_____ Reps _____ Sets _____X Day _____Hold	
77	Notes: *Neuropathy/Hands – Precaution holding weights	78	Notes: *Lymphedema: Do not wrap band around UE or LE

Starting Position

ABDUCTION – WEIGHT – Can do without a weight

Hold a weight with your affected arm at your side. Keeping your elbow straight, raise up your arm to the side.

Starting Position

ABDUCTION – ELASTIC BAND

Fixate an elastic band under a door and hold band with hand farthest away from door at your side. Keeping your elbow straight, raise up your arm to the side.

_____ Reps _____ Sets _____X Day _____Hold		_____ Reps _____ Sets _____X Day _____Hold	
79	Notes: *Lymphedema: Do not wrap band around UE or LE	80	Notes: *Neuropathy/Hands – Precaution holding weights

HORIZONTAL ABDUCTION – BILATERAL - ELASTIC BAND

Hold an elastic band in both hands with your elbows straight in front of your body. Slowly pull your arms apart towards the sides.

Starting Position

90/90 ABDUCTION - WEIGHT

Hold weights at your side with elbows bent to 90 degrees. Raise up your elbows away from your side while maintaining your elbows bent at 90 degrees.

Lateral/Frontal Raise

_____ Reps _____ Sets _____X Day _____Hold	
81	**Notes:** *Neuropathy/Hands – Precaution holding weights

Starting Position

LATERAL RAISES

Hold weights at your side with arms straight. Raise up your elbows away from your side while keeping your elbow straight the entire time.

_____ Reps _____ Sets _____X Day _____Hold	
82	**Notes:** *Neuropathy/Hands – Precaution holding weights

Starting Position

LATERAL RAISES – LEAN FORWARD

Bend slightly at the waist holding weights slightly in front. Raise up your elbows away from your side squeezing shoulder blades together.

_____ Reps _____ Sets _____X Day _____Hold	
83	**Notes:** *Neuropathy/Hands – Precaution holding weights

Starting Position

LATERAL RAISES – LEAN FORWARD - ARM ROTATION

Bend slightly at the waist holding weights slightly in front as shown palms facing your body. Raise up your elbows away from your side squeezing shoulder blades together.

_____ Reps _____ Sets _____X Day _____Hold	
84	**Notes:** *Neuropathy/Hands – Precaution holding weights

FRONTAL RAISE – WEIGHTS – Can do without weights

Hold weights at your side with arms straight. Slowly raise your arms in front of of your body.

Upright Rows

	_____ Reps _____ Sets _____ X Day _____ Hold
85	**Notes:** *Neuropathy/Hands – Precaution holding weights

UPRIGHT ROW – WEIGHTS - Can use kettle bell

Hold weights or kettlebell with both hands at waist height. Lift the weights to chest height as you bend at your elbows.

	_____ Reps _____ Sets _____ X Day _____ Hold
86	**Notes:** *Lymphedema: Do not wrap band around UE or LE

UPRIGHT ROW – ELASTIC BAND

Stand on an elastic band with either one or both feet. Hold band at waist height and raise it up to chest height as you bend at your elbows.

Shoulder Shrugs & Rolls

	_____ Reps _____ Sets _____ X Day _____ Hold
87	**Notes:**

SHRUGS

Raise your shoulders upward towards your ears as shown. Shrug both shoulders at the same time.

	_____ Reps _____ Sets _____ X Day _____ Hold
88	**Notes:** *Neuropathy/Hands – Precaution holding weights

SHRUGS - WEIGHTS

Hold weights in both hands with arms straight. Raise your shoulders upward towards your ears. Shrug both shoulders at the same time.

_____ Reps _____ Sets _____ X Day _____ Hold	_____ Reps _____ Sets _____ X Day _____ Hold
89 Notes:	**90** Notes:

SHOULDER ROLLS

Move your shoulders in a circular pattern so that your are moving in an up, back and down direction. Perform small circles if needed for comfort.
Complete one set and then reverse direction

SHOULDER ROLLS - WEIGHTS

Hold weights in both or one hand. Move your shoulders in a circular pattern so that your are moving in an up, back and down direction.
Complete one set and then reverse direction

Scapular Retraction

_____ Reps _____ Sets _____ X Day _____ Hold	_____ Reps _____ Sets _____ X Day _____ Hold
91 Notes:	**92** Notes:

SCAPULAR RETRACTIONS - BILATERAL

Draw your shoulder blades back and down.

SCAPULAR RETRACTION – SINGLE ARM

With your arm raised up and elbow bent, draw your shoulder blade back and down.

	_____ Reps _____ Sets _____ X Day _____ Hold
93	**Notes:** *Lymphedema: Do not wrap band around UE or LE

ELASTIC BAND SCAPULAR RETRACTIONS WITH MINI SHOULDER EXTENSIONS

Fixate an elastic band to the door and hold with both arms in front of you with your elbows straight. Slowly squeeze your shoulder blades together as you pull the band back. Be sure your shoulders do not rise up.

	_____ Reps _____ Sets _____ X Day _____ Hold
94	**Notes:** *Neuropathy/Hands – Precaution holding weights

PRONE RETRACTION – Can do without weight

Lie face down with your elbows straight. Slowly draw your shoulder blade back towards your spine. Your whole arm should rise including your shoulder blade upward as shown. Your elbow should be straight the entire time.

Scapular Protraction

	_____ Reps _____ Sets _____ X Day _____ Hold
95	**Notes:**

SCAPULAR PROTRACTION - SUPINE - BILATERAL

Lie on your back with your arms extended out in front of your body and towards the ceiling. While keeping your elbows straight, protract your shoulders reaching forward towards the ceiling. Keep your elbows straight the entire time.

	_____ Reps _____ Sets _____ X Day _____ Hold
96	**Notes:** *Neuropathy/Hands – Precaution holding weights

SCAPULAR PROTRACTION - SUPINE - WEIGHT

Lie on your back holding a weight with your arm extended out in front of your body and towards the ceiling. While keeping your elbows straight, protract your shoulders reaching forward towards the ceiling. Keep your elbows straight the entire time.

_____ Reps _____ Sets _____X Day _____Hold		_____ Reps _____ Sets _____X Day _____Hold

97	**Notes:** *Lymphedema: Do not wrap band around UE or LE	**98**	**Notes:**

SCAPULAR PROTRACTION - SUPINE - ELASTIC BAND

Lie on your back and hold elastic band in both hands. Bend the unaffected arm to fixate the band. Extend the target arm out in front of your body and straight up towards the ceiling. While keeping your elbows straight, protract your shoulder blade forward towards the ceiling. Keep your elbows straight the entire time.

SCAPULAR PROTRACTION / TABLE PLANK

Start in a push up position on your hands and leaning up against a table or countertop as shown. Maintain this position as you protract your shoulder blades forward to raise your body upward a few inches. Return to original position.
*Progress by standing further away from the table.

Chest Press

_____ Reps _____ Sets _____X Day _____Hold		_____ Reps _____ Sets _____X Day _____Hold

99	**Notes:** *Lymphedema: Do not wrap band around UE or LE	**100**	**Notes:** *Neuropathy/Hands – Precaution holding weights

CHEST PRESS – SEATED or STANDING - ELASTIC BAND

Hold elastic band with both hands at your side and elbows bent with band wrapped around body or chair. Push the band out in front of your body as you straighten your elbows.

CHEST PRESS – BALL, FLOOR or BENCH- WEIGHTS

Lie on your back with your elbows bent. Slowly raise up your arms towards the ceiling while extending your elbows straight up above your head.

101	_____ Reps _____ Sets _____X Day _____Hold
	Notes:

102	_____ Reps _____ Sets _____X Day _____Hold
	Notes: *Neuropathy/Hands – Precaution holding weights

Starting

Position

DOWEL PRESS – STANDING – Add weight only if equal strength

Hold a dowel/cane at chest height. Slowly push the dowel outwards in front of your body so that your elbows become fully straightened. Return to the original position.

Starting

Position

CHEST PRESS – STANDING or SEATED

Hold weights in both hands with your arms at your side and elbows bent. Push your arms out in front of your body as you straighten your elbows.

Rows

103	_____ Reps _____ Sets _____X Day _____Hold
	Notes: *Neuropathy/Hands – Precaution holding weights

104	_____ Reps _____ Sets _____X Day _____Hold
	Notes: *Neuropathy/Hands – Precaution holding weights

BENT OVER ROWS

Stand, bend over and support yourself with the unaffected arm. Slowly draw up your target arm as you bend your elbow. Keep your back flat the entire time.

ROWS – PRONE – On bed or table

Lie face down with your elbows straight, slowly raise your arms upward while bending your elbows.

	_____ Reps _____ Sets _____ X Day _____ Hold		_____ Reps _____ Sets _____ X Day _____ Hold
105	**Notes:** *Lymphedema: Do not wrap band around UE or LE	**106**	**Notes:** *Lymphedema: Do not wrap band around UE or LE

ROWS - ELASTIC BAND

Fixate the elastic band in the door at elbow level. Hold the elastic band with both hands, draw back the band as you bend your elbows. Keep your elbows near the side of your body.

WIDE ROWS - ELASTIC BAND

Fixate the elastic band in the door and hold the band with both hands. Draw back the band as you bend your elbows squeezing shoulder blades together. Keep your arms about 90 degrees away from the side of your body.

	_____ Reps _____ Sets _____ X Day _____ Hold		_____ Reps _____ Sets _____ X Day _____ Hold
107	**Notes:** *Lymphedema: Do not wrap band around UE or LE	**108**	**Notes:** *Lymphedema: Do not wrap band around UE or LE

LOW ROW – ELASTIC BAND

Fixate the elastic band in the door below elbow level. Hold the elastic band with both hands, draw back the band as you bend your elbows. Keep your elbows near the side of your body.

HIGH ROW – ELASTIC BAND

Fixate the elastic band at the top of the door. Hold the elastic band with both hands, draw back the band as you bend your elbows. Keep your elbows near the side of your body.

Flys

	_____ Reps _____ Sets _____ X Day _____ Hold		_____ Reps _____ Sets _____ X Day _____ Hold
109	**Notes:** *Neuropathy/Hands – Precaution holding weights	**110**	**Notes:** *Neuropathy/Hands – Precaution holding weights

Starting

Position

FLY'S – FLOOR - WEIGHT

Holding weights, lie on your back with your arms horizontally out to the side. Bring your arms up and forward towards the ceiling. Lower your arms back down to the original position. Your elbows should be partially bent the entire time.

FLY'S – BALL or BENCH – WEIGHT

Holding weights, lie on your back on a ball with your arms horizontally out to the side. Bring your arms up and forward towards the ceiling. Lower your arms back down to the original position with elbows partially bent the entire time.

Wall pushups – To progress, move feet further away from wall

	_____ Reps _____ Sets _____ X Day _____ Hold		_____ Reps _____ Sets _____ X Day _____ Hold
111	**Notes:**	**112**	**Notes:**

WALL PUSH UPS

Place your arms out in front of you with your elbows straight so that your hands just reach the wall. Bend your elbows slowly to bring your chest closer to the wall. Straighten your arms pushing your body away from wall. Maintain your feet planted on the ground the entire time.

WALL PUSH UP - BALL

Place a ball on a wall while holding the ball with both hands as shown. Bend your elbows slowly to bring your chest closer to the wall and then straighten your arms pushing your body away from wall. Maintain your feet planted on the ground the entire time.

	_____ Reps _____ Sets _____X Day _____Hold
113	Notes:

WALL PUSH UP - Triceps uneven

Place your arms out in front of you with your elbows straight in an uneven position so that your hands just reach the wall. Bend your elbows slowly to bring your chest closer to the wall and then straighten your arms pushing your body away from wall. Maintain your feet planted on the ground the entire time.

	_____ Reps _____ Sets _____X Day _____Hold
114	Notes:

WALL PUSH UP – Hands inverted

Place your arms out in front of you with your elbows straight and hands inverted just reaching the wall. Bend your elbows slowly to bring your chest closer to the wall and then straighten your arms pushing your body away from wall. Maintain your feet planted on the ground the entire time.

	_____ Reps _____ Sets _____X Day _____Hold
115	Notes:

WALL PUSH UP - Narrow

Place your arms out in front of you with your elbows straight and hands close togther just reaching the wall. Bend your elbows slowly to bring your chest closer to the wall and then straighten your arms pushing your body away from wall. Maintain your feet planted on the ground the entire time.

	_____ Reps _____ Sets _____X Day _____Hold
116	Notes:

WALL PUSH UP – Wide

Place your arms out in front of you with your elbows straight and your arms and hands far apart just reaching the wall. Bend your elbows slowly to bring your chest closer to the wall and then straighten your arms pushing your body away from wall. Maintain your feet planted on the ground the entire time.

Push ups

	_____ Reps _____ Sets _____X Day _____Hold		_____ Reps _____ Sets _____X Day _____Hold
117	**Notes:**	**118**	**Notes:**

Starting

Position

PUSH UPS - BALL

Start in a kneeling position with an exercise ball in front of you. Slowly walk yourself out with your arms so that the ball is positioned under your legs. Then perform push ups. *Progress by moving ball back towards thighs

PUSH UP - MODIFIED

Lie face down and use your arms and push yourself up. Keep your knees in contact with the floor and maintain a straight back the entire time.

	_____ Reps _____ Sets _____X Day _____Hold		_____ Reps _____ Sets _____X Day _____Hold
119	**Notes:**	**120**	**Notes:**

Starting

Position

PUSH UP

Lie face down, use your arms and push yourself. Keep your toes in contact with the floor and maintain a straight back the entire time.

PUSH UP -DIAMOND

Lie face down and place your hands on the floor in the shape of a diamond with your thumbs and index fingers.
Use your arms and push yourself up.. Keep your toes in contact with the floor and maintain a straight back the entire time.

_____ Reps _____ Sets _____ X Day _____ Hold		_____ Reps _____ Sets _____ X Day _____ Hold
121	Notes:	**122**

PUSH UP – MODIFIED - BOSU - UNSTABLE

Perform push-ups with your hands on a Bosu. Keep your knees in contact with the floor and maintain a straight back the entire time.

PUSH UP – BOSU - UNSTABLE

Perform push-ups with your hands on top of a Bosu. Keep your toes in contact with the floor and maintain a straight back the entire time.

_____ Reps _____ Sets _____ X Day _____ Hold		_____ Reps _____ Sets _____ X Day _____ Hold
123	Notes:	**124**

PUSH UP – MODIFIED – INVERTED BOSU - UNSTABLE

Perform push-ups while holding an inverted Bosu. Try and maintain the Bosu platform as level as you can. Keep your knees in contact with the floor and maintain a straight back the entire time.

PUSH UP – INVERTED BOSU - UNSTABLE

Perform push-ups while holding an inverted Bosu. Try and maintain the Bosu platform as level as you can. Keep your toes in contact with the floor and maintain a straight back the entire time.

BALANCE – CORE – STANDING LE STRENGTH

Basics
- Requires LE strengthening for progression
- Perform exercises 2-3x a week
- Should be performed at beginning of exercise routine or can be the main exercise routine for endurance with increased repetitions or strength with resistance.

Duration, Frequency, Intensity, Sets and Reps
- Balance – 1 set, 2-4 repetitions for hold of 5-60 seconds
- Endurance – Less than 30 second rests in between sets
  - Static - 1 set, 5-10 repetitions as tolerated
  - Dynamic – 1 set, 3-10 reps for 10-30+ second hold as tolerated
- Strengthening – Add resistance with bands or weights (*see Strengthening for more information*)
  - Static – 2-3 sets, 3-12 reps – slow controlled movements
  - Dynamic – 1-3 sets, 2-4 reps

Static Balance Progression:
1. Bilateral – Both feet on the ground
2. Unilateral – One foot on the ground
3. Arm Movement – Overhead, can do arm exercises (*See Arm Strengthening for exercises*)
4. Trunk rotation – Rotate with or without arm movement
5. Eyes Shut (lack of visual cues – sensory removal)
6. Head Turns, hand/eye tracking, shifting focal point (vestibular – sensory alteration)
7. Reading (coordination)
8. Unstable – progression
   Repeat above on unstable surface such as balance pad, pillow, balance disc or Bosu.

Decrease Base of Support (BOS) Progression:
- Wide BOS
- Narrow Bos
- Staggered/Split Stance/Semi-tandem
- Tandem Stance
- Single Leg Stance

SOLID GROUND:
1. Support: Hold onto chair, counter, sink or another stationary object.
2. No Support: Stand next to stable surface if needed for security.
   - Can start with 1-2 hands and as you become more stable, decrease the number of fingers used for support. For example, take away the thumb and hold with 4 fingers, 3 fingers, 2 fingers, 1 finger and then without support.
3. Resistance: Add ankle weights on use elastic band for resistance

UNSTABLE SURFACE: Balance pad, Bosu, Half foam roll, Pillow or Other unstable surface
1. Support: Hold onto chair, counter or another stationary object.
2. No Support: Stand next to stable surface if needed for security.
   - Can start with 1-2 hands and as you become more stable, decrease the number of fingers used for support. For example, take away the thumb and hold with 4 fingers, 3 fingers, 2 fingers, 1 finger and then without support.
3. Resistance: Add ankle weights on use elastic band for resistance

Peripheral Neuropathy **Caution Balancing on Uneven Surface**	• Peripheral neuropathy can be a side effect of diabetes or may be as a result of damage to the peripheral nerves. These nerves carry information from the brain to other parts of the body. • Feet or lower extremity – Caution standing on uneven surface, such as a Bosu ball or balance pads due to decreased sensation in feet. Increased risk of falling. • Hands – Caution with holding dumbbells or grasping resistance bands.

EXERCISE	EXERCISE NUMBER	NOTES
Balance		
WIDE BOS DECREASING TO NARROW BOS	1	
NARROW BOS	2	
ARM MOVEMENT	3	
TRUNK ROTATION	4	
EYES SHUTS	5	
HEAD TURNS	6	
READING ALOUD	7	
BALANCE PAD	8	
SPLIT STANCE – SEMI TANDEM	9	
SPLIT STANCE - *Progression*	10	
TANDEM- SHARPENED ROMBERG STANCE	11	
TANDEM STANCE - Progression	12	
SINGLE LEG STANCE (SLS)	13	
SINGLE LEG STANCE (SLS) - *Progression*	14	
SLS – LEG FORWARD	15	
SLS – LEG BACKWARDS	16	
SLS – LEG FORWARD / OPPOSITE ARM UP	17	
SLS – LEG BACKWARDS / OPPOSITE ARM UP	18	
SLS - REACH FORWARD	19	
SLS - REACH TWIST	20	
SINGLE LEG TOE TAP	21	
SINGLE LEG STANCE - CLOCKS	22	
BALL ROLLS - HEEL TOE	23	
BALL ROLLS - LATERAL	24	
SQUAT	25	
SIT TO STAND	26	

EXERCISE Balance	EXERCISE NUMBER	NOTES
SQUATS – WALL WITH BALL	27	
SQUATS WITH WEIGHTS	28	
MINI SQUAT - UNSTABLE SUPPORT - FOAM PAD	29	
SQUATS - SINGLE LEG	30	
SIDE TO SIDE WEIGHT SHIFT	31	
FORWARD AND BACKWARDS WEIGHT SHIFTS	32	
SPLIT STANCE WEIGHT SHIFT SIDE TO SIDE	33	
SPLIT STANCE WEIGHT SHIFT FORWARD AND BACKWARDS	34	
WALL FALLS - FORWARD - BALANCE DRILL	35	
WALL FALLS - LATERAL - BALANCE DRILL	36	
WALL FALLS - BACKWARDS - BALANCE DRILL	37	
WALL FALLS - SINGLE LEG - FORWARD - BALANCE DRILL	38	
WALL FALLS - SINGLE LEG - LATERAL - BALANCE DRILL	39	
WALL FALLS - SINGLE LEG - MEDIAL - BALANCE DRILL	40	
WALL FALLS - SINGLE LEG - BACKWARDS - BALANCE DRILL	41	
FALL LATERAL - STEP RECOVERY	42	
FALL FORWARD - STEP RECOVERY	43	
FALL BACKWARD - STEP RECOVERY	44	
TOE TAP ABDUCTION	45	
HIP ABDUCTION - STANDING	46	
HIP EXTENSION – STANDING	47	
HIP FLEXION - STANDING – STRAIGHT LEG RAISE	48	
HIP / KNEE FLEXION - SINGLE LEG	49	
STANDING MARCHING	50	

EXERCISE	EXERCISE NUMBER	NOTES
Balance		
HAMSTRING CURL	51	
TOE RAISES	52	
TOE RAISES IR AND ER	53	
ONE LEGGED TOE RAISE	54	
SINGLE LEG BALANCE FORWARD	55	
SINGLE LEG BALANCE LATERAL	56	
SINGLE LEG BALANCE RETRO	57	
SINGLE LEG STANCE RETROLATERAL	58	
SQUAT	59	
SINGLE LEG SQUAT	60	
LUNGE – STATIC	61	
LUNGE FORWARD/BACKWARD	62	
FOUR CORNER MARCHING IN PLACE	63	
FOUR CORNER MARCHING IN PLACE WITH HEAD TURNS	64	
WALKING ON HEELS FORWARD AND BACKWARDS	65	
WALKING ON TOES FORWARD AND BACKWARDS	66	
TANDEM STANCE AND WALK – FORWARD AND BACKWARDS	67	
RUNNING MAN	68	
HOP STICK - FORWARD	69	
HOP STICK - BACKWARDS	70	
MINI LATERAL LUNGE	71	
SIDE STEPPING	72	
HOP STICK - LATERAL	73	
SINGLE LEG DEAD LIFT	74	

EXERCISE	EXERCISE NUMBER	NOTES
Balance		
CONE TAPS - SINGLE LEG STANCE	75	
CONE TAPS - SINGLE LEG STANCE - UNSTABLE	76	
FIGURE 8 AROUND CONES	77	
FIGURE 8 AROUND CONES – FOOT OR HAND TAP	78	
BALANCE DOUBLE LEG STANCE - WIDE	79	
BALANCE DOUBLE LEG STANCE - NARROW	80	
TANDEM STANCE	81	
TANDEM WALK	82	
SINGLE LEG STANCE - ABDUCTION	83	
SINGLE LEG STANCE - ABDUCTION	84	
SINGLE LEG STANCE – FORWARD KICK	85	
SINGLE LEG STANCE – HAMSTRING CURL	86	
SINGLE LEG SQUAT – LEG FORWARD	87	
SINGLE LEG SQUAT – LEG BACKWARDS	88	
TOE TAP OR HEEL PLACEMENT	89	
PULL UP FOOT TOUCHES ON STEP	90	
ALTERNATING SUSTAINED FOOT TOUCHES ON STEP	91	
STEP UP AND OVER	92	
FORWARD SWING THROUGH STEP	93	
SIDE STEPPING - *REPEAT STEPS 89-93 from a side approach.*	94	

BALANCE PROGRESSION- STATIC – See WARNING above Re: Peripheral Neuropathy

Hip Width/Narrow Stance >>>>> Staggered Stance >>>>> Tandem Stance   >>>>> Single-Leg Stance

1. Hold onto a chair, counter or other steady object.
2. Continue steps 2-8 holding on to a sturdy object.
3. Can start with 1-2 hands and as you become more stable, decrease the number of fingers used for support. For example, take away the thumb and hold with 4 fingers, 3 fingers, 2 fingers, 1 finger and then without support.
4. When feeling comfortable, take away support staying close to object for security
5. When able to complete with decreased support, add balance pad or unstable surface completing 2-8 as above.

HIP WIDTH OR WIDE BASE OF SUPPORT (BOS) > NARROW BASE OF SUPPORT (BOS)

STAGGERED STANCE – SPLIT STANCE

TANDEM STANCE

SINGLE LEG STANCE

	_____ Reps _____ Sets _____X Day _____Hold		_____ Reps _____ Sets _____X Day _____Hold
1	Notes:	**2**	Notes:

WIDE BOS DECREASING TO NARROW BOS

Continue steps 2-8 holding on to a sturdy object and then progress with decreased support as outlined above.

NARROW BOS

Stand with your feet together Count to 10. Increase time up to 60 seconds as tolerated maintaining your balance in this position.

	_____ Reps _____ Sets _____X Day _____Hold		_____ Reps _____ Sets _____X Day _____Hold
3	Notes:	**4**	Notes:

ARM MOVEMENT

Examples:
- Throw ball up in arm and catch
- Play catch with partner
- Reach hands above head and then down by side
- Do standing arm exercises (_See Arm Strengthening for examples_)

TRUNK ROTATION – reach side to side

Examples:
- Reach side to side within BOS
- Reach side to side and forward out of BOS

	_____ Reps _____ Sets _____X Day _____Hold		_____ Reps _____ Sets _____X Day _____Hold
5	Notes:	**6**	Notes:

EYES SHUTS - Lack of visual cues – _Sensory Removal_

Stand with eyes shut and count to 10. Increase time up to 60 seconds as tolerated.

HEAD TURNS - Vestibular – _Sensory Alteration_

Examples:
- Turn head slowly from side to side
- Move head up and down slowly
- Put one finger out in front of face at arm's length moving in outward/inward direction and move head to follow with eyes. Slow hand tracking.
- Shift focal point to different objects in the room
- _Can add head turns with eyes closed_

	_____ Reps _____ Sets _____X Day _____Hold		_____ Reps _____ Sets _____X Day _____Hold
7	Notes:	**8**	Notes:

READING ALOUD - _Coordination / Cognitive Task_

Hold reading material, such as a book, paper, tablet, or magazine in one or both hands.   Read out loud and progress to moving your head and the object on occasion to the side or up/down.

BALANCE PAD or another unstable surface

Place balance pad, Bosu, pillow or other unstable surface by a chair or counter for support. Stand on the pad.

****REPEAT STEPS 2-8 on unstable surface****

	_____ Reps _____ Sets _____X Day _____Hold
9	Notes:

SPLIT STANCE – SEMI TANDEM

Place one foot forward and the opposite foot to the back and slightly out to the side. Count to 10. Increase time up to 60 seconds as tolerated maintaining your balance in this position.

	_____ Reps _____ Sets _____X Day _____Hold
10	Notes:

SPLIT STANCE

FOLLOW STEPS 2-8 AS SEEN WITH NARROW BOS AS OUTLINED IN BALANCE PROGRESSION

1. HOLD STEADY OBJECT PROGRESSING TO NO SUPPORT
2. STAND FOR 10-60 SECONDS
3. ARM MOVEMENT
4. TRUNK ROTATION
5. EYES SHUT
6. HEAD TURNS
7. READING
8. **UNSTABLE**

REPEAT ABOVE ON UNSTABLE SURFACE SUCH AS BALANCE PAD, PILLOW, BALANCE DISC, HALF FOARM ROLL OR BOSU.

	_____ Reps _____ Sets _____X Day _____Hold
11	Notes:

TANDEM- SHARPENED ROMBERG STANCE

Place the heel of one foot so that it touches the toes of the other foot. Count to 10. Increase time up to 60 seconds as tolerated maintaining your balance in this position.

	_____ Reps _____ Sets _____X Day _____Hold
12	Notes:

TANDEM STANCE

FOLLOW STEPS 2-8 AS SEEN WITH NARROW BOS AS OUTLINED IN BALANCE PROGRESSION

1. HOLD STEADY OBJECT PROGRESSING TO NO SUPPORT
2. STAND FOR 10-60 SECONDS
3. ARM MOVEMENT
4. TRUNK ROTATION
5. EYES SHUT
6. HEAD TURNS
7. READING
8. **UNSTABLE**

REPEAT ABOVE ON UNSTABLE SURFACE SUCH AS BALANCE PAD, PILLOW, BALANCE DISC, HALF FOARM ROLL OR BOSU.

_____ Reps _____ Sets _____X Day _____Hold		_____ Reps _____ Sets _____X Day _____Hold	
13	Notes:	**14**	Notes:

SINGLE LEG STANCE (SLS)

Stand on one foot. Count to 10 > 60 seconds as tolerated maintaining your balance in this position. Maintain a slightly bent knee on the stance side.

SINGLE LEG STANCE

FOLLOW STEPS 2-8 AS SEEN WITH NARROW BOS AS OUTLINED IN BALANCE PROGRESSION

1. HOLD STEADY OBJECT PROGRESSING TO NO SUPPORT
2. STAND FOR 10-60 SECONDS
3. ARM MOVEMENT
4. TRUNK ROTATION
5. EYES SHUT
6. HEAD TURNS
7. READING
8. **UNSTABLE**

REPEAT ABOVE ON UNSTABLE SURFACE SUCH AS BALANCE PAD, PILLOW, BALANCE DISC, HALF FOARM ROLL OR BOSU.

Single Leg Stance (SLS) with Arm and/or Leg Movements- *Progress to Balance Pad*

_____ Reps _____ Sets _____X Day _____Hold		_____ Reps _____ Sets _____X Day _____Hold	
15	Notes:	**16**	Notes:

SLS – LEG FORWARD

Stand on one leg and maintain your balance. Hold your leg out in front of your body and then return to the original position. Repeat on opposite side. Maintain a slightly bent knee on the stance side.

SLS – LEG BACKWARDS

Stand on one leg and maintain your balance. Hold your leg in the back of your body and then return to original position. Repeat on opposite side. Maintain a slightly bent knee on the stance side.

	_____ Reps _____ Sets _____ X Day _____ Hold
17	Notes:

SLS – LEG FORWARD / OPPOSITE ARM UP

Stand on one leg and maintain your balance. Hold your leg out in front of your body and opposite arm up over your head. Return to the original position. Repeat on opposite side. Maintain a slightly bent knee on the stance side.

	_____ Reps _____ Sets _____ X Day _____ Hold
18	Notes:

SLS – LEG BACKWARDS / OPPOSITE ARM UP

Stand on one leg and maintain your balance. Hold your leg out in front of your body and opposite arm up over your head. Return to the original position. Repeat on opposite side. Maintain a slightly bent knee on the stance side.

	_____ Reps _____ Sets _____ X Day _____ Hold
19	Notes:

SLS - REACH FORWARD

Stand on one leg and maintain your balance. Reach forward with your opposite arm as far as you can without losing your balance and then return to original position. Repeat on opposite side. Maintain a slightly bent knee on the stance side.

	_____ Reps _____ Sets _____ X Day _____ Hold
20	Notes:

SLS - REACH TWIST

Stand on one leg and maintain your balance. Reach forward and across your body with your opposite arm as far as you can without losing your balance and then return to original position. Repeat on opposite side. Maintain a slightly bent knee on the stance side.

	_____ Reps _____ Sets _____ X Day _____ Hold
21	Notes:

SINGLE LEG TOE TAP

Start by standing on one leg and maintain your balance. Tap the opposite foot on a slightly raised object, such as a box or balance pad. To progress, increase the height of object, such as a stair step or cone. Can alternate feet or repeat on same side for several repetitions and then repeat on opposite side.

	_____ Reps _____ Sets _____ X Day _____ Hold
22	Notes:

SINGLE LEG STANCE - CLOCKS

Start by standing on one leg and maintain your balance. Image a clock on the floor where your stance leg is in the center. Lightly touch position 1 as illustrated with the opposite foot. Then return that leg to the starting position. Next, touch position 2 and return. Maintain a slightly bent knee on the stance side.

	_____ Reps _____ Sets _____ X Day _____ Hold
23	Notes:

BALL ROLLS - HEEL TOE

In a standing position, place one foot on a ball and roll it forward and back in a controlled motion from heel to toe while maintaining your balance.

	_____ Reps _____ Sets _____ X Day _____ Hold
24	Notes:

BALL ROLLS - LATERAL

In a standing position, place one foot on a ball and roll it side to side in a controlled motion from the inner side of your foot to the outer side of your foot while maintaining your balance.

Squats	
_____ Reps _____ Sets _____X Day _____Hold	_____ Reps _____ Sets _____X Day _____Hold
25 Notes:	**26** Notes:

25

SQUAT – Can use chair or counter for support and chair behind if needed.

Stand with feet shoulder width apart (in front of a stable support for balance if needed.) Bend your knees and lower your body towards the floor. Your body weight should mostly be directed through the heels of your feet. Return to a standing position. Knees should bend in line with toes and not pass the front of the foot.

26

SIT TO STAND - Can use armchair to push off if needed

Start by scooting close to the front of the chair. Lean forward at your trunk and reach forward with your arms and rise to standing. (You may use a chair with arms to push off if needed and progress as tolerated).
Use your arms as a counterbalance by reaching forward when in sitting and lower them as you approach standing.

_____ Reps _____ Sets _____X Day _____Hold	_____ Reps _____ Sets _____X Day _____Hold
27 Notes:	**28** Notes:

27

SQUATS – WALL WITH BALL

Place either a small ball or therapy ball between you and the wall. Bend your knees and lower your body towards the floor. Return to a standing position. Knees should bend in line with toes and not pass the front of the foot.

28

SQUATS WITH WEIGHTS

Hold dumbbells or other weights in both hands by your side. Bend your knees and lower your body towards the floor. Return to a standing position. Knees should bend in line with toes and not pass the front of the foot

	_____ Reps _____ Sets _____ X Day _____ Hold		_____ Reps _____ Sets _____ X Day _____ Hold
29	Notes:	**30**	Notes:

MINI SQUAT - UNSTABLE SUPPORT - FOAM PAD

Start with your feet shoulder-width apart, toes pointed straight ahead and standing on a balance pad. Next, bend your knees to approximately 30 degrees of flexion to perform a mini squat as shown. Then, return to original position. Knees should not pass the front of the foot.

SQUATS - SINGLE LEG

While standing on one leg in front of a stable support for assisted balance, bend your knee and lower your body towards the floor. Return to a standing position.
Knees should not pass the front of the foot.

Weight Shifts, Wall Falls, Balance Recovery (Balance Drills)

	_____ Reps _____ Sets _____ X Day _____ Hold		_____ Reps _____ Sets _____ X Day _____ Hold
31	Notes:	**32**	Notes:

SIDE TO SIDE WEIGHT SHIFT
Stand next to stable surface if needed for support.

Keep feet shoulder width apart. Lean from side to side maintaining balance. _May stand in hallway with walls on both sides._
*Advance to using balance pad

FORWARD AND BACKWARDS WEIGHT SHIFTS
Stand next to stable surface if needed for support.

Keep feet shoulder width apart. Lean from body forward and then backwards maintaining balance. _May stand in hallway with wall in front and in back._
 *Advance to using balance pad

_____ Reps _____ Sets _____ X Day _____ Hold		_____ Reps _____ Sets _____ X Day _____ Hold
33	Notes:	**34**	Notes:

SPLIT STANCE WEIGHT SHIFT SIDE TO SIDE
Stand next to stable surface if needed for support.

Stand in a split stance position. Lean side to side maintaining balance. *May stand in hallway with wall on both sides.*

SPLIT STANCE WEIGHT SHIFT FORWARD AND BACKWARDS Stand next to stable surface if needed for support.

Stand in a split stance position. Lean forward and backwards maintaining balance. *May stand in hallway with wall in front and in back.*

_____ Reps _____ Sets _____ X Day _____ Hold		_____ Reps _____ Sets _____ X Day _____ Hold
35	Notes:	**36**	Notes:

WALL FALLS - FORWARD - BALANCE DRILL

Stand facing wall, a couple feet away from the wall. Slowly and controlled, lean forward towards the wall. Try to control your balance to prevent falling forward. Keep leaning forward gradually until eventually you do lose your balance and fall. Use your arms to catch yourself. Push yourself back upright.

WALL FALLS - LATERAL - BALANCE DRILL

Stand to the side next to a wall, a couple feet away from the wall. Slowly and controlled, lean to the side towards the wall. Try to control your balance to prevent falling sideways. Keep leaning to the side gradually until eventually you do lose your balance and fall. Use your arm to catch yourself. Push yourself back upright.

	_____ Reps _____ Sets _____ X Day _____ Hold
37	**Notes:**

WALL FALLS - BACKWARDS - BALANCE DRILL

Stand facing away from a wall. Slowly and controlled, lean backward towards the wall. Try to control your balance to prevent falling backwards. Keep leaning backwards gradually until eventually you do lose your balance and fall. Use your upper back to catch the fall. Push yourself back upright.

	_____ Reps _____ Sets _____ X Day _____ Hold
38	**Notes:**

WALL FALLS - SINGLE LEG - FORWARD - BALANCE DRILL

Stand on one leg facing a wall, a couple feet away from the wall. Slowly and controlled, lean forward towards the wall. Try to control your balance to prevent falling forward. Keep leaning forward gradually until eventually you do lose your balance and fall. Use your arms to catch yourself. Push yourself back upright.

	_____ Reps _____ Sets _____ X Day _____ Hold
39	**Notes:**

WALL FALLS - SINGLE LEG - LATERAL - BALANCE DRILL

Stand on one leg with a wall a couple feet off to the side of that leg. Slowly and controlled, lean to the side towards the wall. Try to control your balance to prevent falling to the side. Keep leaning gradually towards the wall until eventually you lose your balance and fall. Use your arms to catch yourself. Push yourself back upright.

	_____ Reps _____ Sets _____ X Day _____ Hold
40	**Notes:**

WALL FALLS - SINGLE LEG - MEDIAL - BALANCE DRILL

Stand on one leg with a wall a couple feet off to the opposite side of that leg as shown. Slowly and controlled, lean sideways towards the wall. Try to control your balance to prevent falling to the side. Keep leaning gradually towards the wall until eventually you lose your balance and fall. Use your arms to catch yourself. Push yourself back upright.

_____ Reps _____ Sets _____ X Day _____ Hold		_____ Reps _____ Sets _____ X Day _____ Hold

41	Notes:	42	Notes:

WALL FALLS - SINGLE LEG - BACKWARDS - BALANCE DRILL

Stand on one leg facing away from a wall. Slowly and controlled, lean backward towards the wall. Try and control your balance to prevent falling backwards. Keep leaning backwards gradually until eventually you do lose your balance and fall. Use your upper back to catch the fall. Push yourself back upright.

FALL LATERAL - STEP RECOVERY
Stand next to stable surface if needed for support.

Start in a standing position with feet apart. Slowly lean to the side and try and prevent losing your balance. Continue to lean to the side until eventually you lose your balance and need to take a step to prevent falling.

_____ Reps _____ Sets _____ X Day _____ Hold		_____ Reps _____ Sets _____ X Day _____ Hold

43	Notes:	44	Notes:

FALL FORWARD - STEP RECOVERY
Stand next to stable surface if needed for support.

Start in a standing position with feet apart. Slowly lean forward and try and prevent losing your balance. Continue to lean forward until eventually you lose your balance and need to take a step to prevent falling.

FALL BACKWARD - STEP RECOVERY
Stand next to stable surface if needed for support.

Start in a standing position with feet apart. Slowly lean back and try and prevent losing your balance. Continue to lean backwards until eventually you lose your balance and need to take a step to prevent falling.

LEG EXERCISES > BALANCE > RESISTANCE

SOLID GROUND:
1. **Support:** Hold onto chair, counter, sink or another stationary object
2. **No Support:** Stand next to stable surface if needed for support
3. **Resistance:** Add ankle weights on use elastic band for resistance

UNSTABLE SURFACE: Balance pad, Bosu, Half foam roll, Pillow or Other unstable surface
1. **Support:** Hold onto chair, counter or another stationary object.
2. **No Support:** Stand next to stable surface if needed for support.
3. **Resistance:** Add ankle weights on use elastic band for resistance

Peripheral Neuropathy – See beginning of section for Caution on Unstable Surface

	_____ Reps _____ Sets _____X Day _____Hold	_____ Reps _____ Sets _____X Day _____Hold
45	Notes:	**46** Notes:

TOE TAP ABDUCTION

Standing upright and move your leg out to the side and tap your toe on the ground. Return to starting position and repeat.

HIP ABDUCTION - STANDING – Can add ankle weights or elastic band.

Standing upright, raise your leg out to the side. Keep your knee straight and maintain your toes pointed forward the entire time. Return to starting position and repeat. Maintain a slow, controlled movement throughout.

	_____ Reps _____ Sets _____X Day _____Hold			_____ Reps _____ Sets _____X Day _____Hold
47	Notes:		**48**	Notes:

HIP EXTENSION – STANDING - Can add ankle weights or band.

Standing upright, balance on one leg and move your other leg in a backward direction. Do not swing the leg and tighten the buttock at end range. Keep your trunk stable and without arching or bending forward during the movement. Return to starting position and repeat. Maintain a slow, controlled movement throughout.

HIP FLEXION - STANDING – STRAIGHT LEG RAISE - Can add ankle weights or band.

Standing upright, balance on one leg and lift your other leg forward with a straight knee as shown. Return to starting position and repeat. Maintain a slow, controlled movement throughout.

	_____ Reps _____ Sets _____X Day _____Hold			_____ Reps _____ Sets _____X Day _____Hold
49	Notes:		**50**	Notes:

HIP / KNEE FLEXION - SINGLE LEG - Can add ankle weights

Standing upright, lift your foot and knee up, set it down. Repeat. Maintain a slow, controlled movement throughout.

STANDING MARCHING- Can add ankle weights

Standing upright, draw up your knee, set it down and then alternate to your other side. Maintain a slow, controlled movement throughout.

_____ Reps _____ Sets _____ X Day _____ Hold	_____ Reps _____ Sets _____ X Day _____ Hold

51   Notes:

52   Notes:

HAMSTRING CURL - Can add ankle weights.

Standing upright, balance on one leg while bending the knee of the opposite leg towards the buttocks. Return to starting position and repeat. Maintain a slow, controlled movement throughout.

TOE RAISES - Can add hand weights.

Standing upright, go up on your toes slowly towards the ceiling and then return to the starting position. Maintain a slow, controlled movement throughout.

_____ Reps _____ Sets _____ X Day _____ Hold	_____ Reps _____ Sets _____ X Day _____ Hold

53   Notes:

54   Notes:

IR   **ER**

TOE RAISES IR AND ER - Can add hand weights.

IR (Internal Rotation)
Standing upright, rotate feet/legs inward and go up on your toes slowly towards the ceiling and then return to the starting position. Maintain a slow, controlled movement throughout.
ER (External Rotation)
Standing upright, rotate feet/legs outward and go up on your toes slowly towards the ceiling and then return to the starting position.

ONE LEGGED TOE RAISE - Can add hand weights.

Standing upright and balance on one leg. Go up on your toes on the opposite leg towards the ceiling and then return to the starting position. Maintain a slow, controlled movement throughout.

BOSU – Can use chair for stability

_____ Reps _____ Sets _____X Day _____Hold	_____ Reps _____ Sets _____X Day _____Hold
55 **Notes:**	**56** **Notes:**

SINGLE LEG BALANCE FORWARD

Stand on a Bosu with one leg and maintain your balance. Hold your opposite leg out in front of your body and then return to original position. Maintain a slightly bent knee on the stance side.

SINGLE LEG BALANCE LATERAL

Stand on a Bosu with one leg and maintain your balance. Hold your opposite leg out to the side of your body and then return to original position. Maintain a slightly bent knee on the stance side.

_____ Reps _____ Sets _____X Day _____Hold	_____ Reps _____ Sets _____X Day _____Hold
57 **Notes:**	**58** **Notes:**

SINGLE LEG BALANCE RETRO

Stand on a Bosu Ball with one leg and maintain your balance. Hold your opposite leg back behind your body and then return to original position. Maintain a slightly bent knee on the stance side.

SINGLE LEG STANCE RETROLATERAL

Stand on a Bosu Ball with one leg and maintain your balance. Hold your opposite leg back behind and across your body and then return to original position. Maintain a slightly bent knee on the stance side.

_____ Reps _____ Sets _____ X Day _____ Hold	_____ Reps _____ Sets _____ X Day _____ Hold
59 Notes:	**60** Notes:

SQUAT

While standing and maintaining your balance on a Bosu, squat and return to a standing position. Knees should bend in line with the 2nd toe and not pass the front of the foot.

SINGLE LEG SQUAT

While standing and balancing on a Bosu with one leg, bend your knee and lower your body towards the ground. Return to a standing position. Your stance knee should bend in line with the 2nd toe and not pass the front of the foot.

Lunges

_____ Reps _____ Sets _____ X Day _____ Hold	_____ Reps _____ Sets _____ X Day _____ Hold
61 Notes:	**62** Notes:

Starting Position

LUNGE – STATIC

Start in standing position with back leg straight and front leg with flexed/bent knee. Lean forward on front knee keeping knee in line with foot and back leg remaining straight. Return to starting position and repeat for several repetitions and then repeat on opposite side. *Make sure front knee does not go past the foot.

Backward   Starting Position   Forward

LUNGE FORWARD/BACKWARD

Start in standing (*middle picture*).
Backward: Keep one foot planted and step back with the opposite foot. Return to original position - repeat. *Forward:* Keep one foot planted and step forward with the opposite foot. Return to original position - repeat.

DYNAMIC MOVEMENTS

_____ Reps _____ Sets _____X Day _____Hold		_____ Reps _____ Sets _____X Day _____Hold
63	Notes:	**64**	Notes:

FOUR CORNER MARCHING IN PLACE

Marching in place, move your body clockwise stopping at each corner for several seconds and move to the next corner. After completing the square, march counterclockwise.

FOUR CORNER MARCHING IN PLACE WITH HEAD TURNS

With Head and Body Moving Simultaneously
March in place to four corners, as previous exercise (#63). Move your head and body moving simultaneously as you complete the square.
With Head Turn And Then Body Turn.
March in place to four corners, as previous exercise (#63). Turn head and then body as you complete the square.

_____ Reps _____ Sets _____X Day _____Hold		_____ Reps _____ Sets _____X Day _____Hold
65	Notes:	**66**	Notes:

WALKING ON HEELS FORWARD AND BACKWARDS – May walk along kitchen counter or wall until feeling steady.

Standing up tall, walk forward on heels. After feeling secure with a forward motion, try walking backwards on heels.

WALKING ON TOES FORWARD AND BACKWARDS – May walk along kitchen counter or wall until feeling steady.

Standing up tall, walk forward on up on toes. After feeling secure with a forward motion, try walking backwards up on toes.

_____ Reps _____ Sets _____ X Day _____ Hold

67 | Notes:

TANDEM STANCE AND WALK – FORWARD AND BACKWARDS

Maintaining your balance, stand with one foot directly in front of the other so that the toes of one foot touches the heel of the other. Progress by taking steps with your heel touching your toes with each step.
**Progress by walking backwards with your toe touching your heel with each step. Can also add head turns.

_____ Reps _____ Sets _____ X Day _____ Hold

68 | Notes:

RUNNING MAN

Stand and balance on one leg. Lean forward as you bring your other leg back behind you to tap the floor. Bring the same side arm forward as shown during the movement. Return to starting position and repeat.

_____ Reps _____ Sets _____ X Day _____ Hold

69 | Notes:

HOP STICK - FORWARD

Stand on one leg and then hop forward onto the other leg. Maintain your balance the entire time. Increase the difficulty by hoping forward further or higher.

_____ Reps _____ Sets _____ X Day _____ Hold

70 | Notes:

HOP STICK - BACKWARDS

Stand on one leg and then hop backward onto the other leg. Maintain your balance the entire time. Increase the difficulty by hoping back further or higher.

	_____ Reps _____ Sets _____ X Day _____ Hold
71	Notes:

MINI LATERAL LUNGE

Step to the side and balance on the leg. Next return to the original position. Repeat in the opposite direction. Your knees should be bent about 30 degrees.

	_____ Reps _____ Sets _____ X Day _____ Hold
72	Notes:

SIDE STEPPING – May step along kitchen counter or in hallway for support.

Step to the side continuing for length of room or counter – repeat in opposite direction.

	_____ Reps _____ Sets _____ X Day _____ Hold
73	Notes:

HOP STICK - LATERAL

Stand on one leg and then hop to the side onto the other leg. Maintain your balance the entire time. Increase the difficulty by hoping to the side further and higher.

	_____ Reps _____ Sets _____ X Day _____ Hold
74	Notes:

SINGLE LEG DEAD LIFT

While standing on one leg, bend forward with arms in front towards the ground as you extend your leg behind you and then return to the original position. Keep your legs straight and maintain your balance the entire time.

	_____ Reps _____ Sets _____X Day _____Hold		_____ Reps _____ Sets _____X Day _____Hold
75	Notes:	76	Notes:

CONE TAPS - SINGLE LEG STANCE

Place 3-5 cones or cups around you as shown. Balance on a slightly bent knee. Lower yourself down to tap the top of a cone with your finger. Return to original position and repeat touching a different cone. Advance exercise with smaller cones/cups and or faster speed.

CONE TAPS - SINGLE LEG STANCE - UNSTABLE

Place 3-5 cones or cups around you. Balance on an unstable surface such as a foam pad with a slightly bent knee. Lower yourself down to tap the top of a cone. Return to original position and repeat touching a different cone. Advance exercise with smaller cones/cups and or faster speed.

	_____ Reps _____ Sets _____X Day _____Hold		_____ Reps _____ Sets _____X Day _____Hold
77	Notes:	78	Notes:

FIGURE 8 AROUND CONES

Set up 4-8 cones on the floor about 12 inches apart, although can vary to increase or decrease difficulty. Weave in and out of cones and then turn and repeat.

FIGURE 8 AROUND CONES – FOOT OR HAND TAP

Follow #75 figure around 4- 8 cones. To increase difficulty, you can tap each cone with your foot or lean over and tap with your hand.

HALF ROLLER (static and dynamic) – FLAT SIDE UP OR DOWN

	_____ Reps _____ Sets _____ X Day _____ Hold			_____ Reps _____ Sets _____ X Day _____ Hold
79	Notes:		**80**	Notes:

BALANCE DOUBLE LEG STANCE - WIDE

Place a half foam roll on the ground in a side-to-side direction. Stand on the foam roll with your feet spread apart and maintain your balance.

BALANCE DOUBLE LEG STANCE - NARROW

Place a half foam roll on the ground in a side-to-side direction. Stand on the foam roll with your feet together and maintain your balance.

	_____ Reps _____ Sets _____ X Day _____ Hold			_____ Reps _____ Sets _____ X Day _____ Hold
81	Notes:		**82**	Notes:

TANDEM STANCE

Place a half foam roll on the ground in a forward-back direction. Stand on the foam roll in tandem stance (with your heel and toe touching as shown) and maintain your balance.

TANDEM WALK

Place a half foam roll on the ground in a forward-back direction. Stand on the foam roll and begin tandem walking (heel-toe pattern walking as shown). Once you get to the end of the roll, either turn around or tandem walk backward.

	_____ Reps _____ Sets _____ X Day _____ Hold
83	**Notes:**

SINGLE LEG STANCE - ABDUCTION

Place a half foam roll on the ground in a side-to-side direction. Balance on one leg and move the opposite leg to the side.

	_____ Reps _____ Sets _____ X Day _____ Hold
84	**Notes:**

SINGLE LEG STANCE - ABDUCTION

Place a half foam roll on the ground in a forward-back direction. Balance on one leg with the opposite leg to the side.

	_____ Reps _____ Sets _____ X Day _____ Hold
85	**Notes:**

SINGLE LEG STANCE – FORWARD KICK

Place a half foam roll on the ground in a forward-back direction. Balance on one leg and move the opposite leg forward.

	_____ Reps _____ Sets _____ X Day _____ Hold
86	**Notes:**

SINGLE LEG STANCE – HAMSTRING CURL

Place a half foam roll on the ground in a forward-back direction. Balance on one leg and with the opposite leg, bend the knee backwards as shown.

_____ Reps _____ Sets _____X Day _____Hold		_____ Reps _____ Sets _____X Day _____Hold
87	Notes:	**88**	Notes:

SINGLE LEG SQUAT – LEG FORWARD

Place a half foam roll on the ground in a forward-back direction. Balance on one leg with a slight bend in the supporting knee and move the opposite leg forward. Straighten supporting knee and repeat.

SINGLE LEG SQUAT – LEG BACKWARDS

Place a half foam roll on the ground in a forward-back direction. Balance on one leg with a slight bend in the supporting knee and with the opposite leg, move the leg backwards as shown with bent knee. Straighten supporting knee and repeat.

STAIR STEP – *To progress, increase step height*

_____ Reps _____ Sets _____X Day _____Hold		_____ Reps _____ Sets _____X Day _____Hold
89	Notes:	**90**	Notes:

TOE TAP OR HEEL PLACEMENT

While standing with both feet on the floor, place one foot on the top of the step. Next, return the foot back to the floor and then repeat with the other leg.
You can either put your foot up for several repetitions or alternate.

PULL UP FOOT TOUCHES ON STEP

Whie standing with both feet on the ground, put one foot on the step. Push through the foot straightening the knee until the opposite foot is off the ground. Lower the foot back to the starting position. Repeat with the opposite foot for several repetitions.

	_____ Reps _____ Sets _____X Day _____Hold
91	Notes:

ALTERNATING SUSTAINED FOOT TOUCHES ON STEP

Whie standing with both feet on the ground, put one foot on the step. Push through the foot straightening the knee until the opposite foot is also on the step. Step off backwards to the starting position. Repeat with the opposite foot for several repetitions.

	_____ Reps _____ Sets _____X Day _____Hold
92	Notes:

STEP UP AND OVER

Step up onto the step and then onto the ground on the other side. Turn around and repeat.
Repeat several repetitions on one side and then the other or alternate legs.

	_____ Reps _____ Sets _____X Day _____Hold
93	Notes:

FORWARD SWING THROUGH STEP

Step up onto the step without stopping on the top, swing opposite leg through and onto the floor on the other side.

	_____ Reps _____ Sets _____X Day _____Hold
94	Notes:

SIDE STEPPING

******REPEAT STEPS 89-93 from a side approach******

EXERCISE Agility/Reactivity/Speed	EXERCISE NUMBER	NOTES
Four Square Drills	1	
Dots	2	
Ladder Drills	3	
Box Drills	4	
Cones	5	
Hurdles	6	

Agility/Reactivity/Speed

According to the Twist Conditioning workbook, "Agility is the ability to link several fundamental movement skills into a multidirectional pattern. Reaction skills are the 'whole body' responsiveness to external stimuli, as well as muscle and joint internal reactivity. Quickness is the ability to explosively initiate movement from a stationary position, as well as shifting the gears of speed". *(Twist, Peter, Twist Agility, Quickness and & Reactivity Workbook, 2009, pg 16)*

Agility is a combination of acceleration, deceleration, coordination, power, strength and dynamic balance. With agility training, always keep your head in a neutral position looking straight ahead no matter which way you turn. "Powerful arm movement during transitional and directional changes is essential in order to reacquire a high rate of speed". *(Brown & Ferrigno, 2005, pp 73-74)*

Agility exercises can be done with cones, hurdles, dots or squares on the floor, box drills, Bosu or ladders. Agility can also be high impact or explosive movements. If you are not comfortable with this in the beginning or have any contraindications, stick with low impact movements. In other words, if you are jumping over hurdles, keep them low to the ground and jump over with one leg leading for low impact and jump with both legs for high impact.

If you are doing box drills or Bosu, please do NOT JUMP off backwards.

AGILITY / SPEED / REACTIVITY

4 Square Drills

Dots

Ladder

Box Drills – Box should be no higher than the middle of your shin. This can be done on Bosu for balance.

Alt Tap Box With Foot	Down Up Both Feet Together	Quickly Move Side to Side	Down Up Both Feet Together

Cones

Hurdles – can run or jump over hurdles

Endurance / Aerobic Capacity

Aerobic - with oxygen: Muscular and Cardiovascular

Many repetitions with sub-maximal weight (weight that is less than the maximum you can lift).

Muscular endurance is the ability of the muscle or group of muscles to sustain repeated contractions against resistance for an extended period of time. This is needed to build muscle. (See *Strengthening*). Cardiovascular endurance is the ability of the heart, lungs and blood vessels to deliver oxygen to working muscles and tissues, as well as the ability of those muscles and tissues to utilize that oxygen. This is needed to help endure long runs or sustained activity, as with biking or running. In short, endurance or aerobic exercises increase the heart rate and respiratory rate.

As far as long-term performance goes, there are two types of muscle fibers that can determine the likelihood of success: slow and fast twitch, which may determine whether you are more likely to be a powerlifter or sprinter (*fast twitch*), or a marathon runner (*slow twitch*). Your ability depends on the distribution of these fibers in the body. In other words, you could have a certain percentage of slow twitch in your biceps, but a different percentage in your quadriceps. There is some controversy over whether you can change the percentage or distribution of these fibers with endurance training or training for a specific event, although you may be able to change the glycolytic capacity.

Type of Fibers	*Slow twitch fibers:* Have a high aerobic capacity and are resistant to fatigue. People that have a higher percentage of slow twitch fibers tend to have better endurance abilities.
	Fast twitch fibers: Contract faster than slow twitch, and thus fatigue faster. People that have a higher percentage of fast twitch fibers tend to have better sprinting or muscle building abilities.

The following research is from the: **MAYO CLINIC**

Mayo Clinic - *https://www.mayoclinic.org/healthy-lifestyle/fitness/in-depth/aerobic-exercise/art-20045541*
Regular aerobic activity, such as walking, bicycling or swimming, can help you live longer and healthier. Need motivation? See how aerobic exercise affects your heart, lungs and blood flow.

How your body responds to aerobic exercise
- During aerobic activity, you repeatedly move large muscles in your arms, legs and hips. You'll notice your body's responses quickly.
- You'll breathe faster and more deeply. This maximizes the amount of oxygen in your blood. Your heart will beat faster, which increases blood flow to your muscles and back to your lungs.
- Your small blood vessels (capillaries) will widen to deliver more oxygen to your muscles and carry away waste products, such as carbon dioxide and lactic acid.
- Your body will even release endorphins, natural painkillers that promote an increased sense of well-being.

What aerobic exercise does for your health
Regardless of age, weight or athletic ability, aerobic activity is good for you. As your body adapts to regular aerobic exercise, you'll get stronger and fitter.
Consider the following 10 ways that aerobic activity can help you feel better and enjoy life to the fullest.

Aerobic activity can help you:

1. **Keep excess pounds at bay**
   Combined with a healthy diet, aerobic exercise helps you lose weight and keep it off.

2. **Increase your stamina**
   You may feel tired when you first start regular aerobic exercise. But over the long term, you'll enjoy increased stamina and reduced fatigue.

3. **Ward off viral illnesses**

Aerobic exercise activates your immune system in a good way. This may leave you less susceptible to minor viral illnesses, such as colds and flu.

4. **Reduce your health risks**
    Aerobic exercise reduces the risk of many conditions, including obesity, heart disease, high blood pressure, type 2 diabetes, metabolic syndrome, stroke and certain types of cancer.
    Weight-bearing aerobic exercises, such as walking, help decrease the risk of osteoporosis.

5. **Manage chronic conditions**
    Aerobic exercise may help lower blood pressure and control blood sugar. If you have coronary artery disease, aerobic exercise may help you manage your condition.

6. **Strengthen your heart**
    A stronger heart doesn't need to beat as fast. A stronger heart also pumps blood more efficiently, which improves blood flow to all parts of your body.

7. **Keep your arteries clear**
    Aerobic exercise boosts your high-density lipoprotein (HDL), the "good," cholesterol, and lowers your low-density lipoprotein (LDL), the "bad," cholesterol. This may result in less buildup of plaques in your arteries.

8. **Boost your mood**
    Aerobic exercise may ease the gloominess of depression, reduce the tension associated with anxiety and promote relaxation.

9. **Stay active and independent as you age**
    Aerobic exercise keeps your muscles strong, which can help you maintain mobility as you get older. Studies have found that regular physical activity may help protect memory, reasoning, judgment and thinking skills (cognitive function) in older adults, and may improve cognitive function in young adults.

10. **Live longer**
    Studies show that people who participate in regular aerobic exercise live longer than those who don't exercise regularly.

Take the first step

Ready to get more active? Great. Just remember to start with small steps. If you've been inactive for a long time or if you have a chronic health condition, get your doctor's OK before you start. When you're ready to begin exercising, start slowly. You might walk five minutes in the morning and five minutes in the evening.

The next day, add a few minutes to each walking session. Pick up the pace a bit, too. Soon, you could be walking briskly for at least 30 minutes a day and reaping all the benefits of regular aerobic activity.

Other options for aerobic exercise could include cross-country skiing, aerobic dancing, swimming, stair climbing, bicycling, jogging, elliptical training or rowing.

Mayo Clinic - *https://www.mayoclinic.org/healthy-lifestyle/fitness/in-depth/aerobic-exercise/art-20045541*

Calories

Calorie: A unit of food energy. The word calorie is ordinarily used instead of the more precise, scientific term kilocalorie. A kilocalorie represents the amount of energy required to raise the temperature of a liter of water 1' centigrade at sea level. Technically, a kilocalorie represents 1,000 true calories of energy. *(MedicineNet.com)*

Calories are a measurement tool, like inches or cups. Calories measure the energy a food or beverage provides from the carbohydrate, fat, protein, and alcohol* it contains. Calories give you the fuel or energy you need to work and play – even to rest and sleep! When choosing what to eat and drink, it's important to get the right mix – enough nutrients without too many calories. Paying attention to calories is an important part of managing your weight. The amount of calories you need are different if you want to gain, lose, or maintain your weight. Tracking what and how much you eat, and drink can help you better understand your calorie intake over time. Each person's body may have different needs for calories and exercise. A healthy lifestyle requires balance in the foods you eat, the beverages you drink, the way you do daily activities, adequate sleep, stress management, and in the amount of activity in your daily routine. *(ChooseMyPlate.gov & CDC)*

Example of Activities and Calories Burned (*ChooseMyPlate.gov*)
A 154-pound man who is 5' 10" will use up (burn) about the number of calories listed doing each activity below. Those who weigh more will use more calories; those who weigh less will use fewer calories. The calorie values listed include both calories used by the activity and the calories used for normal body functioning during the activity time.

EXAMPLE	Approximate calories used (burned) by a 154-pound man	
MODERATE physical activities:	In 1 hour	In 30 minutes
Hiking	370	185
Light gardening/ yard work	330	165
Dancing	330	165
Golf (walking and carrying clubs)	330	165
Bicycling (less than 10 mph)	290	145
Walking (3.5 mph)	280	140
Weight training (general light workout)	220	110
Stretching	180	90
VIGOROUS physical activities:	In 1 hour	In 30 minutes
Running/ jogging (5 mph)	590	295
Bicycling (more than 10 mph)	590	295
Swimming (slow freestyle laps)	510	255
Aerobics	480	240
Walking (4.5 mph)	460	230
Heavy yard work (chopping wood)	440	220
Weightlifting (vigorous effort)	440	220
Basketball (vigorous)	440	220

References

Also, Some Good Books, Websites & DVD'

ACE Idea Fitness Journal: *Martina M. Cartwright, PhD, RD http://www.ideafit.com/fitness-library/protein-today-are-consumers-getting-too-much-of-a-good-thing?ACE_ACCESS=ebec6bcf61abff08f7b1d8b27c555758*

ACE Senior Fitness Manual, *American Council on Exercise* (2014)

American Physical Therapy Association, (APTA), 2007. *Basic Science for Animal Physical Therapy: Canine, 2nd edition*

Arleigh J Reynolds, DVM, PhD - *www.absasleddogracing.org.uk/newgang/src/gangline/role.htm*

Australian Institute of Sports - *http://www.ausport.gov.au*

BodyBuilder.com

Brown & Ferrigno, (2005). *Training for Speed, Agility and Quickness*, Champaign, IL: Human Kinetics.

Bryant, C & Green, D, editors (2003), *Ace Personal Trainer Manual, 3rd ed.*, San Diego, CA: American Council on Exercise (ACE)

ChooseMyPlate.gov

Examine.com

ExRx.net

Feher & Szunyoghy (1996). *Cyclopedia Anatomicae,* Tess Press

Gillette, R (2002). Temperature Regulation of the Dog. Retrieved June 2011 from *http://www.sportsvet.com/11Nwsltr.PDF*

Gillette, R (2008). *Feeding the Canine Athlete for Optimal Performance.* Retrieved September 25, 2008 from *www.sports vet.com/Art3.html.*

Glucose (Wikipedia) - *http://en.wikipedia.org/wiki/Glucose*

Glycemic Index (Wikipedia) - *http://en.wikipedia.org/wiki/Glycemic_index*

LiveStrong.com

Mayo Clinic - *https://www.mayoclinic.org/healthy-lifestyle/fitness/in-depth/aerobic-exercise/art-20045541*

MedicineNet.com

Myofascial Release: (Wikipedia) - https://en.wikipedia.org/wiki/Myofascial_release

Rikli, Roberta and Jones, Jessie (2013) *Senior Fitness Test Manual, 2nd Ed.,*

Strength Training: (Wikipedia) *http://en.wikipedia.org/wiki/Strength_training*

Twist, Peter (2009). *Twist Agility, Quickness and & Reactivity Workbook.* British Columbia: Twist Conditioning, Inc. University of Maryland Medical Center.com

Workout Australia

Thank You to:

My Husband Burt
Model
For his support through my battle with cancer and while writing this and previous books.
Also, for the patience and hours he put in modeling for this book.

My Daughter Kayla
For giving me artistic inspiration and providing artwork for my previous books.

My Grandchildren Skyler and Soren
Just Because

God
For giving me the strength to overcome cancer and the wisdom to write these books.

Certifications, Continuing Education and License

Physical Therapist Assistant – L/PTA – 30 years in both Home Therapy and Short-Term Rehab facilities

ACE Certified Personal Trainer – CPT
- o **Functional Training Specialist**
- o **Therapeutic Exercise Specialist**
- o **Senior Fitness Specialist**
- o **Nutrition and Fitness Specialist**

©Klose Education
- o **Certified Lymphedema Therapist – CLT**
- o **Strength After Breast Cancer – Strength ABC**
- o **Breast Cancer Rehabilitation**

©Cancer Exercise Specialist Institute – CETI
- o **Cancer Exercise Specialist – CES**
- o **Breast Cancer Recovery BOSU(R) Specialist Advanced Qualification**
- o **Pilates Mat Certificate**

©MedFit
- o **Medical Fitness Specialist**
- o **Parkinson's Disease Fitness Specialist**
- o **Arthritis Fitness Specialist**

©Pink Ribbon Program

©The BioMechanics Method - Corrective Exercise Specialist

©ISSA - DNA-Based Fitness Coach

Lost Temple Fitness

www.ingramcontent.com/pod-product-compliance
Lightning Source LLC
Chambersburg PA
CBHW052108020426
42335CB00021B/2678